Injury & Trauma Sourcebook

Learning Disabilities Sourcebook, 4th Edition

Leukemia Sourcebook

Liver Disorders Sourcebook

Medical Tests Sourcebook, 4th Edition

Men's Health Concerns Sourcebook, 4th Edition

Mental Health Disorders Sourcebook, 5th Edition

Mental Retardation Sourcebook

Movement Disorders Sourcebook, 2nd Edition

Multiple Sclerosis Sourcebook

Muscular Dystrophy Sourcebook

Obesity Sourcebook

Osteoporosis Sourcebook

Pain Sourcebook, 3rd Edition

Pediatric Cancer Sourcebook

Physical & Mental Issues in Aging Sourcebook

Podiatry Sourcebook, 2nd Edition

Pregnancy & Birth Sourcebook, 3rd Edition

Prostate & Urological Disorders Sourcebook

Prostate Cancer Sourcebook

Rehabilitation Sourcebook

Respiratory Disorders Sourcebook, 2nd Edition

Sexually Transmitted Diseases Sourcebook, 5th Edition

Sleep Disorders Sourcebook, 3rd Edition

Smoking Concerns Sourcebook

Sports Injuries Sourcebook, 4th Edition

Stress-Related Disorders Sourcebook, 3rd Edition

Stroke Sourcebook, 2nd Edition

Surgery Sourcebook, 2nd Edition

Thyroid Disorders Sourcebook

Transplantation Sourcebook

Traveler's Health Sourcebook

Urinary Tract & Kidney Diseases & Disorders Sourcebook, 2nd Edition

Vegetarian Sourcebook

Women's Health Concerns Sourcebook, 3rd Edition

Workplace Health & Safety Sourcebook

Worldwide Health Sourcebook

Teen Health Series

Abuse & Violence Information for Teens

Accident & Safety Information for Teens

Alcohol Information for Teens, 2nd Edition

Allergy Information for Teens

Asthma Information for Teens, 2nd Edition

Body Information for Teens

Cancer Information for Teens, 2nd Edition

Complementary & Alternative Medicine Information for Teens

Diabetes Information for Teens, 2nd Edition

Diet Information for Teens, 3rd Edition

Drug Information for Teens, 3rd Edition

Eating Disorders Information for Teens, 2nd Edition

Fitness Information for Teens, 3rd Edition

Learning Disabilities Information for Teens

Mental Health Information for Teens, 3rd Edition

Pregnancy Information for Teens, 2nd Edition

Sexual Health Information for Teens, 3rd Edition

Skin Health Information for Teens, 2nd Edition

Sleep Information for Teens

Sports Injuries Information for Teens, 3rd Edition

Stress Information for Teens

Suicide Information for Teens, 2nd Edition

Tobacco Information for Teens

D1443506

Eye Care
SOURCEBOOK

Fourth Edition

Health Reference Series

Fourth Edition

Eye Care
SOURCEBOOK

Basic Consumer Health Information about Vision and Disorders Affecting the Eyes and Surrounding Structures, Including Facts about Hyperopia, Myopia, Presbyopia, Astigmatism, Cataracts, Macular Degeneration, Glaucoma, and Other Disorders of the Cornea, Retina, Macula, Conjunctiva, and Optic Nerve

Along with Guidelines for Recognizing and Treating Eye Emergencies, Advice about Protecting the Eyes at Work, Home, and Play, Tips for Living with Low Vision, a Glossary of Terms Related to the Eyes and Eye Disorders, and a Directory of Resources for Further Information

Edited by
Sandra J. Judd

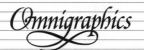

155 W. Congress, Suite 200, Detroit, MI 48226

Bibliographic Note

Because this page cannot legibly accommodate all the copyright notices, the Bibliographic Note portion of the Preface constitutes an extension of the copyright notice.

Edited by Sandra J. Judd

Health Reference Series

Karen Bellenir, *Managing Editor*
David A. Cooke, MD, FACP, *Medical Consultant*
Elizabeth Collins, *Research and Permissions Coordinator*
Cherry Edwards, *Permissions Assistant*
EdIndex, Services for Publishers, *Indexers*

* * *

Omnigraphics, Inc.

Matthew P. Barbour, *Senior Vice President*
Kevin M. Hayes, *Operations Manager*

* * *

Peter E. Ruffner, *Publisher*

Copyright © 2012 Omnigraphics, Inc.

ISBN 978-0-7808-1228-4

E-ISBN 978-0-7808-1229-1

Library of Congress Cataloging-in-Publication Data

Eye care sourcebook : basic consumer health information about vision and disorders affecting the eyes and surrounding structures, including facts about hyperopia, myopia, presbyopia, astigmatism, cataracts, macular degeneration, glaucoma, and other disorders of the cornea, retina, macula, conjunctiva, and optic nerve; along with guidelines for recognizing and treating eye emergencies, advice about protecting the eyes at work, home, and play, tips for living with low vision ... / edited by Sandra J. Judd. -- 5th ed.
       p. cm.
   Includes bibliographical references and index.
   Summary: "Provides basic consumer health information about the diagnosis and treatment of eye diseases and disorders and the prevention of eye injuries, along with tips for coping with low vision. Includes index, glossary of related terms, and other resources"-- Provided by publisher.
   ISBN 978-0-7808-1228-4 (hardcover : alk. paper) 1. Eye--Diseases--Popular works. 2. Eye--Care and hygiene--Popular works. I. Judd, Sandra J.
   RE51.O64 2012
   617.7--dc23
                                                            2012000391

Table of Contents

Visit www.healthreferenceseries.com to view *A Contents Guide to the Health Reference Series*, a listing of more than 16,000 topics and the volumes in which they are covered.

Part III: Understanding and Treating Disorders of the Cornea, Conjunctiva, Sclera, Iris, and Pupil

Part IV: Understanding and Treating Disorders of the Macula, Optic Nerve, Retina, Vitreous, and Uvea

Part V: Eye Injuries and Disorders of the Surrounding Structures

Part VI: Congenital and Other Disorders That Affect Vision

Part VIII: Additional Help and Information

Preface

About This Book

Low vision or blindness affects more than three million Americans aged forty years and over. This number is expected to double by 2030, due to the increasing epidemics of diabetes and other chronic diseases and the rapidly aging U.S. population. Furthermore, an estimated sixty-one million adults in the United States are at high risk for serious vision loss, yet only half have visited an eye doctor within the past twelve months. Few know the warning signs of serious eye disorders, and fewer still know that the effects of many of these disorders could be lessened or eliminated entirely with a doctor's care.

Eye Care Sourcebook, Fourth Edition provides information about common vision and eye-related problems and how they are diagnosed and treated. It includes facts about cataracts, corneal disorders, macular degeneration, glaucoma and other disorders of the optic nerve, retinal disorders, and refractive and eye movement disorders. It describes congenital and hereditary disorders that affect vision, and infectious diseases, traumatic injuries, and other disorders with eye-related complications. It also provides tips for recognizing and treating eye emergencies and suggestions to help prevent eye injuries. The book concludes with a summary of tips for living with low vision, a glossary of terms related to eye disorders, and a directory of resources for further help and information.

How to Use This Book

This book is divided into parts and chapters. Parts focus on broad areas of interest. Chapters are devoted to single topics within a part.

Part I: Eye and Eye Care Basics explains how the eyes work and describes the most common methods of diagnosing vision and other eye-related problems. It offers suggestions for maintaining healthy eyes and discusses common pediatric and age-related vision concerns. Finally, it describes ongoing research in the field of vision disorders.

Part II: Understanding and Treating Refractive, Eye Movement, and Alignment Disorders describes common disorders affecting the eyes' refractive ability, ability to move, and alignment, including astigmatism, hyperopia (farsightedness), myopia (nearsightedness), presbyopia, and strabismus. It provides details about the different types of eyeglasses and contact lenses used to treat refractive disorders and describes how to fit them and care for them properly. The section concludes with a discussion of the most common types of refractive surgery.

Part III: Understanding and Treating Disorders of the Cornea, Conjunctiva, Sclera, Iris, and Pupil discusses cataracts and other corneal disorders such as corneal abrasions, corneal ulcers and infections, and pterygium and provides a detailed description of treatments such as cataract surgery and corneal transplant. It also discusses conjunctivitis, pinkeye, dry eye, episcleritis, and other common disorders of the conjunctiva and describes the methods used to diagnose and treat these disorders.

Part IV: Understanding and Treating Disorders of the Macula, Optic Nerve, Retina, Vitreous, and Uvea provides information about macular degeneration and other macular disorders, glaucoma, optic nerve atrophy, and other disorders of the optic nerve, retinal detachment, retinopathy of prematurity, and other disorders of the retina, and disorders of the vitreous and uvea, including floaters, vitreous detachment, uveitis, and iritis. It details the signs and symptoms of these disorders and explains how they are diagnosed and treated.

Part V: Eye Injuries and Disorders of the Surrounding Structures discusses how to recognize and treat eye emergencies, including chemical burns, foreign objects in the eye, and blowout fractures, and how to prevent these injuries. It includes a description of recommended forms of workplace and sports eye protection. It also discusses the most common disorders of the eyelids and tear ducts, including blepharospasm, chalazion, eyelid tumors, and blocked tear ducts.

Part VI: Congenital and Other Disorders That Affect Vision describes the most common hereditary and other congenital disorders affecting vision, including albinism, color blindness, and Down syndrome. It provides information about infectious diseases, such as herpes, toxoplasmosis, and trachoma, that affect the eyes, and describes diseases and injuries, including diabetes, multiple sclerosis, acquired immune deficiency syndrome, strokes, and traumatic brain injury, that have eye-related complications.

Part VII: Living with Low Vision defines what is meant by the terms "low vision," "legal blindness," and "night blindness" and provides tips for coping with vision loss. It offers suggestions for home modification to improve safety and provides tips for driving safely and traveling independently with vision loss. The section concludes with a discussion of the laws regarding employment of people with low vision.

Part VIII: Additional Help and Information includes a glossary of terms related to eyes and eye disorders and a directory of resources for further help and support.

Bibliographic Note

This volume contains documents and excerpts from the following U.S. government agencies: Centers for Disease Control and Prevention; Federal Trade Commission; National Cancer Institute; National Eye Institute; National Highway Traffic Safety Administration; National Human Genome Research Institute; National Institute of Neurological Disorders and Stroke; National Institutes of Health Office of Rare Diseases; U.S. Department of Agriculture; U.S. Environmental Protection Agency; U.S. Food and Drug Administration; and the U.S. Occupational Safety and Health Administration.

In addition, this volume contains copyrighted documents from the following organizations: About.com; Access Media Group, LLC (All AboutVision.com); A.D.A,M., Inc.; Alström Syndrome International; AMD Alliance International; American Association for Pediatric Ophthalmology and Strabismus; American Foundation for the Blind; American Optometric Association; American Society of Ophthalmic Plastic and Reconstructive Surgery; Baby Center LLC; California School for the Blind; Cleveland Clinic; Cornea Research Foundation of America; Eyecare Trust; Fort Worth Eye Associates; Foundation Fighting Blindness; Georgetown University Medical Center; Glaucoma Research Foundation; Indiana University News; Indiana University School of Optometry; Lighthouse International; Macular Degeneration Partnership; MAGIC

Foundation; Minnesota Optometric Association; National Down Syndrome Society; National Keratoconus Foundation; National Organization for Albinism and Hypopigmentation; National Stroke Association; Nemours Foundation; North American Neuro-Ophthalmology Society; Optometric Physicians of Washington; ParentGuide News; Penn Eye Care/Scheie Eye Institute; Prevent Blindness America; Remedy Health Media; St. Luke's Cataract and Laser Institute; University of Illinois Eye Center; Uveitis Information Group; Virtual Medical Centre; Vision for Tomorrow Foundation; Vision Help; and Your-eye-sight.org.

Acknowledgements

Thanks go to the many organizations, agencies, and individuals who have contributed materials for this *Sourcebook* and to medical consultant Dr. David Cooke and prepress services provider WhimsyInk. Special thanks go to managing editor Karen Bellenir and permissions coordinator Liz Collins for their help and support.

About the Health Reference Series

The *Health Reference Series* is designed to provide basic medical information for patients, families, caregivers, and the general public. Each volume takes a particular topic and provides comprehensive coverage. This is especially important for people who may be dealing with a newly diagnosed disease or a chronic disorder in themselves or in a family member. People looking for preventive guidance, information about disease warning signs, medical statistics, and risk factors for health problems will also find answers to their questions in the *Health Reference Series*. The *Series*, however, is not intended to serve as a tool for diagnosing illness, in prescribing treatments, or as a substitute for the physician/patient relationship. All people concerned about medical symptoms or the possibility of disease are encouraged to seek professional care from an appropriate healthcare provider.

A Note about Spelling and Style

Health Reference Series editors use *Stedman's Medical Dictionary* as an authority for questions related to the spelling of medical terms and the *Chicago Manual of Style* for questions related to grammatical structures, punctuation, and other editorial concerns. Consistent adherence is not always possible, however, because the individual volumes within the *Series* include many documents from a wide variety of different producers and copyright holders, and the editor's primary goal is to present material from each source as accurately as is possible following the terms specified by each document's producer. This sometimes means that information in different chapters or sections may follow other guidelines and alternate spelling authorities. For example, occasionally a copyright holder may require that eponymous terms be shown in possessive forms (Crohn's disease *vs.* Crohn disease) or that British spelling norms be retained (leukaemia *vs.* leukemia).

Locating Information within the Health Reference Series

The *Health Reference Series* contains a wealth of information about a wide variety of medical topics. Ensuring easy access to all the fact sheets, research reports, in-depth discussions, and other material contained within the individual books of the series remains one of our highest priorities. As the *Series* continues to grow in size and scope, however, locating the precise information needed by a reader may become more challenging.

A Contents Guide to the Health Reference Series was developed to direct readers to the specific volumes that address their concerns. It presents an extensive list of diseases, treatments, and other topics of general interest compiled from the Tables of Contents and major index headings. To access *A Contents Guide to the Health Reference Series*, visit www.healthreferenceseries.com.

Medical Consultant

Medical consultation services are provided to the *Health Reference Series* editors by David A. Cooke, MD, FACP. Dr. Cooke is a graduate of Brandeis University, and he received his M.D. degree from the University of Michigan. He completed residency training at the University of Wisconsin Hospital and Clinics. He is board-certified in Internal Medicine. Dr. Cooke currently works as part of the University of Michigan Health System and practices in Ann Arbor, MI. In his free time, he enjoys writing, science fiction, and spending time with his family.

Our Advisory Board

We would like to thank the following board members for providing guidance to the development of this series:

Dr. Lynda Baker, Associate Professor of Library and Information Science, Wayne State University, Detroit, MI

Nancy Bulgarelli, William Beaumont Hospital Library,
Royal Oak, MI

Karen Imarisio, Bloomfield Township Public Library,
Bloomfield Township, MI

Karen Morgan, Mardigian Library, University of
Michigan-Dearborn, Dearborn, MI

Rosemary Orlando, St. Clair Shores Public Library,
St. Clair Shores, MI

Health Reference Series *Update Policy*

The inaugural book in the *Health Reference Series* was the first edition of *Cancer Sourcebook* published in 1989. Since then, the *Series* has been enthusiastically received by librarians and in the medical community. In order to maintain the standard of providing high-quality health information for the layperson the editorial staff at Omnigraphics felt it was necessary to implement a policy of updating volumes when warranted.

Medical researchers have been making tremendous strides, and it is the purpose of the *Health Reference Series* to stay current with the most recent advances. Each decision to update a volume is made on an individual basis. Some of the considerations include how much new information is available and the feedback we receive from people who use the books. If there is a topic you would like to see added to the update list, or an area of medical concern you feel has not been adequately addressed, please write to:

Editor
Health Reference Series
Omnigraphics, Inc.
155 W. Congress, Suite 200
Detroit, MI 48226
E-mail: editorial@omnigraphics.com

Part One

Eye and Eye Care Basics

Chapter 1

How the Eyes Work

Chapter Contents

Section 1.1

Anatomy of the Eye

You may have heard the analogy that our eyes work like cameras:
Light enters the camera through the shutter and is focused by the
lens to produce a sharp image on the film at the back of the camera.
The film with the captured image is then sent to a lab to be developed
and printed.

Our eyes work in much the same manner: Light enters our eye
through the pupil (shutter) and is focused by the lens to produce a
sharp image on the retina (film) at the back of the eye. The image
captured on the retina is then sent via the optic nerve to the brain
(lab) to be developed and "printed" by the mind's eye.

Choroid: The vascular layer of the eye lying between the retina and
the sclera, it provides nourishment to outer layers of the retina.

Cornea: The transparent tissue that covers the iris and pupil at the
front of the eye. It helps focus incoming light.

Fovea: Central pit in the macula that produces sharpest vision.

Lens: The clear biconvex (curved on both sides) lens of the eye helps
focus light through the vitreous to the retina.

Macula: The small central layer of tissue in the retina, responsible
for central vision.

Optic nerve: Largest sensory nerve of the eye, it carries visual information from the retina to the brain.

Iris: Pigmented tissue lying behind the cornea that gives color to the
eye (e.g., blue or brown eyes) and contracts or expands to let more or
less light into the eye through the pupil.

Pupil: The variable-sized black circular opening in the center of the
iris regulating the amount of light that enters the eye.

Retina: The lining of the rear two-thirds of the eye, it converts images from the eye's optical system into electrical impulses sent along the optic nerve to the brain.

Retinal pigment epithelium: The pigment cell layer just outside the retina that nourishes retinal visual cells; it is firmly attached to underlying choroid and overlying retinal visual cells and composed of one layer of cells that are densely packed with pigment granules.

Sclera: Opaque, fibrous, protective outer layer of the eye ("white of the eye") that is directly continuous with the cornea in front and with the sheath covering the optic nerve behind.

Vitreous: Transparent, colorless gel that fills the rear two-thirds of the interior of the eyeball, between the lens and the retina.

Section 1.2

How We See

Reprinted from "Healthy Eyes: How We See," National Eye Institute, National Institutes of Health. The complete text of this document can be found online at http://www.nei.nih.gov/healthyeyes/howwesee.asp; accessed March 14, 2011.

There are many different parts of the eye that help to create vision. Light passes through the cornea, the clear, dome-shaped surface that covers the front of the eye. The cornea bends—or refracts—this incoming light. The iris, the colored part of the eye, regulates the size of the pupil, the opening that controls the amount of light that enters the eye. Behind the pupil is the lens, a clear part of the eye that further focuses light, or an image, onto the retina. The retina is a thin, delicate, photosensitive tissue that contains the special "photoreceptor" cells that convert light into electrical signals. These electrical signals are processed further, and then travel from the retina of the eye to the brain through the optic nerve, a bundle of about one million nerve fibers. We "see" with our brains; our eyes collect visual information and begin this complex process.

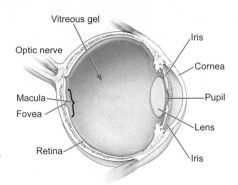

Figure 1.1. *Diagram of the Eye*

Section 1.3

What Is 20/20 Vision?

20/20 vision is a term used to express normal visual acuity (the clarity or sharpness of vision) measured at a distance of twenty feet. If you have 20/20 vision, you can see clearly at twenty feet what should normally be seen at that distance. If you have 20/100 vision, it means that you must be as close as twenty feet to see what a person with normal vision can see at one hundred feet.

20/20 does not necessarily mean perfect vision. 20/20 vision only indicates the sharpness or clarity of vision at a distance. There are other important vision skills, including peripheral awareness or side vision, eye coordination, depth perception, focusing ability, and color vision that contribute to your overall visual ability.

Some people can see well at a distance, but are unable to bring nearer objects into focus. This condition can be caused by hyperopia (farsightedness) or presbyopia (loss of focusing ability). Others can see items that are close, but cannot see those far away. This condition may be caused by myopia (nearsightedness).

A comprehensive eye examination by a doctor of optometry can diagnose those causes, if any, that are affecting your ability to see well. In most cases, your optometrist can prescribe glasses, contact lenses, or a vision therapy program that will help improve your vision. If the reduced vision is due to an eye disease, the use of ocular medication or other treatment may be used.

Chapter 2

Maintaining Eye Health

Chapter Contents

Section 2.1

Simple Tips for Healthy Eyes

Reprinted from the Centers for Disease
Control and Prevention, June 18, 2010.

Your eyes are an important part of your health. You can do many things to keep them healthy and make sure you're seeing your best. Follow these simple guidelines for maintaining healthy eyes well into your golden years.

Have a comprehensive dilated eye exam. You might think your vision is fine or that your eyes are healthy, but visiting your eye care professional for a comprehensive dilated eye exam is the only way to really be sure. When it comes to common vision problems, some people don't realize they could see better with glasses or contact lenses. In addition, many common eye diseases, such as glaucoma, diabetic eye disease, and age-related macular degeneration, often have no warning signs. A dilated eye exam is the only way to detect these diseases in their early stages.

During a comprehensive dilated eye exam, your eye care professional places drops in your eyes to dilate, or widen, the pupil to allow more light to enter the eye—the same way an open door lets more light into a dark room. This process enables your eye care professional to get a good look at the back of the eyes and examine them for any signs of damage or disease. Your eye care professional is the only one who can determine if your eyes are healthy and if you're seeing your best.

Know your family's eye health history. Talk to your family members about their eye health history. It's important to know if anyone has been diagnosed with an eye disease or condition, since many are hereditary. This information will help to determine if you're at higher risk for developing an eye disease or condition.

Eat right to protect your sight. You've heard that carrots are good for your eyes. But eating a diet rich in fruits and vegetables—particularly dark leafy greens, such as spinach, kale, or collard greens—is important for keeping your eyes healthy, too.[1] Research has also shown there are eye health benefits from eating fish high in omega-3 fatty acids, such as salmon, tuna, and halibut.

Maintain a healthy weight. Being overweight or obese increases your risk of developing diabetes and other systemic conditions, which can lead to vision loss, such as diabetic eye disease or glaucoma. If you're having trouble maintaining a healthy weight, talk to your doctor.

Wear protective eyewear. Wear protective eyewear when playing sports or doing activities around the home. Protective eyewear includes safety glasses and goggles, safety shields, and eye guards specially designed to provide the correct protection for the activity in which you're engaged. Most protective eyewear lenses are made of polycarbonate, which is ten times stronger than other plastics. Many eye care providers sell protective eyewear, as do some sporting goods stores.

Quit smoking or never start. Smoking is as bad for your eyes as it is for the rest of your body. Research has linked smoking to an increased risk of developing age-related macular degeneration, cataract, and optic nerve damage, all of which can lead to blindness.[2,3]

Be cool and wear your shades. Sunglasses are a great fashion accessory, but their most important job is to protect your eyes from the sun's ultraviolet rays. When purchasing sunglasses, look for ones that block out 99 to 100 percent of both ultraviolet A (UV-A) and ultraviolet B (UV-B) radiation.

Give your eyes a rest. If you spend a lot of time at the computer or focusing on any one thing, you sometimes forget to blink and your eyes can get fatigued. Try the 20-20-20 rule: Every twenty minutes, look away about twenty feet in front of you for twenty seconds. This short exercise can help reduce eyestrain.

Clean your hands and your contact lenses—properly. To avoid the risk of infection, always wash your hands thoroughly before putting in or taking out your contact lenses. Make sure to disinfect contact lenses as instructed and replace them as appropriate.

Practice workplace eye safety. Employers are required to provide a safe work environment. When protective eyewear is required as a part of your job, make a habit of wearing the appropriate type at all times, and encourage your coworkers to do the same.

References

1. Age-Related Eye Disease Study Research Group. The relationship of dietary carotenoid with vitamin A, E, and C intake with age-related macular degeneration in a case-control study. *Archives of Ophthalmology* 2007;125(9):1225–32.

2. Age-Related Eye Disease Study Research Group. Risk factors associated with age-related nuclear and cortical cataract. *Ophthalmology* 2001;108(8):1400–1408.

3. U.S. Department of Health and Human Services, Office of the Surgeon General. *The Health Consequences of Smoking: A Report of the Surgeon General* (Washington, D.C., 2004).

Section 2.2

Vitamins and Your Sight

"Scientists Link Nutrition and Eye Health,"
United States Department of Agriculture, January 15, 2004.
Reviewed by David A. Cooke, MD, FACP, December 2011.

About sixteen million people in the United States over age forty-five report some vision loss. This group may find hope in a growing body of evidence that diet can influence eye health. The Agricultural Research Service (ARS) has several scientists studying the possibility of reducing—by way of dietary modification—the risk of two common sight-robbing disorders: cataract formation and age-related macular degeneration.

About twenty years ago, scientists were hard-pressed to find published research studies on correlations between nutrition and risk of eye disease. But steady efforts by government and academic researchers over the years have led to a clearly established discipline of ophthalmologic nutrition and epidemiology.

A Cloudy Matter

For baby boomers reaching an age at which steady vision can no longer be taken for granted, many are wishing they'd worn sunglasses when young. Sunlight is somewhat of a natural enemy to the eye's lens.

"Lens cells make a specific, predominant set of proteins called crystallins," says bio-organic chemist Allen Taylor. He is chief of the Laboratory for Nutrition and Vision Research at the Jean Mayer United States Department of Agriculture (USDA) Human Nutrition Research Center on Aging (HNRCA) at Tufts University in Boston, Massachusetts. "Those proteins act like fiber-optics, allowing light to pass through the lens and onto the retina," he says. They must function over decades with little opportunity for repair.

Red, blue, green, yellow, and ultraviolet (UV) wavelengths penetrate the transparent lens. But UV light appears to be particularly damaging to the lens, and blue light appears to damage the retina—a complex, sensory membrane that lines the eye and receives the images formed by the lens. Normal byproducts of metabolism, called oxygen free radicals, also cause damage. If not neutralized by an antioxidant, over time such oxidation damages the lipids, proteins, and other components of the lens. The result is a clouding of the lens in a gradual slide from transparent to opaque. These opacities are called cataracts.

Antioxidants are compounds in foods that help maintain healthy cells and tissues in the eye and other organs. Inside the lens are high levels of vitamins C and E as well as some lutein and zeaxanthin. The latter two fall within a class of phytochemicals called carotenoids, and they are concentrated in the retina.

"As damaged proteins gather, they result in lens opacities," says Taylor. His research suggests that protective, antioxidant-rich nutrition could be the least costly and most practical means to delay cataracts. "The accumulation of oxidized or modified proteins we've observed is consistent with the failure of protective systems to keep pace with the insults that damage lens proteins," he says. The protective systems include protein-digesting enzymes, which may seek out and destroy damaged proteins, as well as antioxidants, which can lessen initial damage and may keep protective enzymes functioning longer.

In economic and human terms, damage to lens proteins is costly. About half of those over seventy-five in the United States will experience a visually significant cataract. The costs of cataract-related disability and cataract surgery now total $6 billion annually worldwide.

Various Causes

Three distinguishable areas of the lens can be affected by cataracts: the nuclear, cortical, and posterior subcapsular (PSC) areas. The nuclear and cortical areas are associated with age-related cataracts, while the PSC area is associated with diabetes-related cataracts.

Nuclear lens opacity has been the most widely studied of the three lens areas. Paul F. Jacques, Taylor, and colleagues reported in 2001 that antioxidant nutrients play a role in the prevention of nuclear cataracts. Jacques is chief of HNRCA's Nutritional Epidemiology Program.

The scientists looked at 478 nondiabetic women from Boston, aged fifty-three to seventy-three years and not previously diagnosed with cataracts. These women were sampled from the Nutrition and Vision Project (NVP), a substudy of the federally funded Nurses' Health Study. Researchers conducted eye exams to study the relationship between newly diagnosed nuclear opacities and nutrient intake over time. Food intake was assessed from multiple food frequency questionnaires completed over thirteen to fifteen years.

The study showed that women with the highest intakes of vitamins C and E, riboflavin, folate, beta carotene, lutein, and zeaxanthin had a lower prevalence of nuclear opacification than did those with the lowest intakes of those nutrients. Moreover, those who used vitamin C supplements for ten or more years were 64 percent less likely to have nuclear opacification than those who never used vitamin C supplements.

Taylor, Jacques, and colleagues reported similar findings in 2002 when they looked for cataracts in the cortical and PSC regions of the lens in some NVP participants. Those findings support a role for vitamin C in reducing the risk of cortical cataracts in women younger than sixty. The data also indicated that women who consumed higher amounts of carotenoids had a lower risk of PSC cataracts if they had never smoked.

In the same NVP population, women who regularly took vitamin E had less progression of eye lens damage, as Taylor reported during the 2003 Association for Research in Vision and Ophthalmology proceedings in Fort Lauderdale, Florida. "The increase in nuclear opacification—over five years of follow-up after their initial examination—was 30 percent lower among women who used vitamin E supplements for at least ten years than among those who had never used vitamin E supplements," says Jacques.

Another recently completed study explored the relationship between body mass index, waist circumference, diabetes, and the presence of age-related cataracts in women. The study supports other findings that diabetes is a strong risk factor for PSC opacities and that abdominal fat and obesity may also be associated with PSC. Several variables complicate a comprehensive evaluation of the existing evidence linking nutrition and age-related vision loss. "Definitions of cataract may differ from one study to another, and the various methods for assessing the intake or status of nutrients, such as antioxidants, certainly complicate matters," says Jacques. "There are several questions that still need to be resolved."

At this point, what scientists do know is that oxidative damage within the eye is harmful to several eye tissues.

The Yellow Spot

Among Americans who are fifty-five or older, age-related macular degeneration (AMD) is reported to be a leading cause of blindness and vision impairment. According to the National Eye Institute (NEI), more than 1.6 million Americans in that age group have advanced AMD. Some experts estimate up to 7 million more may be at the intermediate stage. They see fine now, but they are at high risk for developing the advanced form, which causes vision loss.

Among the causes of AMD, scientists describe a breakdown of light-sensitive cells within the retina. The focus is on a three-millimeter-wide yellow spot, called the macula lutea, toward the back and center of the eye. The macula plays a key role in the central part of visual images. But as the eye ages, oxidized proteins, or debris called drusen, begin to pile up and cause trouble. Taylor and other scientists are seeking to unravel the mystery of why this process happens.

Scientists have long known that the yellow color, or pigment, inside the macula comes from the carotenoids lutein and zeaxanthin. Many scientists believe that these plant chemicals help protect the eye by absorbing blue light and neutralizing free radicals. But as the body ages, the importance of carotenoids in the macula may increase because of the lifelong exposure to damaging light.

These two carotenoids circulate in the food supply and in blood plasma at a ratio of about one part zeaxanthin to about six or seven parts lutein. As blood passes by the macula through retinal blood vessels, these pigments pass through the macula's outer layer to rest in high concentrations inside its center. Perhaps most interesting is that people with macular degeneration have been found to have lower levels of zeaxanthin and lutein in the macula than people without—which supports the premise that these antioxidants provide some protection.

Absorbing Research

Nutritional biochemist Elizabeth J. Johnson, who is with HNRCA's Carotenoids and Health Laboratory, is now leading a study aimed at determining differences in the body's absorption and use—known as bioavailability—of lutein from eggs, spinach, and supplements.

After study volunteers—healthy adult men—consumed cooked spinach, eggs, and lutein supplements, Johnson measured levels of lutein and triglyceride-rich lipoproteins in their blood serum. The study, which is supported by the Egg Nutrition Center in Washington, D.C., used eggs from chickens that had been fed marigold petals, which are high in lutein. Consumption of these eggs considerably increased the lutein in volunteers' blood.

"After volunteers ate eggs as a source of lutein, their blood serum level of lutein was two to three times greater than it was after they ate the same amount of lutein from other sources," says Johnson. These preliminary results provide compelling evidence that eggs can be a more bioavailable source of lutein than more conventional sources, such as spinach and supplements. "We don't know why the lutein in egg yolks is more bioavailable, but we think it's due to other components in the yolks, such as lecithins."

The "designer" eggs used in the study had about six times—about 1.5 milligrams—the lutein of standard eggs. Still, spinach has about 11 milligrams per two-ounce serving. "Even though the lutein in the eggs is a comparatively tiny amount, it goes right into the blood-stream," says Johnson.

She has also studied and will soon report the effects of lutein and zeaxanthin supplementation on carotenoid levels in the blood, adipose (fat) tissue, and macula of monkeys. That research has led to new findings about the source of an important form of zeaxanthin, called meso zeaxanthin. Curiously, that form is found in the macula, but not in food or blood. It may be better than lutein at reducing damage from light entering the eye. Johnson believes meso zeaxanthin could actually be formed from lutein once it's inside the macula itself.

Diminishing Risk

In 2001, NEI researchers reported results from the seven-year Age-Related Eye Disease Study, or AREDS. Results showed that people lowered their risk of developing advanced AMD by about 25 percent when they took a high-dose combination of vitamins C and E, beta-carotene, and zinc for more than six years.

NEI defines high risk as having intermediate or advanced AMD in one eye. In those with advanced AMD, the nutrients reduced their risk of further vision loss by about 19 percent. NEI concluded that while the nutrients will not restore vision already lost from the disease, they may play a key role in helping high-risk people keep their remaining vision.

Lutein supplements were not available at the study's inception, but NEI is starting to study it now. "Lutein is compelling because of evidence that it neutralizes free radicals," says Johnson. "Since it's in the macula, it's right where it needs to be to protect against damage." In the meantime, during regular examinations, eye doctors can see the telltale signs of early, intermediate, and advanced AMD.

The AREDS supplements had no significant effect on cataract development or progression. But intervention was only for about six years, and some people in the control group had already taken, or continued to take, antioxidant supplements.

Cataract surgery is the most expensive outpatient surgery covered by Medicare. While some see surgery as a stopgap intervention for cataracts, there is as yet no known surgical remedy for AMD, making optimal nutrition all the more attractive.

Researchers focusing on eye health today agree that for some, nutrition will play an important role in lessening the risk of developing these sight-robbing eye disorders.

Section 2.3

Fish and Eye Health

Is there anything you can do to protect your eyes against age-related macular degeneration? The importance of omega-3 fatty acids, found in fatty fish and other foods, in heart disease prevention is well documented. Now research suggests that eating oily fish can help slow or prevent age-related macular degeneration. Read what the experts have found.

The causes of age-related macular degeneration—both non-neovascular (also known as nonexudative, atrophic, or dry) and neovascular (also called exudative or wet)—are unknown, although there are known risk factors for both forms of the disease.

Increasing age, farsightedness, cigarette smoking (and possibly exposure to secondhand smoke), a light-colored iris, obesity, and a family history of age-related macular degeneration all raise the risk of both types. In addition, high blood pressure appears to be linked to a greater risk of neovascular age-related macular degeneration, as are high levels of C-reactive protein, a marker of inflammation in the body.

Studies published in the *Archives of Ophthalmology* (Volume 124, page 981) point to fish oil as a potent anti-inflammatory, protecting high-risk individuals against age-related macular degeneration.

Eating oily fish like salmon, herring, tuna, and mackerel one to three times a week appears to cut the risk of age-related macular degeneration, according to two studies. In a study at the University of Sydney Eye Clinic in Australia, researchers followed nearly three thousand men and women for five years. Those who ate fish once a week had a 40 percent reduced risk of early age-related macular degeneration compared with those who ate fish only once a month; those who ate fish three times a week had a reduced risk of late age-related macular degeneration.

In another study of almost seven hundred male twins by researchers at the Massachusetts Eye and Ear Infirmary and Harvard Medical School, those who ate fish at least twice a week lowered their risk of age-related macular degeneration by 45 percent compared with people who ate fish less than once a week.

Researchers believe the protection stems from the omega-3 fatty acids that are plentiful in oily fish. Other studies have shown that omega-3's reduce inflammation that results from free radicals, molecules that damage healthy cells, including those in the retina.

Section 2.4

Smoking and Eye Health

Introduction to Smoking and Eye Health

It is well known that the tobacco smoke generated by smoking a cigarette, pipe, or other tobacco product can cause damage to the individual who is smoking, and also to the people exposed to the smoke.

The health conditions most commonly associated with tobacco smoke exposure are cancers and cardiovascular disorders. However, there is now a significant body of evidence showing an increased risk of a number of eye disorders, not only in those who smoke, but also in those who are frequently exposed to tobacco smoke.

What Is Tobacco Smoke?

Tobacco smoke is the smoke generated from smoking tobacco. There are two types of tobacco smoke:

- **Sidestream smoke:** Sidestream smoke is the smoke which comes from the tip of a burning cigarette. It contributes about 80 percent of tobacco smoke–related air pollution, and is forty-six times more toxic than mainstream smoke.

- **Mainstream smoke:** Mainstream smoke is the smoke which comes from the filter of a burning cigarette, or is inhaled and exhaled by the smoker.

Tobacco smoke contains over four thousand substances, including many known carcinogens, irritants, and inflammatory agents.

What Conditions Are Associated with Exposure to Tobacco Smoke?

Children

While children do not typically smoke cigarettes (at least until adolescence), many are exposed to environmental tobacco smoke, either because their parents smoke at home or in the car, or because they find themselves in environments where adults are smoking. This is commonly known as passive smoking.

Passive smoking has negative effects on the eyes of children exposed to tobacco smoke. The eye diseases and conditions associated with exposure to tobacco smoke in children include:

- **Strabismus:** Strabismus is a condition in which the eyes become misaligned (e.g., crossed eyes). Maternal smoking during pregnancy is associated with a 6.55 times increased risk of strabismus among children.

- **Allergic conjunctivitis:** Allergic conjunctivitis is a condition in which the conjunctiva becomes inflamed due to the presence of an allergen. While no studies have been conducted specifically to assess the relationship between allergic conjunctivitis and tobacco smoke exposure, a number of studies of allergic reactions in children have reported that the risk of developing allergic conjunctivitis increased by about 20 percent in children who are exposed to environmental tobacco smoke.

Adults

In adults, smoking cigarettes is associated with the following eye diseases and disorders:

- **Cataract:** There is strong evidence that smoking, particularly pipe smoking, increases the risk of cataracts (clouding of the lens of the eye). A review of twenty-seven studies examining the association between cigarette smoking and cataract reported a three times increased risk of nuclear cataract, and also evidence of an association between smoking and subcapsular posterior cataract. While studies have not yet demonstrated an association between environmental tobacco smoke exposure and cataract, it remains a potential risk factor.

- **Uveitis:** Uveitis is a condition characterized by inflammation of the uvea (middle section) of the eye. While no studies have been conducted in humans, laboratory studies using rats have determined that endotoxin (a chemical found in tobacco smoke) can induce an inflammatory response and acute uveitis. Thus it is plausible that tobacco-smoke exposure can increase the risk of uveitis in smokers and those exposed to environmental tobacco smoke.

- **Age-related macular degeneration:** Smoking is a clearly established risk factor for age-related macular degeneration (the deterioration of vision with age). Data from three large cross-sectional studies estimated a three times increased risk of age-related macular degeneration in smokers compared to nonsmokers. A review of studies examining the association between age-related macular degeneration and smoking reported that smoking actually causes age-related macular degeneration, rather than just being indirectly associated with the condition. That review also reported that the more people smoked, the more likely they were to develop age-related macular degeneration. The association between environmental tobacco smoke exposure and age-related macular degeneration is less clear, and studies to date have presented conflicting results. These conflicting results may be because each of the studies used a different definition of passive smoking.

- **Graves ophthalmopathy (thyroid eye disease):** Graves ophthalmopathy, also called thyroid eye disease, is a condition characterized by inflammation of the eye and fat in the eye socket. Studies have provided strong evidence of an association between thyroid eye disease and how much an individual smokes. Smokers with thyroid eye disease had poorer outcomes than nonsmokers. Data suggests that environmental tobacco smoke exposure increases the risk of Graves ophthalmopathy, although the data is limited.

- **Ocular surface disorders:** Smoking has been linked to an increase in disorders of the eye's ocular surface which result in symptoms such as itchiness, redness, and irritation of the eyes. Changes to the eye's ocular surface associated with smoking include changes to the lipid layer of the tear film, reduced tear secretion, and reduced corneal and conjunctival sensitivity. Passive smoking can also increase the risk of these disorders. Ocular surface disorders include atopic keratoconjunctivitis and allergic conjunctivitis.

Preventing Tobacco Smoke–Associated Eye Disorders

Reducing or eliminating exposure to environmental tobacco smoke and stopping smoking are the key ways to prevent tobacco smoke–associated eye disorders.

Note

1. Smoking cessation guidelines for Australian general practice [online]. Canberra, ACT: Australian Government Department of Health and Ageing; 2004 [cited 11 January 2011].

References

Lois N, Abdelkader E, Reglitz K, et al. Environmental tobacco exposure and eye disease. *Br J Ophthalmol*. 2008;92(10):1304–10.

Stone RA, Wilson LB, Ying GS, et al. Associations between childhood refraction and parental smoking. *Invest Ophthalmol Vis Sci*. 2006;47(10):4277–87.

Cumming RG, Mitchell P. Alcohol, smoking and cataracts: The Blue Mountains Eye Study. *Arch Ophthalmol*. 1997;115(10):1296–1303.

Kelly SP, Thornton J, Edwards R, et al. Smoking and cataract: Review of causal association. *J Cataract Refract Surg*. 2005;31(12):2395–2404.

Smith W, Assink J, Klein R, et al. Risk factors for age-related macular degeneration: Pooled findings from three continents. *Ophthalmology*. 2001;108(4):697–704.

Thornton J, Edwards R, Mitchell P, et al. Smoking and age-related macular degeneration: A review of association. *Eye*. 2005;19(9):935–44.

Klein R, Klein BE, Linton KL, DeMets DL. The Beaver Dam Eye Study: The relation of age-related maculopathy to smoking. *Am J Epidemiol*. 1993;137(2):190–200.

Smith W, Mitchell P, Leeder SR. Smoking and age-related maculopathy. The Blue Mountains Eye Study. *Arch Ophthalmol*. 1996;114(12):1518–23.

Khan JC, Thurlby DA, Shahid H, et al. Smoking and age-related macular degeneration: The number of pack years of cigarette smoking is a major determinant of risk for both geographic atrophy and choroidal neovascularisation. *Br J Ophthalmol*. 2006;90(1):75–80.

Thornton J, Kelly SP, Harrision RA, Edwards R. Cigarette smoking and risk of thyroid eye disease: A systematic review. *Eye.* 2007;21(9):1135–45.

Edwards R, Thornton J, Ajit R, et al. Cigarette smoking and primary open angle glaucoma: A systematic review. *J Glaucoma.* 2008;17(7):558–66.

Section 2.5

Safe Use of Cosmetics

Introduction to Cosmetics and the Eyes

Facial cosmetics and cleansers can sometimes pass through the eyelids and come into contact with the eye's surface. Applicators or fingers used to apply eye cosmetics may also sometimes accidentally touch the eye's surface during the application process. As many cosmetics contain chemicals, and their applicators can house unseen dirt and bacteria, exposure of the eyes' surface to cosmetics and cosmetic applicators can cause eye disorders.

However, eye disorders caused by cosmetic use can be avoided if the right cosmetics are purchased, stored, and applied in a hygienic manner. There are many measures which cosmetic users can take to reduce their risk of developing a cosmetics-related eye disorder.

Eye Disorders Associated with Cosmetic Use

The eye disorders associated with cosmetic use are most commonly minor irritations and infections. However, more serious infections and irritations have also occurred following use of eye cosmetics, and minor irritations and infections may become more serious if left untreated.

Swelling or Inflammation of the Eye Area

The use of eyelash dyes is associated with swelling and inflammation of the eye area. In two very serious cases in the United States in the 1930s, one woman was permanently blinded and another died from the use of eyelash dyes.

The eyes may also become swollen or irritated when some other eye cosmetics are applied, or if they become infected by cosmetics, applicators, or fingers during the application process.

Conjunctivitis

Severe conjunctivitis, a condition in which the conjunctiva (covering of the eyeball) becomes inflamed, is associated with the application of some cosmetic products, in particular eyelash dyes.

Dermatitis

There have also been reports of severe cases of dermatitis affecting the eyelid and causing pain and discomfort in the eye area following the application of eyelash dyes.

How to Prevent Eye Disorders When You Use Cosmetics

There are a range of measures which can be taken to protect the eyes from exposure to cosmetic products and their applicators. Individuals who use cosmetics should become familiar with and implement these measures to protect their eyes from infections and irritations.

Don't Share Eye Cosmetics

Eye cosmetics or their applicators are exposed to the user's bacteria when they are used. An individual who shares their cosmetics may therefore become exposed to the bacteria of others who have used the same product. Cosmetic users should not share their cosmetics with friends or use single-use applicators if they do. Individuals who use cosmetics should also be aware that "tester" cosmetics which allow sampling of cosmetic products in stores are particularly dangerous because they are often shared by a large number of people. Individuals who decide to use testers should use a single-use applicator.

Take Care When Applying Eye Cosmetics

It is easy to poke an applicator or finger in the eye when applying cosmetics and this can scratch the eyeball or introduce bacteria into the eye. It is therefore important to take care when applying cosmetics. In particular, eye cosmetics should not be applied in a moving vehicle or other situation where a sudden bump may cause an applicator to poke the eye.

Avoid Cosmetics Containing Irritants

Many cosmetics contain chemicals and in some cases these will irritate the eyes. This is particularly likely if the cosmetic product is not specifically designed for use on the eyes but is applied to the eye area anyway (e.g., lip liner applied as eyeliner). Use of cosmetics that are not specifically developed for eye application should therefore be avoided. However, irritation can also occur with products designed specifically for use with eyes.

There have been numerous reports of cases of severe eye irritations such as conjunctivitis and dermatitis of the eyelid following the application of eyelash tints and dyes. Individuals who wish to avoid these eye disorders should avoid the use of permanent eyelash tints and dyes.

There is evidence that solvent-based mascaras (e.g., those which use petroleum distillate to maintain product consistency) cause contact dermatitis, whereas stearate-based mascaras do not.

Kohl, an ingredient commonly found in eyeliners, is known to have high concentrations of lead, and while this does not directly affect the eye, it can affect an individual's health more broadly.

Individuals should check product labels and avoid cosmetics containing solvents, kohl, and other substances to which they are hypersensitive.

Keep Cosmetics (and the Hands and Tools That Apply Them) Clean

Avoiding dirt and bacteria is an important way to avoid eye disorders. In order to avoid dirt and bacteria on hands and cosmetics which may contact the eye, cosmetic users should:

- keep cosmetics and their applicators clean and ensure they do not become covered with dirt or dust;

- discard cosmetics which are exposed to dirt or applied during an eye infection;

- wash their hands prior to applying cosmetics and ensure that any instruments which they use to assist in the application process are clean;

- store cosmetics at room temperature, as high temperatures may destroy the preservatives which protect them against bacteria; and

- use cosmetics as they are. Cosmetics should not be tampered with (e.g., water should not be added if the product becomes dry), as this may introduce bacteria.

Avoid Using Cosmetics When the Eyes Are Infected or Irritated

Cosmetics should not be used while the eyes are infected or irritated, as cosmetic use may make the infection worse. If the eyes become irritated while cosmetics are applied, they should be removed immediately and any unused portion of the product should be disposed of.

Face Washing to Remove Cosmetics

It is important that cosmetic users thoroughly remove cosmetics and dirt from their faces everyday. This can be done using facial cleansing solutions (including soaps), facial cleansing instruments, (e.g. exfoliating brushes), or a combination of the two. The best way to cleanse the face will depend on the individual's skin type. The best cosmetic removal technique will depend on the type of cosmetic used and its properties, such as if it was waterproof or water soluble.

Many soaps which are highly fragranced and suitable for cleaning the body are unsuitable for the sensitive skin of the face. However, there are a range of soap-free facial cleansing bars (e.g., beauty bar soaps) and solutions which have been developed for use on the face. They typically have a higher pH (that is, they are not as acidic as regular soap), and are thus less likely to cause irritation to the skin of the eyes and face. They may not be suitable for individuals with very oily skin, who may need to use a facial scrub or facial cloth to achieve oil removal.

Waterproof cosmetics must be removed using special facial cleansing solutions. As many of these cleansing solutions contain chemicals which may irritate the eye (e.g., cause contact dermatitis), it is safer to use cosmetic products which are not waterproof, and can therefore be removed with water alone. Contact lens users should ensure they remove their lenses prior to cleaning cosmetics from the eye area.

References

United States Food and Drug Authority. Eye cosmetics and eyebrow/eyelash dyes. 2001. [cited 2009 May 15] available at: http://www.cfsan.fda.gov/~dms/cos-821.html

Kaiserman, I. Severe allergic blepharoconjuntivitis induced by a dye for eyelashes and eyebrows. *Ocular Immunol & Infamm.* 2003;11(2):149–51.

Texeira, M. Wachter, L. Ronsyn, E. Goossens, A. Contact allergy to para-phenylenediamin in a permanent eyelash dye. *Contact Dermatitis* 2006;55(2):92–94.

Gallardo, M. Randleman, J. Price, K. et al. Ocular Argyosis after long-term self-application of eyelash tint. *Am J Ophthalmol.* 2006;141(1):198–200.

Wessman, L.J. Mascaras may cause irritant contact dermatitis. *Int J Cosmetic Sci.* 2002;24(5):281–85.

Al Hazzaa, S.A. Krahn, P.M. Kohl: a hazardous eyeliner. *Int Ophthalmol.* 1995;19(2):83–88.

National Industrial Chemicals Notification and Assessment Scheme, Cosmetic Guidelines 2007 [online]. Australian Government Department of Health and Ageing. 2 December 2008. [cited 15 May 2009]. Available from URL: http://www.nicnas.gov.au/

Draelos, Z.D. Special considerations in eye cosmetics. *Clin Dermatol.* 2001;19:424–30.

American Academy of Dermatology. Cutting through the clutter: making the most of your facial cleansing routine, 2005 [cited 2009, May 23], available from: http://www.prnewswire.com/gh/cnoc/comp/638376.html

Chapter 3

*Vision Disorders:
A Statistical Picture*

Chapter Contents

Section 3.1

Fast Facts about Vision Disorders

"Fast Facts," Centers for Disease Control and
Prevention, November 5, 2009.

Approximately fourteen million individuals aged twelve years and older have visual impairment, among which more than 80 percent could be corrected to good vision with refractive correction.

As of 2004, blindness or low vision affects more than 3.3 million Americans aged forty years and older; this number is predicted to double by 2030 due to the increasing epidemics of diabetes and other chronic diseases and our rapidly aging U.S. population.

Approximately 6.8 percent of children younger than eighteen years in the United States have a diagnosed eye and vision condition.

In 2001, about two million Americans sustained eye injuries that required medical attention.

An estimated sixty-one million adults in the United States are at high risk for serious vision loss, but only half have visited an eye doctor in the past twelve months.

The annual economic impact of major vision problems among the adult population forty years and older is more than $51 billion.

Vision disability is one of the top ten disabilities among adults eighteen years and older and one of the most prevalent disabling conditions among children.

Early detection and timely treatment of eye conditions such as diabetic retinopathy has been found to be efficacious and cost effective.

The National Commission on Prevention Priorities has identified vision screening among adults aged sixty-five years and older as one of the top ten priorities among effective clinical preventive services.

Vision loss causes a substantial social and economic toll for millions of people including significant suffering, disability, loss of productivity, and diminished quality of life.

National and state data show that more than half of adult Americans did not seek eye care are due to lack of awareness or costs, which often were exacerbated by lack of adequate health insurance.

More than 70 percent of survey respondents from National Eye Health Education Program (NEHEP) 2005 Public Knowledge, Attitudes, and Practices survey consider that the loss of their eyesight would have the greatest impact on their day-to-day life; however, less than 11 percent knew that there are no early warning signs of glaucoma and diabetic retinopathy.

Section 3.2

The Burden of Vision Loss

Excerpted from "The Burden of Vision Loss," Centers for Disease Control and Prevention, September 25, 2009.

Population Estimates

More than 3.4 million (3 percent) Americans aged forty years and older are either legally blind (having visual acuity [VA] of 20/200 or worse or a visual field of less than 20 degrees) or are visually impaired (having VA of 20/40 or less) (Eye Diseases Prevalence Research Group, 2004). The Federal Interagency Forum on Aging Related Statistics (2008) estimates that 17 percent of the population age sixty-five and older report "vision trouble." Twenty-one million Americans report functional vision problems or eye conditions that may compromise vision (Pleis & Lethbridge-Çejku, 2007). Older people are more likely to experience vision loss because of age-related eye diseases. State-level data are available from the Vision Loss and Access to Eye Care Module of the Behavioral Risk Factors Surveillance System (BRFSS). A 2006 Centers for Disease Control and Prevention (CDC) study revealed that self-reported vision loss (a little, moderate, or extreme difficulty) ranged from 14.3 percent to 20.5 percent among five states. The Vision Module of the BRFSS allows states to estimate population and describe the characteristics of people aged forty years and older who experience vision loss. Despite the magnitude of the population at risk for vision loss as well as the grave consequences of vision loss and blindness, many individuals do not benefit from available cost-effective early detection, timely treatments, and interventions to promote health.

Vision Loss among Top Ten Disabilities

An analysis of the 1999 Survey of Income and Program Participation (CDC, 2001) revealed blindness or vision problems to be among the top ten disabilities among adults aged eighteen years and older. Vision loss has serious consequences for the individual as well as those who care for and about people who have compromised vision because it impedes the ability to read, drive, prepare meals, watch television, and attend to personal affairs. Reduced vision among mature adults has been shown to result in social isolation, family stress, and ultimately a greater tendency to experience other health conditions or die prematurely (Ellwein, Friedlin, McBean, & Lee, 1996).

Estimated Growth in Population

During the next three decades, the population of adults with vision impairment and age-related eye diseases is estimated to double because of the rapidly aging U.S. population. In addition, the epidemic of diabetes as well as other chronic diseases will contribute to an increasing population of people who experience vision loss.

A recent CDC investigation (Saaddine, Honeycutt, Narayan, Zhang, Klein, & Boyle, 2008) revealed that eye diseases associated with diabetes are likely to surge during the next four decades, reflecting overall changes in the population as well as improved treatment of diabetes and survival among those who experience diabetes. The number of people who experience diabetic retinopathy is expected to triple between 2005 and 2050 from 5.5 million to 16 million people.

Table 3.1. Estimated Growth in Vision Impairment and Age-Related Eye Diseases by 2020

Disorder	Current Estimates (in millions)	2020 Projections (in millions)
Advanced Age-Related Macular Degeneration (with Associated Vision Loss)	1.8[a]	2.9
Glaucoma	2.2	3.3
Diabetic Retinopathy	4.1	7.2
Cataract	20.5	30.1

Note: a Another 7.3 million people are at substantial risk for vision loss from age-related macular degeneration (AMD).
Source: National Eye Institute, *Archives of Ophthalmology*, 122(4): 444–676. Available from URL: http://www.nei.nih.gov/eyedata/pbd_tables.asp.

References

Bailey RN, Indian RW, Zhang X, Geiss LS, Duenas MR, & Saaddine JB. Visual impairment and eye care among older adults—five states, 2005. *MMWR* 2006;55(49):1321–25.

Eye Diseases Prevalence Research Group. Causes and prevalence of visual impairment among adults in the United States. *Archives of Ophthalmology* 2004;122:477–85.

Federal Interagency Forum on Aging-Related Statistics. *Older Americans 2008: Key Indicators of Wellbeing.* Washington, DC: U.S. Government Printing Office 2008.

Pleis JR, Lethbridge-Çejku M. Summary health statistics for U.S. adults: National Health Interview Survey, 2006. National Center for Health Statistics. *Vital Health Stat* 2007;10(235).

Ellwein LB, Friedlin V, McBean AM, Lee PP. Use of eye care services among the 1991 Medicare population. *Ophthalmology* 1996;103:1732–43.

Saaddine JB, Honeycutt AA, Venkat Narayan KM, Zhang X, Klein R, and Boyle, JP. (2008). Projection of diabetic retinopathy and other major eye diseases among people with diabetes mellitus. *Archives of Ophthalmology* 2008;126(12):1740–47.

Section 3.3

Prevalence of Vision Disorders Across the Lifespan

From "Health Across Lifespan," Centers for Disease
Control and Prevention, September 28, 2009.

Infancy and Childhood (Birth to Age Eighteen)

In the United States, the most prevalent disabling childhood conditions are vision disorders, including amblyopia, strabismus, and significant refractive errors. Early detection increases the likelihood of effective treatment; however, less than 15 percent of all preschool children receive an eye exam, and less than 22 percent of preschool children receive some type of vision screening. Vision screening for children scored on par with breast cancer screening for women. Other eye diseases affecting this age group include retinopathy of prematurity (ROP), congenital defects, diabetic retinopathy (DR), and cancers such as retinoblastoma.

Adults Younger Than Age Forty

Vision impairments in people younger than age forty are mainly caused by refractive errors, which affect 25 percent of children and adolescents, and accidental eye injury. Approximately one million eye injuries occur each year, and 90 percent of these injuries are preventable. More than half (52 percent) of all patients treated for eye injuries are between ages eighteen and forty-five and almost 30 percent of those are aged thirty to forty years (McGwin, Aiyuan, & Owsley, 2005). Additionally, diabetes affects this age group and is the leading cause of blindness among the working-age group twenty to seventy-four. Racial disparities occur in prevalence and incidence of some eye conditions. For example, among specific high-risk groups such as African Americans, early signs of glaucoma may begin in this age group, particularly if there is a family history for glaucoma. Lifestyle choices adopted during this period may adversely affect vision and eye health in later years (e.g., smoking, sunlight exposure).

Adults Older Than Age Forty

American adults aged forty years and older are at greatest risk for eye diseases; as a result, extensive population-based study data are available for this age group. The major eye diseases among people aged forty years and older are cataract, diabetic retinopathy, glaucoma, and age-related macular degeneration. These diseases are often asymptomatic in the early treatable stages. The prevalence of blindness and vision impairment increases rapidly with age among all racial and ethnic groups, particularly after age seventy-five (Prevent Blindness America, 2002). Although aging is unavoidable, evidence is mounting to show the association between some modifiable risk factors (i.e., smoking, ultraviolet light exposure, avoidable trauma, etc.) and these leading eye diseases affecting older Americans. Additional modifiable factors that might lend themselves to improved overall ocular health include a diet rich in antioxidants and maintenance of normal levels of blood sugar, lipids, total cholesterol, body weight, and blood pressure combined with regular exercise.

References

Bailey RN, Indian RW, Zhang X, Geiss LS, Duenas MR, Saaddine JB (2006). Visual impairment and eye care among older adults—five states. *MMWR* 2005:55:49;1321–25.

Centers for Disease Control and Prevention. Prevalence of disabilities and associated health conditions among adults—United States. *MMWR* 2001:50(7):120–25.

Prevent Blindness America, National Eye Institute. *Vision Problems in the U. S.—Prevalence of Adult Vision Impairment and Age-Related Eye Disease in America.* Schaumburg, IL: Prevent Blindness America, 2002.

McGwin G, Aiyuan X, Owsley C. Rate of eye injury in the United States. *Arch of Ophthalmol* 2005:123;970–76.

Yawn BP, Kurland M, Butterfield L, Johnson B. Barriers to seeking care following school vision screening in Rochester, Minnesota, *J Sch Health* 1998:68:8;319–24.

Chapter 4

What You Should Know about Regular Eye Exams

Chapter Contents

Section 4.1

Recommended Intervals for Regular Eye Exams

"Eye Exam Costs and When to Have an Eye Exam,"
reprinted with permission from www.AllAboutVision.com.
© 2011 Access Media Group LLC. All rights reserved.

Common questions about eye exams include: How much does an eye exam cost? How frequently should I have my eyes examined? What should I bring with me to my exam?

These guidelines can help you prepare for your next (or first) eye exam.

Eye Exam Costs

Eye exams are available through several different venues, including an independent eye doctor's office, the eye department of a multidisciplinary medical clinic, a group eye care practice (optometrists, ophthalmologists, or both), and at an optical retailer or optical shop that also offers eye exams by an affiliated optometrist.

Also, large retailers like Walmart, Costco, and Target have optical departments where you can undergo an eye exam.

The cost of an eye exam can vary significantly, based on where you get your exam and other factors, including:

- whether the exam is performed by an optometrist or an ophthalmologist;
- the tests that are included in the exam;
- whether the exam includes a contact lens fitting or other contact lens–related services.

Generally, eye exam costs can range from less than $50 (usually at a retail store or optical chain) to $100 or more (usually at a medical clinic or private eye doctor's office). Also, eye exams for contact lenses nearly always cost more than routine eye exams to update your eyeglasses prescription.

When comparing how much an eye exam costs, be sure you are comparing "apples to apples." A comprehensive eye exam should include at least the following:

- A review of your personal and family health history and any history of eye problems

- Evaluation of your distance and near vision with an eye chart

- Evaluation for the presence of nearsightedness, farsightedness, astigmatism, and presbyopia

- Near vision testing to determine if you have presbyopia and need progressive lenses or bifocals

- Evaluation of your eyes' ability to work together as a team

- An eye pressure test and examination of the optic nerve to rule out glaucoma

- Examination of the interior of your eyes to rule out other eye problems, such as cataracts and macular degeneration

Contact lens exams typically include additional tests and procedures to those noted above.

Be sure to ask what tests are included when you obtain information about eye exam costs. Some locations will advertise a low exam fee, but upon arrival you may be informed you must pay extra if you want certain procedures—such as pupil dilation, retinal photos, etc.—that may be included in a higher exam fee quoted elsewhere.

Certain "intangibles" should be considered when you compare eye exam costs, such as the professionalism and friendliness of the doctor and his or her staff, the level of training of the doctor's assistants, how long you must wait to be seen, the cleanliness of the office, advanced (vs. outdated) exam equipment used, and the convenience of the office location and hours of operation.

It's also a good idea when choosing an eye doctor to ask friends for referrals and to "shop around" first via a personal visit to the office before scheduling an exam.

Many vision insurance plans, including Medicare, cover at least a portion of eye exam services. Check to see what your benefits are and what doctors participate in your plan before you make an appointment. Then be sure to give the doctor's office your insurance information when scheduling your exam to avoid any misunderstandings about your coverage.

When to Have Your Eyes Examined

Most eye care experts recommend that you have a complete eye exam every one to three years, depending on your age, risk factors, and whether you currently wear corrective lenses.

Children

Routine eye exams are essential for children to be ready to learn in school, and experts say more than 80 percent of information children receive in classrooms is presented visually.

According to the American Optometric Association (AOA), children generally should have their first eye exam at six months of age, another exam at age three, and again at the start of school. Risk-free children should then continue to have their eyes examined every two years until age eighteen.

Children with risk factors for vision problems may need their first eye exam earlier than six months of age and may need more frequent eye exams throughout childhood. Examples of risk factors include:

- history of premature birth or low birth weight;
- infection of mother during pregnancy (examples: rubella, venereal disease, herpes, acquired immunodeficiency syndrome [AIDS]);
- developmental delays;
- turned or crossed eyes (strabismus);
- family history of eye disease;
- high refractive error or anisometropia;
- other physical illness or disease.

Also, children who currently wear eyeglasses or contact lenses should have annual eye exams, according to the American Optometric Association (AOA).

Unfortunately, many American children don't receive the eye care they need, and children in poor families are at the greatest risk of undetected vision problems. According to the National Commission on Vision and Health (NCVH), 83 percent of families earning less than twice the federal poverty level include children who have not had an eye exam in the last year.

Currently, fifteen states do not require any form of vision screenings or exams for children prior to them beginning school, resulting in "a public health emergency for millions of children," according to NCVH. Even in states that have requirements for vision screenings for schoolchildren, researchers found that screenings failed to detect vision problems in one-third of children who had them, and most of the children who fail vision screenings don't receive the follow-up vision care they need, NCVH says.[1]

Adults

To maintain a lifetime of healthy vision, the AOA recommends a comprehensive eye exam every two years for adults ages eighteen to sixty, and annual exams for seniors age sixty-one and older.

"At risk" adults should have more frequent exams. Risk factors for adults include:

- a family history of eye disease (glaucoma, macular degeneration, etc.);
- diabetes or high blood pressure;
- a visually demanding occupation or one that may pose hazards to the eyes;
- taking prescription or nonprescription drugs that may have visual or eye-related side effects;
- previous eye injuries or eye surgery.

Also, adults who wear contact lenses should have annual eye exams, according to the AOA.

If you have any doubt how often you (or your children or parents) should have your eyes examined, ask your eye care professional for guidance.

Who Should I See For My Eye Exam?

There are three different kinds of eye care professionals: ophthalmologists, optometrists, and opticians. Who you should see depends on your needs.

Ophthalmologists are medical doctors (MDs or DOs) who specialize in eye care. Not only do they prescribe eyeglasses and contacts, but they also perform eye surgery and treat medical conditions of the eye. Ophthalmologists are eye doctors who have completed medical school and have undergone additional post-graduate training in medical and surgical eye care.

Optometrists also are eye doctors who diagnose vision problems and treat medical conditions of the eye with eye drops and other medicines. Optometrists generally attend four years of optometry school after college to attain their Doctor of Optometry (OD) degree. They prescribe glasses, contacts, low vision aids, vision therapy, and medication to treat eye diseases, but, with a few exceptions, optometrists typically are not trained or licensed to perform eye surgery.

Opticians are not eye doctors. They are eye care professionals who fit, adjust, and repair glasses and teach patients how to apply, remove, and care for contact lenses. In some cases, specially trained opticians fit contact lenses. Opticians generally receive their training either "on the job" by apprenticeship or from technical schools.

What Should I Bring with Me to My Eye Exam?

It is important to bring information to your eye exam that will alert your eye doctor to risks you may have for eye or vision problems.

In particular, bring a list of any prescription or nonprescription medications you are currently taking or that you took on a regular basis in the past. Include vitamins, herbs, and other nontraditional remedies you may use. Include the dosages you take for each medicine or other substance, and how long you have been taking them.

If you currently wear corrective lenses, bring all pairs of eyeglasses you wear routinely. If you wear contacts that were prescribed elsewhere, bring a copy of your most recent contact lens prescription.

Also, be sure to bring a copy of your vision insurance card and any other medical insurance cards you have if you are seeking insurance coverage for a portion of your fees.

Finally, prepare and bring a list of questions or concerns that you would like to discuss with the doctor. And if you are interested in specialty services such as contact lens fitting or laser surgery evaluation, be sure to mention this—both when you schedule your exam and when you check in on exam day.

Notes

1. New evidence-based research shows that universal comprehensive eye exams would help more children succeed in school. *National Commission on Vision & Health*, August 2009.

Section 4.2

Limitations of Vision Screening Programs

Vision screening programs are intended to help identify children or adults who may have undetected vision problems and refer them for further evaluation. However, they can't be relied on to provide the same results as a comprehensive eye and vision examination.

Screenings can take many forms. Often schools provide periodic vision screenings for their students. A pediatrician or other primary care physician may do a vision screening as part of a school physical. When applying for a driver's license, chances are your vision will be screened. Many times vision screenings are part of local health fairs put on by hospitals, social service agencies or fraternal groups like the Lions and Elks Clubs.

While vision screenings can uncover some individuals with vision problems, they can miss more than they find. This is a major concern about vision screening programs.

Current vision screening methods cannot be relied upon to effectively identify individuals in need of vision care. In some cases, vision screening may actually serve as an unnecessary barrier to an early diagnosis of vision problems. They can create a false sense of security for those individuals who "pass" the screening, but who actually have a vision problem, thereby delaying further examination and treatment. Vision screening programs may also result in unnecessary referral for further evaluation of persons who are found not to have an eye or vision problem.

Undetected and untreated vision problems can interfere with a child's ability to learn in school and participate in sports or with an adult's ability to do their job or to drive safely. The earlier a vision problem is diagnosed and treated, the less it will impact an individual's quality of life.

What are the limitations of vision screening programs?

To understand why vision screenings may not find a vision problem, we need to look at the factors that can limit their effectiveness:

- **Limited testing:** Many vision screenings test only for distance visual acuity. While the ability to see clearly in the distance is important, it does not give any indication of how well the eyes focus up close, or work together. It also does not give any information about the health of the eyes. Some screenings may also include a plus lens test for farsightedness and a test of eye coordination. However, even these additional screening tests will fail to detect many vision problems.

- **Untrained personnel:** Oftentimes a vision screening is conducted by administrative personnel or volunteers who have little training. While well intentioned, these individuals do not have the knowledge to competently assess screening results.

- **Inadequate testing equipment:** Even when done in a pediatricians' or primary care physicians' office, the scope of vision screening may be limited by the type of testing equipment available. Factors such as room lighting, testing distances, and maintenance of the testing equipment can also affect test results.

There is often misunderstanding about what passing a vision screening means. The information obtained from a vision screening can be compared to the information obtained from a blood pressure measurement. Because your blood pressure may be in the normal range, it cannot indicate that you do not have other health problems. It provides a single measure of one aspect of your overall health. Just like a complete physical is needed to evaluate total health, only a comprehensive eye and vision examination can evaluate your overall eye health and vision status.

How is a comprehensive eye and vision examination different from a vision screening?

A comprehensive eye and vision examination can only be conducted by an optometrist or ophthalmologist, who has the specialized training needed to make a definitive diagnosis and prescribe treatment. In addition, a comprehensive adult eye and vision examination includes:

- patient and family health history;

- visual acuity measurement;

- preliminary tests of visual function and eye health including depth perception, color vision, peripheral vision, and response of the pupils to light;

- assessment of refractive status to determine the presence of nearsightedness, farsightedness, or astigmatism;

- evaluation of eye focusing, eye teaming, and eye movement abilities;

- eye health examination;

- additional tests as needed.

Vision screening programs can't substitute for regular professional vision care. Periodic eye and vision examinations are needed to fully evaluate eye health and vision.

Even if a child or adult passes a vision screening, they shouldn't assume that they don't have an eye health or vision problem. Professional examinations are the only effective way to confirm or rule out the presence of any eye disease or vision problem. The American Optometric Association recommends the following frequency of eye and vision examinations by age.

Table 4.1. Recommended Frequency of Eye and Vision Examinations

Patient Age	Examination Interval	
	Asymptomatic/ Risk Free	At Risk
Birth to twenty-four months	At six months of age	At six months of age or as recommended
Two to five years	At three years of age	At three years of age or as recommended
Six to eighteen years	Before first grade and every two years thereafter	Annually or as recommended
Eighteen to sixty years	Every two years	Every one to two years or as recommended
Sixty-one and older	Annually	Annually or as recommended

Chapter 5

Screening and Diagnostic Tests for Vision and Other Eye-Related Problems

Chapter Contents

Section 5.1

Comprehensive Eye and Vision Examination

Periodic eye and vision examinations are an important part of preventive health care. Many eye and vision problems have no obvious signs or symptoms. As a result, individuals are often unaware that problems exist. Early diagnosis and treatment of eye and vision problems are important for maintaining good vision and eye health, and when possible, preventing vision loss.

A comprehensive adult eye and vision examination may include, but is not limited to, the following tests. Individual patient signs and symptoms, along with the professional judgment of the doctor, may significantly influence the testing done.

Patient History

A patient history helps to determine any symptoms the individual is experiencing, when they began, the presence of any general heath problems, medications taken, and occupational or environmental conditions that may be affecting vision. The doctor will ask about any eye or vision problems you may be having and about your overall health. The doctor will also ask about any previous eye or health conditions of you and your family members.

Visual Acuity

Visual acuity measurements evaluate how clearly each eye is seeing. As part of the testing, you are asked to read letters on distance and near reading charts. The results of visual acuity testing are written as a fraction such as 20/40.

When testing distance vision, the top number in the fraction is the standard distance at which testing is done, twenty feet. The bottom number is the smallest letter size you were able to read. A person with 20/40 visual acuity would have to get within twenty feet of a letter that should be seen at forty feet in order to see it clearly. Normal distance visual acuity is 20/20.

Preliminary Tests

Preliminary testing may include evaluation of specific aspects of visual function and eye health such as depth perception, color vision, eye muscle movements, peripheral or side vision, and the way your pupils respond to light.

Keratometry

This test measures the curvature of the cornea, the clear outer surface of the eye, by focusing a circle of light on the cornea and measuring its reflection. This measurement is particularly critical in determining the proper fit for contact lenses.

Refraction

Refraction is conducted to determine the appropriate lens power needed to compensate for any refractive error (nearsightedness, farsightedness, or astigmatism). Using an instrument called a phoroptor, your optometrist places a series of lenses in front of your eyes and measures how they focus light using a handheld lighted instrument called a retinoscope. The doctor may choose to use an automated instrument that automatically evaluates the focusing power of the eye. The power is then refined by patient's responses to determine the lenses that allow the clearest vision.

This testing may be done without the use of eye drops to determine how the eyes respond under normal seeing conditions. In some cases, such as for patients who can't respond verbally or when some of the eyes' focusing power may be hidden, eye drops are used. The drops temporarily keep the eyes from changing focus while testing is done.

Eye Focusing, Eye Teaming, and Eye Movement Testing

Assessment of accommodation, ocular motility, and binocular vision determines how well the eyes focus, move, and work together. In order to obtain a clear, single image of what is being viewed, the eyes must effectively change focus, move, and work in unison. This testing will look for problems that keep your eyes from focusing effectively or make using both eyes together difficult.

47

Eye Health Evaluation

External examination of the eye includes evaluation of the cornea, eyelids, conjunctiva, and surrounding eye tissue using bright light and magnification.

Evaluation of the lens, retina, and posterior section of the eye may be done through a dilated pupil to provide a better view of the internal structures of the eye.

Measurement of pressure within the eye (tonometry) is performed. Normal eye pressures range from 10 to 21 millimeters of mercury (mm Hg), averaging about 14 to 16 mm Hg. Anyone with eye pressure greater than 22 mm Hg is at an increased risk of developing glaucoma, although many people with normal pressure also develop glaucoma.

Supplemental Testing

Additional testing may be needed based on the results of the previous tests to confirm or rule out possible problems, to clarify uncertain findings, or to provide a more in-depth assessment.

At the completion of the examination, your optometrist will assess and evaluate the results of the testing to determine a diagnosis and develop a treatment plan. He or she will discuss with you the nature of any visual or eye health problems found and explain available treatment options. In some cases, referral for consultation with, or treatment by, another optometrist or other healthcare provider may be indicated.

If you have questions regarding any eye or vision conditions diagnosed, or treatment recommended, don't hesitate to ask for additional information or explanation from your doctor.

Section 5.2

Visual Acuity Test

Excerpted from "Visual Acuity Test,"
© 2011 A.D.A.M., Inc. Reprinted with permission.

The visual acuity test is used to determine the smallest letters a person can read on a standardized chart (Snellen chart) or a card held fourteen to twenty feet away.

How the Test Is Performed

This test may be done in a healthcare provider's office, a school, a workplace, or elsewhere.

You will be asked to remove your glasses or contact lenses and stand or sit twenty feet from the eye chart. You will keep both eyes open.

Gently cover one eye with the palm of your hand, a piece of paper, or a paper cup while you read out loud the smallest line of letters you can see on the chart. Numbers or pictures are used for people who cannot read, especially children.

If you are not sure of the letter, you may guess. This test is done on each eye, one at a time. If needed, it is repeated while you wear your glasses or contacts. You may also be asked to read letters or numbers from a card held fourteen inches from your face. This will test your near vision.

How to Prepare for the Test

No special preparation is necessary for this test.

How the Test Will Feel

There is no discomfort.

Why the Test Is Performed

The visual acuity test is a routine part of an eye examination or general physical examination, particularly if there is a change in vision or a problem with vision.

In children, the test is performed to screen for vision problems. Vision problems in young children can often be corrected or improved. Undetected or untreated problems may lead to permanent vision damage.

There are other ways to check vision in very young children, or in people who do not know their letters or numbers.

Normal Results

Visual acuity is expressed as a fraction:

- The top number refers to the distance you stand from the chart. This is usually twenty feet.

- The bottom number indicates the distance at which a person with normal eyesight could read the same line you correctly read.

For example, 20/20 is considered normal. 20/40 indicates that the line you correctly read at twenty feet away can be read by a person with normal vision from forty feet away.

Even if you miss one or two letters on the smallest line you can read, you are still considered to have vision equal to that line.

What Abnormal Results Mean

Abnormal results may be a sign that you need glasses or contacts, or it may mean that you have an eye condition that needs further evaluation by a healthcare provider.

Risks

There are no risks.

References

Colenbrander A. Measuring vision and vision loss. In: Tasman W, Jaeger EA, eds. *Duane's Ophthalmology. 15th ed.* Philadelphia, Pa: Lippincott Williams & Wilkins; 2009:chap 51.

Miller D, Schor P, Magnante P. Optics of the normal eye. In: Yanoff M, Duker JS, eds. *Ophthalmology. 3rd ed.* St. Louis, MO: Mosby Elsevier; 2008:chap 2.6.

American Academy of Ophthalmology Preferred Practice Patterns Committee. *Preferred Practice Guidelines. Comprehensive Adult Medical Eye Evaluation.* San Francisco, CA: American Academy of Ophthalmology, 2010. Accessed January 17, 2011.

Section 5.3

Refraction Test

Do you have trouble identifying faces at a distance? Do you have trouble reading small print at near? Do you have difficulty seeing at all distances? You need an eye exam, which will include an eye refraction exam … let's look closer.

An eye refraction exam involves the use of an instrument called the phoroptor. This instrument has dials and knobs that your eye doctor can spin and move in order to change the lenses you see through and thus check for such refractive errors and eye problems as:

- myopia;

- hyperopia;

- astigmatism;

- presbyopia;

- amblyopia.

Your eye doctor will place the phoroptor in front of your face and plug in a prescription in the instrument as a starting point.

This starting point can be found any number of ways:

- using your old eyeglasses prescription if you see well through them;

- using the auto-refraction numbers measured by the technician during pre-testing;

- using a procedure called retinoscopy, during which your eye doctor uses an instrument with a light to neutralize the movement of a beam of light reflecting off your retina.

Your eye doctor will move the instrument back and forth and side to side while adding lenses until the beam of light stops moving. This finding can then serve as an accurate starting point for refining your prescription.

The refraction exam will then involve many choices provided by your eye doctor in the effort to refine and fine-tune your eyeglasses prescription. Your eye doctor will probably isolate a line of letters (or other figures) on an eye test chart for you to look at during this part of the eye exam.

First, your eye doctor will find the spherical component of your prescription. During this part of the eye exam, your eye doctor will add or take away either minus lenses (for myopia) or plus lenses (for hyperopia) until you see the clearest. Once the best spherical lens is found that gives you the clearest vision, your eye doctor may check for astigmatism, if you have it.

First, the axis will be fine-tuned by having you choose the clearer of two choices as your eye doctor spins the axis dial gradually.

Once the axis of the astigmatism is found, then your eye doctor will provide choices to fine-tune the power of the astigmatism.

Your vision should be considerably clearer than in the beginning of the exam after this portion of the eye refraction exam.

You will then have to read the smallest line of letters (or other figures) you see through the new prescription in the distance.

Your eye doctor will document this visual acuity in the record along with the numbers of the prescription. But your eye refraction exam does not end there. Your eye doctor will then have you read from a near eye test chart through the new prescription.

If you have difficulty reading at near and you are over forty, then you will be checked for a bifocal prescription.

Your eye doctor will add magnifying plus lenses over your distance prescription until you can achieve 20/20 vision at near, or the best vision you can. Even if you are not over forty, you will be checked for focusing problems and may be prescribed bifocals to help you with near work.

Section 5.4

Color Vision Test

Has your family told you on multiple occasions that your clothes do not match in color? Or have you noticed that your child's clothes consistently do not match in color? Are you unable to tell a difference in the color of traffic lights? You (or your child) may need to go to an eye doctor and have a color blind test.

What should you expect from a color blind test?

A color blind test will help your eye doctor determine if you are able to distinguish between colors. If you are only able to discriminate certain colors and not others, then you have a color deficiency. If you are unable to appreciate any color at all, then you have color blindness. Because color vision ability can vary in severity and can be deficient in certain colors and not others, a color blind test will be used to determine the type, and in some cases, the severity of color deficiency.

A color blind test may be qualitative (i.e., can you see color and if not, which ones can you not see?) or quantitative (i.e., how severe is your color deficiency?). Thus, the quantitative tests try to provide a measure of the severity of color deficiency.

Regardless of which color blind test is used, there are factors that affect test performance such as:

- lighting;
- field size;
- cognitive and emotional issues.

These variables should be controlled as closely as possible in order to minimize error.

What should you expect from a qualitative color blind test?

The most commonly used screening tests for color deficiency in clinical practice are plate tests or pseudoisochromatic plates (PIP). These tests can be used on children and illiterate adults. Most of these plate tests provide very efficient screening of congenital red-green defects. Plate tests generally consist of a series of cards on which is printed a number or pattern in multiple colors against a multicolored background. The figure is easily seen by color normal individuals, but if you have a color deficiency, you may have trouble seeing it.

A second variety of the plate test is PIP II, which is used for identifying acquired color deficiency since it tests for blue-yellow defects, more readily seen in acquired eye diseases or medication toxicity.

Despite their popularity and advantages, plate tests have distinct limitations, such as:

- If the quality of the light source illuminating the plates is not adequate, the efficacy of the test is affected.

- These tests are not effective in grading the severity of the color deficiency and thus give your eye doctor limited information about the extent of color deficiency.

What should you expect from a quantitative color blind test?

A color blind test category that includes a scoring system is that of arrangement tests. These tests were designed by the Navy commander Dean Farnsworth for military use in 1943.

These tests were designed to evaluate color discrimination ability and to classify those tested into groups of protan, deutan, and tritan based on the error axis of the scored results.

The basic design of these tests is to present you with colored caps of fixed saturation (how different cap color is from white) and value (refers to relative lightness or darkness of color) selected from the hue circle.

[Isaac] Newton joined the "orange red" and "violet" ends of the spectrum to create a hue circle, and thus show the spectrum as a continuous gradation of hues from orange red to blue violet, but now the ends are joined by mixed colors red, violet red, red violet, and violet.

You will be asked to arrange randomly placed caps in what you perceive to be a natural order. The color differences between adjacent caps on the Farnsworth-Munsell 100-Hue Test (FM 100-Hue Test) were designed to be very small. The Farnsworth Panel D-15 was designed to have larger color differences.

Your eye doctor will score the test by comparing your arrangement of the caps to the correct arrangement, which is indicated by the numbers written on the back of each cap.

A total error score can be computed for the test and it indicates your aptitude for hue discrimination. A higher score suggests worse discrimination. Your arrangement of caps can also be plotted in order to identify zones or poles of discrimination loss.

Similarly to the plate tests, the arrangement tests have their drawbacks:

- Specific lighting conditions are necessary for the test to be effective.

- The shortened version, or Farnsworth Panel D-15, selects primarily those individuals with severe color discrimination loss. This test is not effective as a screening tool but rather it is a rapid and effective means of identifying severe color deficiency.

Another color blind test category that includes a scoring system involves the use of an instrument called an anomaloscope. This instrument provides a superior clinical method of diagnosing and classifying color deficiency.

You will be asked to view through the eyepiece to see a circle of color, one half of which is yellow light and the other half is a mixture of red and green light. You will be asked to match the color and brightness of the two halves using two knobs. The amount of each color that you use to match the two halves can indicate the particular kind and severity of color deficiency you have.

While this instrument is the benchmark color matching test for diagnosis for red-green deficiency, it has several disadvantages as well:

- The use and maintenance of an anomaloscope can be challenging and requires the expertise of a trained technician.

- This instrument is not readily available in local eye clinics and you will need to go to a special color vision clinic at a university optometry school or to a research facility to be tested with it.

A promising new color blind test is a contribution of military research studies and is called the cone contrast test (CCT). The CCT is inexpensive enough to be used in mainstream clinics, but sensitive and specific enough to diagnose color deficiency as well as determine the type and score the severity of it.

The CCT can be useful in diagnosing congenital color deficiency as well as in monitoring the progression of acquired color deficiency, which can make an impact in your eye doctor's ability to manage such diseases as diabetic retinopathy and glaucoma.

Each cone type is tested separately in decreasing levels of contrast in order to quantify any loss and the type of loss. This test will be available in automated form and the computer will generate a score for each cone type. With a measure each visit, you can see how any decrease in color vision sensitivity will be easier to detect.

Section 5.5

Tonometry

Tonometry is a test to measure the pressure inside your eyes. The test is used to screen for glaucoma.

How the Test Is Performed

There are several methods of testing for glaucoma.

The most accurate method measures the force needed to flatten a certain area of the cornea:

- The surface of the eye is numbed. A fine strip of paper stained with orange dye is touched to the side of the eye. The dye stains the front of the eye to help with the examination.

- The slit-lamp is placed in front of you, and you rest your chin and forehead on a support that keeps your head steady. The lamp is moved forward until the tip of the tonometer just touches the cornea.

- The light is usually a blue circle. The healthcare provider looks through the eyepiece on the lamp and adjusts the tension on the tonometer. There is no discomfort with the test.

A slightly different method uses a handheld device similar in shape to a pencil. Again, you are given numbing eye drops to prevent any discomfort. The device touches the outside of the eye and instantly records eye pressure.

The last method is the noncontact method (air puff). In this method, your chin rests on a padded stand:

- You stare straight into the examining device. The eye doctor shines a bright light into your eye to properly line up the instrument, and then delivers a brief puff of air at your eye.

- The machine measures eye pressure by looking at how the light reflections change as the air hits the eye.

How to Prepare for the Test

Remove contact lenses before the examination. The dye can permanently stain contact lenses.

Inform the healthcare provider if you have corneal ulcers and infections, an eye infection, if you are taking any drugs, or if you have a history of glaucoma in your family.

How the Test Will Feel

If numbing eye drops were used, you should not have any pain. In the noncontact method, you may feel mild pressure on your eye.

Why the Test Is Performed

Tonometry is a test to measure the pressure inside your eyes. The test is used to screen for glaucoma.

People over age forty, especially African Americans, have the highest risk for developing glaucoma. Regular eye exams can help detect glaucoma early. If it is detected early, glaucoma can be treated before too much damage is done.

The test may also be done before and after eye surgery.

Normal Results

A normal result means your eye pressure is within the normal range. The normal eye pressure range is 10–21 mmHg.

Note: Normal value ranges may vary slightly among different laboratories. Talk to your doctor about the meaning of your specific test results.

What Abnormal Results Mean

Abnormal results may be due to:

- glaucoma;
- hyphema;
- trauma to the eye or head.

Risks

If the applanation method is used, there is a small chance the cornea may be scratched (corneal abrasion). This will normally heal itself within a few days.

Alternative Names

Intraocular pressure (IOP) measurement; glaucoma test; applanation

Section 5.6

Other Vision Tests

Reprinted from "Other Tests," "Corneal Shape," "Binocular Function," "Direct Ophthalmoscope," "Binocular Indirect Ophthalmoscopy," "Biomicroscopy (Fundus Lens)," and "Visual Field Testing," written by Luke Lindsell and Gerald Lowther, O.D., PhD. © 2011 The Trustees of Indiana University. All rights reserved. Reprinted with permission. For additional information, visit the website of the Indiana University School of Optometry, www.opt .indiana.edu.

Other Tests

Motility

The doctor will ask you to focus on a near target (most likely their finger) and follow it as he/she traces a broad letter "H." This tests the ability of your eyes to follow the target. It will indicate any problem with the nerve supply to your eye muscles or problems with the muscles themselves.

Pupillary Response

This is another exam used to survey your visual system. A light beam will be directed at and away from your eye to observe if your pupils constrict and dilate as expected.

Cover Test

The first part of this test is the unilateral cover test. While wearing your corrective eyewear, you will be asked to focus on a letter of the distance eye chart. The optometrist will then cover your right eye while watching for a movement of the left eye. Upon removing the occluder, the optometrist will wait for a few seconds to allow your eyes to return to equilibrium then will proceed by covering the left eye. If the eye not being covered moves to fixate the target (with both eyes open one eye is not aimed at the point of interest), that eye was not being used. This is referred to as a strabismus.

The alternating cover test is very similar to the unilateral cover test but the main difference is that the occluder is switched from one eye to the next. If the eye just uncovered moves, this is called a phoria. This means that in the resting position both eyes are not aimed at the target. Consequently, you must use effort to keep both eyes fixated on the target. This can cause eyestrain and headaches. Prisms in your spectacles or visual training may be required.

Near Point of Convergence

The purpose of this test is to inspect your ability to converge your eyes. The practitioner will ask you to focus on a near target. As it is brought closer and closer to your nose, you will be asked when you first see two targets. There is a normal range at which you should be able to see a single target.

Corneal Shape

The shape of the front surface of the eye (the cornea) may be measured with a keratometer. With this device, the patient puts their head in a headrest and the doctor focuses the instrument. A light pattern is reflected off the cornea and by making the proper adjustments, the curvature of the eye surface is measured. This is useful in helping determine the amount of astigmatism, fitting contact lenses, and determining the cause of decreased visual acuity even with the best spectacle prescription.

A more sophisticated device is a corneal topographer. This instrument captures a photograph of a light pattern reflected off the cornea with a video camera. The image is then analyzed with a computer which produces a detailed map of the shape of the eye. This is often used to diagnose certain corneal diseases, aid in contact lens fitting, and in conjunction with refractive surgery techniques.

Binocular Function

Using special prisms or lenses in the phoroptor, the eye care practitioner will test the way the eyes aim when relaxed and the ability to point and hold the eyes on a target. This quantifies the phoria finding described under the cover test section.

A patient's depth perception—called stereopsis—may also be tested. A common test for this is known as the stereo fly test. The patient wears a pair of polaroid spectacles and looks at special photos, one of which is a picture of a fly. If the patient has depth perception the fly will appear to stand off the page. Other photos are used to quantify the degree of stereopsis.

Using special prisms on the phoroptor, the eye care practitioner will test the way the eyes aim when relaxed and the ability to point and hold the eyes on a target. Likewise, the ability to focus up close (accommodation) and the correction for reading is also tested.

Direct Ophthalmoscopy

This is a very safe, noncontact examination of the inside of the eye and retina. The instrument used is a small handheld device called an ophthalmoscope. The head of the tool contains many lenses and projects light through a variably sized aperture. This is attached to a handle which serves as the power source. The beauty of the ophthalmoscope is that it uses the eye as a simple magnifier, producing a magnified image for the eye care physician to view. To obtain the best results from this analysis, lights in the exam room are generally dimmed, allowing the pupil to maximally dilate. If the pupil is still too small, a topical mydriatic solution may be used to aid in dilation. The patient is then asked to fixate on a target. By varying the lenses, the distance from the patient's eye, and aperture size, the doctor can survey the iris, crystalline lens vitreous, retina, and optic disc.

Binocular Indirect Ophthalmoscopy

Like its direct counterpart, binocular indirect ophthalmoscopy is used to inspect the retina. However, with the binocular indirect technique a large area of the retina can be viewed instead of only a small portion, as seen with direct ophthalmoscopy. The device consists of a headband, an optical viewing system, and a controllable illumination source. The lens system has eyepieces which are adjusted depending on the practitioner's distance from the patient. In addition, a condensing lens held in the doctor's hand near the patient's eye is used to generate an image of the retina. With binocular indirect ophthalmoscopy the eye care practitioner has the advantages of a large field of view, bright illumination, a comfortable working distance from the patient, and little periphery view distortion. The pupils are dilated prior to performing this test.

Biomicroscopy (Fundus Lens)

The fundus lens is another noncontact, well-illuminated, retinal evaluation procedure. The fundus lens exam uses a powerful condensing lens to produce a magnified image. A biomicroscope is used, allowing easy illumination and viewing. Similar to the binocular indirect exam, the condensing lens is held in front of the patient's eye. The examination provides a high-quality, highly magnified, 3-D view of the optic disc in addition to detailed inspection of the posterior portion of the eye.

Visual Field Testing

These tests determine if your peripheral vision is normal. The importance of this stems from the fact that visual field testing can detect neurological problems as well as glaucoma and other eye diseases. Typically, this is done with a large white bowl apparatus on which spots of light are projected. The patient fixates on a central spot and then indicates when they see a small spot of light off to the side. The visual field can also be tested using a screen on which a white spot is moved and the patient indicates when the spot disappears.

The Amsler grid also tests the visual field, specifically the central vision capabilities of the patient. The test consists of a black grid on a white background with a central fixation point located in the middle. It is very easy to conduct and provides a fairly good barometer of the health of the macula (region of the retina responsible for our central vision). To take the test you will fixate on the dot in the middle of the grid. If your macula is healthy, the lines should appear straight and clear. By contrast, an unhealthy macula will sometimes view the lines as wavering or will see a blank spot in some areas. These are all indicators of a compromised macula.

Chapter 6

Working with Your Eye Care Doctor

Chapter Contents

Section 6.1

Know Who Is Taking Care of Your Eyes

First, it's important to understand what each type of eye care professional can do for you.

Ophthalmologist

An ophthalmologist is qualified to treat eye diseases, prescribe medications, and perform all types of surgery to improve, or prevent the worsening of, eye and vision-related conditions. An ophthalmologist has graduated from medical school and will have the initials "M.D." (Doctor of Medicine) after his or her name.

Optometrist

An optometrist is qualified to diagnose eye diseases and prescribe eyeglasses, contact lenses, low vision devices, vision therapy, and certain medications to treat eye diseases. An optometrist has graduated from optometry school and will have the initials "O.D." (Doctor of Optometry) after his or her name.

If you do not have an eye doctor, a good way to start is to make an appointment with an optometrist, who can diagnose and treat many common eye problems and is similar to a primary care doctor or practitioner.

If you need surgery or specialty care, an optometrist can refer you to an ophthalmologist or a sub-specialist, such as a retinal specialist, who can address specialized treatments such as those needed for macular degeneration or diabetic retinopathy.

Please note: Some states have passed legislation that allows optometrists to perform certain surgical procedures, such as laser treatment; administer injections, such as local anesthesia or treatment for macular degeneration; and prescribe additional medications. Visit the American Optometric Association website to determine if your state permits optometrists to perform these additional procedures.

Low Vision Specialist

Many optometrists and some ophthalmologists have an additional credential or specialization in low vision testing, diagnosis, and treatment, and are trained to conduct low vision eye examinations and prescribe special low vision optical devices.

If you're experiencing significant vision loss, a low vision specialist can determine whether special optical and nonoptical devices, improved lighting, or other types of specialized services and equipment can help.

Orthoptist

An orthoptist works under the supervision of an ophthalmologist and/or optometrist to evaluate and treat eye disorders with an emphasis on binocular vision (using both eyes to see) and eye movements; much of their work is with children. An orthoptist has a baccalaureate degree in addition to a two-year orthoptic internship. An orthoptist has not graduated from medical school or optometry school.

Optician

An optician fits eyeglasses and, in some states, contact lenses; analyzes and interprets prescriptions written by ophthalmologists or optometrists; and takes eye measurements to ensure that eyeglass prescriptions are correct and fit properly. An optician has not graduated from medical school or optometry school.

Locate an Eye Care Professional in Your Area

- Visit the American Academy of Ophthalmology website and use their "Find an Eye MD" online database to locate an ophthalmologist in your area.

- Visit the American Optometric Association website and use their "Dr. Locator" online database to locate an optometrist in your area.

- Visit the Vision Aware website and use their searchable databases to locate a low vision specialist in your area.

- Ask for a recommendation from family members, friends, or your family doctor.

- Call your local hospitals and ask if they have outpatient ophthalmology departments.

- Check your health insurance plan for listings of approved eye care providers.

- In most cases, it is not recommended that you visit an optician for your initial exam and diagnosis.

If your vision loss can't be corrected and interferes with your everyday living, vision rehabilitation services can help maintain or restore your independent living skills.

Section 6.2

Talking to Your Eye Care Doctor

"Talking to Your Doctor," National Eye Institute,
National Institutes of Health, March 2009.

Today, patients take an active role in their healthcare. You and your doctor will work in partnership to achieve your best possible level of health. An important part of this relationship is good communication. Here are some questions you can ask your doctor to get your discussion started.

About my disease or disorder:

- What is my diagnosis?

- What caused my condition?

- Can my condition be treated?

- How will this condition affect my vision now and in the future?

- Should I watch for any particular symptoms and notify you if they occur?

- Should I make any lifestyle changes?

About my treatment:

- What is the treatment for my condition?
- When will the treatment start, and how long will it last?
- What are the benefits of this treatment, and how successful is it?
- What are the risks and side effects associated with this treatment?
- Are there foods, drugs, or activities I should avoid while I'm on this treatment?
- If my treatment includes taking a medication, what should I do if I miss a dose?
- Are other treatments available?

About my tests:

- What kinds of tests will I have?
- What do you expect to find out from these tests?
- When will I know the results?
- Do I have to do anything special to prepare for any of the tests?
- Do these tests have any side effects or risks?
- Will I need more tests later?

Understanding your doctor's responses is essential to good communication. Here are a few more tips:

- If you don't understand your doctor's responses, ask questions until you do understand.
- Take notes, or get a friend or family member to take notes for you. Or, bring a tape-recorder to assist in your recollection of the discussion.
- Ask your doctor to write down his or her instructions to you.
- Ask your doctor for printed material about your condition.
- If you still have trouble understanding your doctor's answers, ask where you can go for more information.
- Other members of your healthcare team, such as nurses and pharmacists, can be good sources of information. Talk to them, too.

Chapter 7

Pediatric Vision Concerns

Chapter Contents

Section 7.1

Vision Development in Infants and Young Children

"Your Baby's Developing Sight," © 2011 Prevent Blindness America (www.preventblindness.org). Reprinted with permission.

The wonders of the world are often first encountered through the eyes of a child. Yet without good vision, a child's ability to learn about the world becomes more difficult. Vision problems affect one in twenty preschoolers and one in four school-age children. Since many vision problems begin at an early age, it is very important that children receive proper eye care. Untreated eye problems can worsen and lead to other serious problems as well as affect learning ability, personality, and adjustment in school.

Development of Vision

Newborns

The acuity (sharpness of vision) of newborns is less than fully developed. They usually prefer looking at close objects, and are especially attracted to faces and by objects that are brightly colored or of high contrast and moving.

Three Months

By this age, most babies can smoothly follow a moving object and can hold their eyes on it even when the object stops. The colors, details, and moving parts of mobiles in cribs fascinate infants and help stimulate their visual development.

Three to Six Months

By now, the retina of the eye is quite well developed, and the baby's visual acuity is good enough to permit small details to be seen. The infant is able to look from near to far and back to near again. Judgment of distances (depth perception) is also developing.

Six Months

At six months of age, the eye has reached about two-thirds of its adult size. Usually by this stage, the two eyes are fully working together, resulting in good binocular vision. Distance vision and depth perception are still improving.

One Year Old

By the age of one, a child's vision is well on its way toward full development. Coordination of the eyes with the hands and body are naturally practiced by children and can be enhanced by games involving pointing, grasping, tossing, placing, and catching.

Two to Five Years Old

The preschooler is typically eager to draw and look at pictures. Stories connected to pictures, drawings, and symbols often captivate the child and help to coordinate hearing and vision.

Section 7.2

What You Need to Know about Vision Concerns in Children

"Your Child's Vision," January 2011, reprinted with permission from www .kidshealth.org. Copyright © 2011 The Nemours Foundation. This information was provided by KidsHealth, one of the largest resources online for medically reviewed health information written for parents, kids, and teens. For more articles like this one, visit www.KidsHealth.org, or www.TeensHealth.org.

Healthy eyes and vision are a critical part of kids' development. Their eyes should be examined regularly, as many vision problems and eye diseases can be detected and treated early.

Eye Doctors

Be sure to make vision care and eye checks a part of your child's routine medical care.

Different kinds of doctors offer eye care, and the names can be confusing:

- Ophthalmologists are medical doctors (have gone to medical school) who provide comprehensive eye care with medicine and surgery.

- Pediatric ophthalmologists have additional special training to treat kids' eye problems.

- Optometrists provide services that may be similar to ophthalmologists, but they don't perform surgery. Some optometrists specialize in kids' eye problems.

- Opticians fit and adjust eyeglasses.

Eye Exams

Routine medical exams for kids' vision include:

- Newborns should be checked for general eye health by a pediatrician or family physician in the hospital nursery.

- High-risk newborns (including premature infants), those with a family history of eye problems, and those with obvious eye irregularities should be examined by an eye doctor.

- In the first year of life, all infants should be routinely screened for eye health during checkups with their pediatrician or family doctor.

- Around age three and a half, kids should undergo eye health screenings and visual acuity tests (or tests that measure sharpness of vision) with their pediatrician or family doctor.

- Around age five, kids should have their vision and eye alignment evaluated by their doctors. Those who fail either test should be examined by their pediatrician or family doctor.

- After age five, further routine screenings should be done at school or the doctor's office, or after the appearance of symptoms such as squinting or frequent headaches. (Many times, a teacher will realize the child isn't seeing well in class.)

- Kids who wear prescription glasses or contacts should have annual checkups by an eye doctor to screen for vision changes.

Spotting Eye Problems

Signs that a child may have vision problems include:

- constant eye rubbing;
- extreme light sensitivity;
- poor focusing;
- poor visual tracking (following an object);
- abnormal alignment or movement of the eyes (after six months of age);
- chronic redness of the eyes;
- chronic tearing of the eyes;
- a white pupil instead of black.

In school-age children, watch for other signs such as:

- inability to see objects at a distance;
- inability to read the blackboard;
- squinting;

- difficulty reading;

- sitting too close to the TV.

Watch your child for evidence of poor vision or crossed eyes. If you notice any eye problems, have your child examined immediately so that the problem doesn't become permanent.

If caught early, eye conditions often can be reversed.

Common Eye Problems

Several eye conditions can affect kids. Most are detected by a vision screening using an acuity chart during the preschool years:

- Amblyopia ("lazy eye") is poor vision in an eye that may appear to be normal. Two common causes are crossed eyes and a difference in the refractive error between the two eyes. If untreated, amblyopia can cause irreversible visual loss in the affected eye. (By then, the brain's "programming" will ignore signals from that eye.) Amblyopia is best treated during the preschool years.

- Strabismus is a misalignment of the eyes; they may turn in, out, up, or down. If the same eye is chronically misaligned, amblyopia may also develop in that eye. With early detection, vision can be restored by patching the properly aligned eye, which forces the misaligned one to work. Surgery or specially designed glasses also may help the eyes to align.

- Refractive errors mean that the shape of the eye doesn't refract, or bend, light properly, so images appear blurred. Refractive errors also can cause amblyopia. Nearsightedness is the most common refractive error in school-age children; others include farsightedness and astigmatism:

  - Nearsightedness is poor distance vision (also called myopia), which is usually treated with glasses or contacts.

  - Farsightedness is poor near vision (also called hyperopia), which is usually treated with glasses or contacts.

  - Astigmatism is imperfect curvature of the front surface of the eye, which is usually treated with glasses if it causes blurred vision or discomfort.

Other eye conditions require immediate attention, such as retinopathy of prematurity (a disease that affects the eyes of premature babies) and those associated with a family history, including:

- Retinoblastoma is a malignant tumor that usually appears in the first three years of life. The affected eye or eyes may have visual loss and whiteness in the pupil.

- Infantile cataracts can occur in newborns. A cataract is a clouding of the eye's lens.

- Congenital glaucoma in infants is a rare condition that may be inherited. It is the result of incorrect or incomplete development of the eye drainage canals before birth and can be treated with medication and surgery.

- Genetic or metabolic diseases of the eye, such as inherited disorders that make a child more likely to develop retinoblastoma or cataracts, may require kids to have eye exams at an early age and regular screenings.

Be sure to talk to your doctor if your child is at risk for any of these conditions.

Glasses and Contacts

Kids of all ages—even babies—can wear glasses and contacts. Keep these tips in mind for kids who wear glasses:

- Allow kids to pick their own frames.

- Plastic frames are best for children younger than two.

- If older kids wear metal frames, make sure they have spring hinges, which are more durable.

- An elastic strap attached to the glasses will help keep them in place for active toddlers.

- Kids with severe eye problems may need special lenses called high-index lenses, which are thinner and lighter than plastic lenses.

- Polycarbonate lenses are recommended for all kids, especially for kids who play sports. Polycarbonate is a tough, shatterproof, transparent thermoplastic used to make thin, light lenses. However, although they're very impact-resistant, these lenses scratch more easily than plastic lenses.

Infants born with congenital cataracts may need to have their cataracts surgically removed during the first few weeks of life. Some children born with cataracts wear contact lenses after cataract surgery.

Around age ten, kids may express a desire to get contact lenses for cosmetic reasons or convenience if they play sports. Allowing a child to wear contacts depends on his or her ability to insert and remove lenses properly, faithfully take them out as required, and clean them as recommended by the doctor. Contact lens problems are almost always caused by poor habits and bad hygiene.

Your eye doctor can help you decide what type of vision correction is best for your child.

Section 7.3

Signs of Eye Problems in Children

"Signs of Possible Eye Problems in Children," © 2011 Prevent Blindness America (www.preventblindness.org). Reprinted with permission.

If one or more of these signs appear, take your child to an eye doctor right away.

What do your child's eyes look like?

- Eyes don't line up, one eye appears crossed or looks out!

- Eyelids are red-rimmed, crusted, or swollen.

- Eyes are watery or red (inflamed).

How does your child act?

- Rubs eyes a lot.

- Closes or covers one eye.

- Tilts head or thrusts head forward.

- Has trouble reading or doing other close-up work, or holds objects close to eyes to see.

- Blinks more than usual or seems cranky when doing close-up work.

- Things are blurry or hard to see.

- Squints eyes or frowns.

What does your child say?

- "My eyes are itchy," "my eyes are burning," or "my eyes feel scratchy." "I can't see very well."

- After doing close-up work, your child says, "I feel dizzy," "I have a headache," or "I feel sick/nauseous."

- "Everything looks blurry," or "I see double."

Remember, your child may still have an eye problem even if he or she does not complain or has not shown any unusual signs.

Section 7.4

Taking Your Child to the Eye Doctor

"Planning a Trip to the Eye Doctor?" © 2011 Prevent Blindness America
(www.preventblindness.org). Reprinted with permission.

All children, even those with no signs of trouble, should have their eyes checked at regular intervals. Any child who experiences vision problems or shows symptoms of eye trouble should receive a comprehensive eye exam by an optometrist or an ophthalmologist. If you are planning to take your child to the eye doctor, here are some helpful tips:

1. Ask your relatives, friends, and neighbors if they know the name of an eye doctor who is good with children.

2. Schedule the appointment when your child is not likely to be sleepy or hungry. If your child has a "cranky" time of day, schedule around it.

3. Make a list of your questions and bring it with you. Take notes when speaking to the doctor, so that you can refer to them later.

4. Have a plan ready in case you need to spend time in the waiting room. Bring a favorite storybook, coloring book, or small toy that your child can play with quietly. A snack can also help to pass the time.

5. Let your child watch a family member get an eye exam. Have the doctor explain what is being done, step by step, and encourage the child to ask questions.

6. Bring your child's favorite cuddly toy. The doctor can "examine" the bear or doll and holding a toy may keep little hands off of expensive equipment.

7. Relax. Children look to adults for cues: if you seem nervous, your child may become anxious. A trip to the eye doctor should be fun for both of you.

Chapter 8

Adult Vision Concerns

Chapter Contents

Section 8.1

Signs of Eye Problems in Adults

If you notice any signs of potential eye problems, see an eye doctor
for a complete eye exam.

Even if you have no signs, regular eye exams are recommended—
especially for those with some chronic health conditions such as diabetes and high blood pressure. Early detection and treatment can be
the key to preventing sight loss.

Any changes in the appearance of your eyes or vision should be
investigated further. Some examples include:

- unusual trouble adjusting to dark rooms;

- difficulty focusing on near or distant objects;

- squinting or blinking due to unusual sensitivity to light or glare;

- change in color of iris;

- red-rimmed, encrusted, or swollen lids;

- recurrent pain in or around eyes;

- double vision;

- dark spot at the center of viewing;

- lines and edges appear distorted or wavy;

- excess tearing or "watery eyes";

- dry eyes with itching or burning; and

- seeing spots, ghost-like images.

The following may be indications of potentially serious problems
that might require emergency medical attention:

- Sudden loss of vision in one eye

- Sudden hazy or blurred vision

- Flashes of light or black spots

- Halos or rainbows around light

- Curtain-like blotting out of vision

- Loss of peripheral (side) vision

Section 8.2

Vision Concerns in Pregnancy

Can pregnancy affect my vision?

Yes. Changes in hormones, metabolism, fluid retention, and blood circulation can all affect your eyes and your eyesight during pregnancy.

Water retention, for instance, may cause the thickness and curvature of the cornea of your eye to increase slightly. It's a small change, but it could affect how well your glasses or contacts correct your vision. It's also why laser eye surgery isn't recommended during pregnancy and why it's not a good time to be fitted for new contact lenses.

If you experience vision changes during pregnancy, they'll probably be minor. Most women who experience a change find that they're a bit more nearsighted than they were before pregnancy.

If you wear glasses, it's unlikely that you'll need to change your prescription, but it is possible. If you think your vision has changed significantly, have it checked.

Pregnancy isn't a great time to invest in a new pair of glasses, though. In most cases, these changes are temporary and will reverse themselves within several months of delivery.

How else can pregnancy affect my eyes?

You may find that your eyes are drier and more irritated during pregnancy (as well as during breastfeeding). This, along with subtle changes in the shape and thickness of the cornea, may contribute to some difficulty wearing contact lenses that were once comfortable.

Pregnancy can also bring about changes in existing eye conditions—for better or for worse. If you have diabetes, see an ophthalmologist before you get pregnant and again in early pregnancy to get screened for damage to the blood vessels in your retina. This condition, called diabetic retinopathy, often worsens during pregnancy, so you'll need more frequent eye exams while you're pregnant and in the postpartum period.

Glaucoma, on the other hand, sometimes improves during pregnancy, so your medication may need to be adjusted. (If you have glaucoma and are planning a pregnancy, your doctor may be able to lessen your baby's exposure to the medication by starting you off with as low a dose as possible.)

How can I get relief for dry eyes?

Ask your eye doctor about dry-eye remedies. Some over-the-counter solutions are fine to use, but others contain active ingredients that may not be completely safe during pregnancy.

If you use contact lenses, try wearing them for shorter stretches of time. If that doesn't help, switch to glasses until you have your baby.

Make regular breaks from the computer part of your routine. Staring at a computer screen for long periods of time (during which you may not blink as frequently as usual) can exacerbate the dryness and irritation.

Are eye symptoms during pregnancy ever cause for concern?

Yes, eye symptoms can signal specific problems during pregnancy. High blood pressure or preeclampsia, for example, may cause vision disturbances.

Be sure to let your doctor or midwife know immediately if you have any of the following symptoms:

- Double vision

- Blurry vision

- Sensitivity to light

- Temporary loss of vision

- Seeing spots or flashing lights

Also call your caregiver if you notice swelling or puffiness around your eyes—another symptom that may accompany preeclampsia. Eye pain or redness should also prompt a call to your caregiver.

Section 8.3

Normal Changes in the Aging Eye and Their Symptoms

Our eyes function differently when we reach our sixties than they did when we were in our thirties. We simply don't see as well at certain distances. By the time we celebrate our eightieth birthday, our eyesight will have almost certainly declined further. Such changes in vision are perfectly normal, offer few serious risks, and, in general, are easily corrected with eyeglasses or contact lenses.

But how do you know what constitutes a "normal" change in vision strength and what is more serious? To determine the answer, your doctor will want to know your specific symptoms.

The Aging Eye—Normal Changes and Their Symptoms

Symptom: Difficulty reading newsprint or prescription bottles.

What's happening: The most likely culprit is presbyopia, which is the tightening of the muscles of the eye that allow us to focus at close distances. Familiar to almost everyone over forty, this condition occurs naturally and is easily corrected with bifocals or reading glasses.

You may also be experiencing reduced visual acuity. Normal visual acuity is 20/20 for a young person, and 20/40 for an older person. In other words, an older person will normally be able to see at a twenty-foot distance what a younger person sees at a forty-foot distance. Again, this is to be expected and is not a dramatic enough change to prevent you from functioning fairly normally.

Symptom: Increased need for light; dimness makes it difficult to focus on close tasks like sewing or handcrafts.

What's happening: As we grow older, the once-clear lens of the eye grows progressively hazy and yellow, allowing for less light to pass through. An older person normally requires four times more light than a younger person—by age eighty, it might be ten times. To compensate, natural sunlight works best, followed by natural full-spectrum bulbs that imitate sunlight and are now available commercially.

Symptom: "Do these socks match? Are they both black or is one dark blue? I can't quite make out the white plates when they're resting on the white tablecloth."

What's happening: It's common for the aging eye to experience reduced contrast sensitivity, which makes it difficult to differentiate similar patterns and colors. The simple use of bolder contrasts can make your home safer and easier to navigate.

Other normal symptoms of the naturally aging eye:

- Difficulty adapting to changes in light and dark environments
- Difficulty with glare
- Reduced depth perception
- Reduced ability to see colors
- Eye dryness
- Floaters (tiny specks, usually noticeable in bright sunlight)

Is It Serious? The Warning Signs

While we can all expect some decline in vision as we grow older, severe or persistent symptoms could indicate a serious degenerative condition that could lead to low vision, or even blindness. Contact your eye care professional immediately if you experience:

- sudden hazy or blurred vision;
- recurrent pain in or around the eye;
- double vision;
- seeing flashes of light;
- seeing halos around lights;
- unusual, even painful, sensitivity to light or glare;
- changes in the color of the iris;
- sudden development of persistent floaters.

At any age, it's important to have your eyes checked regularly. If symptoms or concerns arise, contact your eye care professional as soon as possible.

Section 8.4

Age-Related Eye Diseases and Conditions

Excerpted from "The Aging Eye: Age-Related Eye Diseases and Conditions," National Eye Institute, National Institutes of Health, 2008.

Since your forties, you have probably noticed that you needed glasses to see up close. You may have more trouble adjusting to glare or distinguishing some colors, particularly shades of blue and green. These changes are a normal part of aging. They alone cannot stop you from enjoying an active lifestyle. They will not stop you from maintaining your independence. In fact, you can live an active life well into your golden years without ever experiencing severe vision loss. But as you age, you should know you are at higher risk of developing age-related eye diseases and conditions.

What Are These Diseases?

These conditions affect different parts of the eye. If not caught early and treated, they can lead to vision loss and even blindness.

Age-Related Macular Degeneration (AMD)

AMD is a common eye disease among people aged sixty and older. It gradually destroys the macula, the part of the eye that provides sharp, central vision needed for seeing objects clearly. It comes in two forms: dry and wet. Each form requires different techniques to be used by eye care professionals to treat the condition.

Cataract

Cataract is a clouding of the eye's lens and is common in older adults and people with diabetes. Vision loss by cataract is successfully

85

restored with surgery. Although cataract surgery is one of the most common procedures performed in the United States today, some people never need it. Many others are able to postpone it for years.

Diabetic Retinopathy

Diabetic retinopathy is the most common condition among people with diabetes. It damages the blood vessels in the retina, usually in both eyes. If you have early-stage retinopathy, your eye care professional may suggest controlling your blood sugar, blood pressure, and cholesterol to prevent the disease from getting worse. For the more advanced stage, you may need laser surgery.

Glaucoma

Glaucoma is not just one disease. It is a group of diseases that are all caused by the same event; fluid in the eye builds up and damages the optic nerve. Your eye care professional can help control glaucoma by prescribing eye drops or pills. Laser surgery is another way to open clogged areas so that the eye fluid drains and eases pressure against the optic nerve. Surgery is another option, but is used only when drops or laser surgery fail to control the pressure.

What Is Low Vision?

People who have age-related eye disease are more likely to develop low vision. Low vision means that, even with regular glasses, contact lenses, medicine, and surgery, everyday tasks are difficult to do. Reading the mail, shopping, cooking, seeing the TV, and writing can seem challenging.

Fortunately, help is available. Low vision specialists can offer a variety of services that help people make the most of their remaining vision.

Chapter 9

Current Vision Research

If you or someone you know is thinking about taking part in a clinical trial, this chapter can answer some of your questions. The National Eye Institute (NEI) conducts or sponsors clinical trials to find new ways to treat or prevent eye disease and vision loss. Clinical trials in vision research have led to new medicines and surgeries that have saved or improved sight for thousands of people.

What Is a Clinical Trial?

Clinical trials involve medical research with people. Most medical research begins with studies in test tubes and in animals. Treatments that show promise in these early studies may then be tried with people. The only sure way to find out whether a new treatment is safe, effective, and better than other treatments is to try it on patients in a clinical trial.

What Kinds of Clinical Trials Are There?

Clinical trials are carried out in three parts, or phases:

- **Phase I:** Researchers first conduct Phase I trials in small numbers of patients and healthy volunteers. If the new treatment is a medicine, researchers also want to find out how much of it can be given safely.

"Clinical Trials in Vision Research," National Eye Institute, National Institutes of Health, May 2011.

- **Phase II:** Researchers conduct Phase II trials in small numbers of patients to find out the effect of a new treatment on an eye disease or disorder.

- **Phase III:** Finally, researchers conduct Phase III trials to find out whether the new treatments work better, the same, or not as well as the standard treatments already being used. Phase III trials also help to determine if new treatments have any side effects. These trials—which may involve hundreds, perhaps thousands, of people around the country—can also compare new treatments with no treatment.

Natural History Studies: How They Differ from Clinical Trials

Unlike clinical trials, in which patient volunteers may receive new treatments, natural history studies provide important information to researchers on how certain eye diseases or conditions develop over time. A natural history study follows patient volunteers to see how factors such as age, sex, race, or family history might make some people more or less at risk for certain eye diseases or disorders. A natural history study may also tell researchers if diet, lifestyle, or occupation affect how a disease or disorder develops and progresses. Results from these studies provide information that helps answer questions such as: How fast will a disease or disorder usually progress? How bad will vision become? Will treatment be needed?

Where Do Clinical Trials Take Place?

The NEI supports clinical trials at about 250 medical centers, hospitals, universities, and doctors' offices across the country. NEI researchers conduct other clinical trials at the National Institutes of Health in Bethesda, Maryland.

How Is a Clinical Trial Conducted?

At each facility taking part in the clinical trial, the principal investigator is the researcher in charge of the study. Most of the people who conduct clinical trials in eye disease are ophthalmologists or optometrists. The clinic coordinator knows all about how the study works and makes all the arrangements for your visits.

All doctors who take part in the study carefully follow a detailed treatment plan called a protocol. This plan fully explains how the doctors will treat you in the study. The protocol ensures that all patients are treated in the same way, no matter where they receive care:

- Clinical trials are controlled. This means that researchers compare the effects of the new treatment with those of the standard treatment. In some cases, when no standard treatment exists, the new treatment is compared with no treatment.

- Patients who get the new treatment are in the treatment group.

- Patients who get the standard treatment or no treatment are in the control group.

- In some clinical trials, patients in the treatment group get a new medicine and patients in the control group get a placebo. A placebo is a harmless substance—a "dummy" pill—that looks like the real treatment but has no effect on the eye disease or disorder. In other clinical trials, where a new surgery or device (not a medicine) is being tested, patients in the control group may receive a sham treatment. This treatment, like a placebo, has no effect on the eye disease or disorder and does not harm patients.

- Researchers assign patients randomly to the treatment or control group. This is like flipping a coin to decide which patients are in each group. Patients do not know ahead of time which group that is. The chance of any patient getting the new treatment is about 50 percent. Patients cannot request to receive the new treatment instead of the placebo or sham treatment. In some clinical trials, where the disease or disorder affects both eyes, one eye may be in the treatment group, and the other eye may be in the control group.

- Patients often do not know until the study is over whether they are in the treatment group or the control group. This is called a masked study. In some trials, neither doctors nor patients know who is getting what treatment. This is called a double masked study. These types of trials help to ensure that what patients or doctors might think about the treatment will not affect the study results.

What Is Expected of Patients in a Clinical Trial?

Patients in a clinical trial are expected to have eye exams and other tests. You may also need to take medications and/or undergo surgery. Depending upon the treatment and the examination procedure, you may need a hospital stay.

You may have to go back to the medical facility later for follow-up examinations. These exams help find out how well the treatment is working. Follow-up studies can take months or years. However, the success of the clinical trial often depends on learning what happens to patients over a long period of time. Only patients who continue to return for follow-up examinations can provide this important long-term information.

What Are the Benefits of Participating in a Clinical Trial?

Participating in a clinical trial can bring many benefits:

- There is the hope that a new treatment will be more effective than the current treatment for an eye disease or disorder. Only about half of the people in a clinical trial get the new treatment. If the new treatment is effective and safer than the current treatment, those patients who do not receive the new treatment during the clinical trial may be among the first to benefit from the new treatment when the study is over.

- If the treatment is effective, it may help to improve vision and control or prevent eye disease or disorder.

- Clinical trial patients receive the highest quality medical care. Experts watch them closely during the study and may continue to follow them after the study is over.

- People who take part in these trials contribute to new knowledge that may help other people with the same eye problems. In cases where certain eye diseases or disorders run in families, your participation may lead to better care for family members.

The Informed Consent

Once you agree to take part in a clinical trial, you will be asked to sign an informed consent. This document explains a clinical trial's risks and benefits, what researchers expect of you, and your rights as a patient.

What Are the Risks?

Clinical trials may involve risks as well as possible benefits:

- Whether or not a new treatment will work cannot be known ahead of time. There is always a chance that a new treatment may not work better than a standard treatment, may not work at all, or may be harmful.

- The treatment you receive may cause side effects that are serious enough to require medical attention.

How Is Patient Safety Protected?

Clinical trials can raise fears of the unknown. Understanding the safeguards that protect patients can ease some of these fears:

- Before a clinical trial begins, researchers must get approval from their hospital's Institutional Review Board (IRB), an advisory group that makes sure a clinical trial is designed to protect patient safety.

- During a clinical trial, doctors will closely watch you to see if the treatment is working and if you are having any side effects. All the results are carefully recorded and reviewed.

- A group of experts—the Data and Safety Monitoring Committee—carefully watches each clinical trial supported by the NEI. This group can recommend that a study be stopped at any time.

- Patients are asked to take part in a clinical trial only if they volunteer and understand the risks and benefits.

What Are a Patient's Rights in a Clinical Trial?

Patients who are eligible for a clinical trial will be given information to help them decide whether to take part. As a patient, you have the right to:

- be told about all known risks and benefits of treatments involved in the study;

- know how the researchers plan to carry out the study, for how long, and where;

- know what is expected of you;

- know any costs involved for you or your insurers;

- be informed about any medical or personal information that may be shared with other researchers directly involved in the clinical trial;

- talk openly with doctors and ask any questions.

After you join a clinical trial, you have the right to do the following things:

- Leave the study at any time. Participation is strictly voluntary. However, you should not enroll if you do not plan to complete the study.

- Receive any new information about the new treatment.

- Continue to ask questions and get answers.

- Maintain your privacy. Your name will not appear in any reports based on the study.

- Be informed of your treatment assignment once the study is completed.

What About Costs?

In some clinical trials, the medical facility conducting the research pays for treatment costs and some other expenses. You or your health insurance may have to pay for some things that are considered part of standard care. These things may include hospital stays, laboratory and other tests, and medical procedures. You also may need to pay for travel between your home and the clinic. For clinical trials conducted at the NEI's medical facility in Bethesda, Maryland, medical care is provided at no cost to patients. You should find out about costs ahead of time. If you have health insurance, find out exactly what it will cover. If you don't have health insurance, or if your insurance company will not cover your costs, talk to the clinic staff about other options for covering the cost of your care.

What Questions Should You Ask Before Deciding to Join a Clinical Trial?

Questions you should ask when thinking about joining a clinical trial include the following:

- What is the purpose of the clinical trial?

- What are the standard treatments for my disease or condition? Why do researchers think the new treatment may be better? What is likely to happen to me with or without the new treatment?

- What tests and treatments will I need? Will I need surgery? Medicines? Hospitalization?

- How long will the treatment last? How often will I have to come back for follow-up exams?

- What are the treatment's possible benefits to my condition? What are the short- and long-term risks? What are the possible side effects?

- Will the treatment be uncomfortable? Will it make me feel sick? If so, for how long?

- How will my health be monitored?

- Where will I need to go for the clinical trial? How will I get there?

- How much will it cost me to be in the study? What costs are covered by the study? How much will my health insurance cover?

- Will I be able to see my own doctor? Who will be in charge of my care?

- Will taking part in the study affect my daily life? Will I have the time to be in it?

- How do I feel about taking part in a clinical trial? Are there family members or friends who may benefit from my contributions to new medical knowledge?

What Clinical Trials Are Being Held? Who Can Take Part in Them?

The NEI conducts or sponsors research on many eye diseases and disorders. Because funding for eye research goes to the medical areas that show promising research opportunities, it is not possible for the NEI to sponsor clinical trials in every eye disease and disorder at all times.

Not everyone can take part in a clinical trial for a specific eye disease or disorder. Each study enrolls patients with certain features or eligibility criteria. These criteria may include the type and stage of disease or disorder, as well as the age and previous treatment history of the patient.

You or your doctor can contact the NEI to find out more about specific clinical trials and their eligibility criteria. If you are interested in joining a clinical trial, your doctor must contact one of the trial's investigators and provide details about your diagnosis and medical history.

The NEI's website lists the clinical trials the NEI is helping to support. Each trial description includes information on its background and purpose, as well as patient eligibility. There is information on how to participate in a trial and how to refer a patient to a trial.

Some Recent Clinical Trials

Treatment for Herpes of the Eye

The Herpetic Eye Disease Study (HEDS) is an example of a Phase III treatment trial. Herpes of the eye, which is controllable but incurable, can produce a painful sore on the eyelid and inflammation of the cornea, the transparent tissue on the surface of the eye. Previous studies showed that once people develop ocular herpes, they have up to a 50 percent chance of having a recurrence. In one part of the HEDS, researchers followed 703 patients who had herpes of the eye during the preceding year, but did not currently have an active case of the disease. Of this number, 357 were treated with the antiviral drug acyclovir by mouth, and 346 received a placebo.

Results: Scientists found that acyclovir reduced by 41 percent the probability that herpes of the eye would return. The findings from this research have helped to change how doctors treat the disease.

Uncovering an Ineffective Treatment

Decompression surgery was once thought to be a sight saver for people with ischemic optic neuropathy, a swelling of the optic nerve. An NEI-sponsored clinical trial examined this surgery in 244 patients.

Results: The operation proved to be neither safe nor effective. In addition, nearly half of those who did not have the surgery had improved eyesight within six months. Because of these results, the NEI stopped the study earlier than expected and mailed a special bulletin to twenty-five thousand doctors.

Saving the Sight of Premature Infants

Retinopathy of prematurity (ROP) occurs when abnormal blood vessels grow and spread throughout the retinas of premature infants. The disorder mostly affects infants who weigh less than three pounds at birth. The NEI sponsored a clinical trial to find out whether a procedure called cryotherapy was a safe and effective treatment to prevent ROP. In this procedure, doctors briefly touch spots on the surface of the eye with an instrument called a cryoprobe. This freezes parts of the retina to stop the growth of abnormal blood vessels.

Results: Fewer of the infants' eyes that were treated with cryotherapy became blind compared with the eyes of untreated infants. Researchers continue to follow these children to gain information about the long-term effects of this treatment.

Laser Treatment for Diabetic Retinopathy

Two NEI-sponsored clinical trials examined the use of laser treatment in patients with diabetic retinopathy, a disease that damages the blood vessels in the retina. About half of the sixteen million Americans with diabetes have this disorder, which is a leading cause of blindness in working-age adults. Laser treatment was given to 4,453 people with diabetes at twenty-five medical centers. One eye of each patient received laser treatment. The other eye was not initially treated.

Results: Laser treatment was very effective in preventing vision loss in more than 90 percent of patients with diabetic retinopathy.

Preventing Blindness in People with Acquired Immunodeficiency Syndrome (AIDS)

Many people with AIDS have an eye infection known as cytomegalovirus (CMV) retinitis. Drugs such as ganciclovir can control the infection and reduce the chance of blindness. In the past, doctors gave the drug through a tube that had to remain in a vein. It took two hours to give each dose. Another way to give ganciclovir is through the use of a tiny implant in the eye. The implant slowly releases the medication for several months. The NEI supported a clinical trial to find out whether this implant was safe and effective.

Results: Almost all of the eyes treated with the implant had complete control of their eye infection and maintained nearly perfect vision. The implant also improved the patients' quality of life by making treatment easier.

Part Two

Understanding and Treating Refractive, Eye Movement, and Alignment Disorders

Chapter 10

Refractive Disorders

Chapter Contents

Section 10.1

Facts about Refractive Errors

Reprinted from the National Eye Institute,
National Institutes of Health, October 2010.

Refractive Errors Defined

What are refractive errors?

Refractive errors occur when the shape of the eye prevents light from focusing directly on the retina. The length of the eyeball (longer or shorter), changes in the shape of the cornea, or aging of the lens can cause refractive errors.

What is refraction?

Refraction is the bending of light as it passes through one object to another. Vision occurs when light rays are bent (refracted) as they pass through the cornea and the lens. The light is then focused on the retina. The retina converts the light-rays into messages that are sent through the optic nerve to the brain. The brain interprets these messages into the images we see.

Frequently Asked Questions about Refractive Errors

What are the different types of refractive errors?

The most common types of refractive errors are myopia, hyperopia, presbyopia, and astigmatism.

Myopia (nearsightedness) is a condition where objects up close appear clearly, while objects far away appear blurry. With myopia, light comes to focus in front of the retina instead of on the retina.

Hyperopia (farsightedness) is a common type of refractive error where distant objects may be seen more clearly than objects that are near. However, people experience hyperopia differently. Some people may not notice any problems with their vision, especially when they are young. For people with significant hyperopia, vision can be blurry for objects at any distance, near or far.

Astigmatism is a condition in which the eye does not focus light evenly onto the retina, the light-sensitive tissue at the back of the eye. This can cause images to appear blurry and stretched out.

Presbyopia is an age-related condition in which the ability to focus up close becomes more difficult. As the eye ages, the lens can no longer change shape enough to allow the eye to focus on close objects clearly.

Risk Factors

Who is at risk for refractive errors?

Presbyopia affects most adults over age thirty-five. Other refractive errors can affect both children and adults. Individuals that have parents with certain refractive errors may be more likely to get one or more refractive errors.

Symptoms and Detection

What are the signs and symptoms of refractive errors?

Blurred vision is the most common symptom of refractive errors. Other symptoms may include the following:

- Double vision
- Glare or halos around bright lights
- Headaches
- Haziness
- Squinting
- Eyestrain

How are refractive errors diagnosed?

An eye care professional can diagnose refractive errors during a comprehensive dilated eye examination. People with a refractive error often visit their eye care professional with complaints of visual discomfort or blurred vision. However, some people don't know they aren't seeing as clearly as they could.

Treatment

How are refractive errors treated?

Refractive errors can be corrected with eyeglasses, contact lenses, or surgery.

Eyeglasses are the simplest and safest way to correct refractive errors. Your eye care professional can prescribe appropriate lenses to correct your refractive error and give you optimal vision.

Contact lenses work by becoming the first refractive surface for light rays entering the eye, causing a more precise refraction or focus. In many cases, contact lenses provide clearer vision, a wider field of vision, and greater comfort. They are a safe and effective option if fitted and used properly. It is very important to wash your hands and clean your lenses as instructed in order to reduce the risk of infection.

If you have certain eye conditions you may not be able to wear contact lenses. Discuss this with your eye care professional.

Refractive surgery aims to change the shape of the cornea permanently. This change in eye shape restores the focusing power of the eye by allowing the light rays to focus precisely on the retina for improved vision. There are many types of refractive surgeries. Your eye care professional can help you decide if surgery is an option for you.

Section 10.2

Astigmatism

Excerpted from "Facts about Astigmatism," National Eye Institute, National Institutes of Health, October 2010.

Astigmatism Defined

What is astigmatism?

Astigmatism is a common type of refractive error. It is a condition in which the eye does not focus light evenly onto the retina, the light-sensitive tissue at the back of the eye.

Causes and Risk Factors

How does astigmatism occur?

Astigmatism occurs when light is bent differently depending on where it strikes the cornea and passes through the eyeball. The cornea of a normal eye is curved like a basketball, with the same degree of roundness in all areas. An eye with astigmatism has a cornea that is curved more like a football, with some areas that are steeper or more rounded than others. This can cause images to appear blurry and stretched out.

Who is at risk for astigmatism?

Astigmatism can affect both children and adults. Some patients with slight astigmatism will not notice much change in their vision. It is important to have eye examinations at regular intervals in order to detect any astigmatism early on for children.

Symptoms and Detection

What are the signs and symptoms of astigmatism?

Signs and symptoms include the following:

- Headaches
- Eyestrain
- Squinting
- Distorted or blurred vision at all distances
- Difficulty driving at night

If you experience any of these symptoms, visit your eye care professional. If you wear glasses or contact lenses and still have these issues, a new prescription might be needed.

How is astigmatism diagnosed?

Astigmatism is usually found during a comprehensive dilated eye exam. Being aware of any changes in your vision is important. It can help in detecting any common vision problems. If you notice any changes in your vision, visit your eye care professional for a comprehensive eye dilated examination.

Can you have astigmatism and not know it?

It is possible to have mild astigmatism and not know about it. This is especially true for children, who are not aware of their vision being other than normal. Some adults may also have mild astigmatism without any symptoms. It's important to have comprehensive dilated eye exams to make sure you are seeing your best.

Treatment

How is astigmatism corrected?

Astigmatism can be corrected with eyeglasses, contact lenses, or surgery. Individual lifestyles affect the way astigmatism is treated.

Eyeglasses are the simplest and safest way to correct astigmatism. Your eye care professional will prescribe appropriate lenses to help you see as clearly as possible.

Contact lenses work by becoming the first refractive surface for light rays entering the eye, causing a more precise refraction or focus. In many cases, contact lenses provide clearer vision, a wider field of vision, and greater comfort. They are a safe and effective option if fitted and used properly. It is very important to wash your hands and clean your lenses as instructed in order to reduce the risk of infection.

If you have certain eye conditions you may not be able to wear contact lenses. Discuss this with your eye care professional.

Refractive surgery aims to change the shape of the cornea permanently. This change in eye shape restores the focusing power of the eye by allowing the light rays to focus precisely on the retina for improved vision. There are many types of refractive surgeries. Your eye care professional can help you decide if surgery is an option for you.

Section 10.3

Hyperopia

Excerpted from "Facts about Hyperopia," National Eye Institute, National Institutes of Health, October 2010.

Hyperopia Defined

What is hyperopia?

Hyperopia, also known as farsightedness, is a common type of refractive error where distant objects may be seen more clearly than objects that are near. However, people experience hyperopia differently. Some people may not notice any problems with their vision, especially when they are young. For people with significant hyperopia, vision can be blurry for objects at any distance, near or far.

Causes and Risk Factors

How does hyperopia develop?

Hyperopia develops in eyes that focus images behind the retina instead of on the retina, which can result in blurred vision. This occurs when the eyeball is too short, which prevents incoming light from focusing directly on the retina. It may also be caused by an abnormally shaped cornea or lens.

Who is at risk for hyperopia?

Hyperopia can affect both children and adults. It affects about 5 to 10 percent of Americans. People whose parents have hyperopia may also be more likely to get the condition.

Symptoms and Detection

What are the signs and symptoms of hyperopia?

The symptoms of hyperopia vary from person to person. Your eye care professional can help you understand how the condition affects you.

Common signs and symptoms of hyperopia include the following:

- Headaches

- Eyestrain

- Squinting

- Blurry vision, especially for close objects

How is hyperopia diagnosed?

An eye care professional can diagnose hyperopia and other refractive errors during a comprehensive dilated eye examination. People with this condition often visit their eye care professional with complaints of visual discomfort or blurred vision.

Treatment

How is hyperopia corrected?

Hyperopia can be corrected with eyeglasses, contact lenses, or surgery.

Eyeglasses are the simplest and safest way to correct hyperopia. Your eye care professional can prescribe lenses that will help correct the problem and help you see your best.

Contact lenses work by becoming the first refractive surface for light rays entering the eye, causing a more precise refraction or focus. In many cases, contact lenses may provide clearer vision, wider field of vision, and greater comfort. They are a safe and effective option if fitted and used properly. However, contact lenses may not be the best option for everyone.

If you have certain eye conditions you may not be able to wear contact lenses. Discuss this with your eye care professional.

Refractive surgery aims to permanently change the shape of the cornea, which will improve refractive vision. Surgery can decrease or eliminate dependency on wearing eyeglasses and contact lenses. There are many types of refractive surgeries and surgical options should be discussed with an eye care professional.

Section 10.4

Myopia

Excerpted from "Facts about Myopia," National Eye
Institute, National Institutes of Health, October 2010.

Myopia Defined

What is myopia?

Myopia, also known as nearsightedness, is a common type of refractive error where close objects appear clearly, but distant objects
appear blurry.

What is high myopia?

High myopia is a severe form of the condition. In high myopia, the
eyeball stretches and becomes too long. This can lead to holes or tears
in the retina and can also cause retinal detachment. Abnormal blood
vessels may grow under the retina and cause changes in vision. People
with high myopia need comprehensive dilated eye exams more often.
Early detection and timely treatment can help prevent vision loss.

Causes and Risk Factors

How does myopia develop?

Myopia develops in eyes that focus images in front of the retina
instead of on the retina, which results in blurred vision. This occurs
when the eyeball becomes too long and prevents incoming light from
focusing directly on the retina. It may also be caused by an abnormally
shaped cornea or lens.

Who is at risk for myopia?

Myopia can affect both children and adults. The condition affects
about 25 percent of Americans. Myopia is often diagnosed in children
between eight and twelve years of age and may worsen during the
teen years. Little change may occur between ages twenty to forty, but

sometimes myopia may worsen with age. People whose parents have myopia may be more likely to get the condition.

Symptoms and Detection

What are the signs and symptoms of myopia?

Some of the signs and symptoms of myopia include the following:

- Headaches
- Eyestrain
- Squinting
- Difficulty seeing distant objects, such as highway signs

How is myopia diagnosed?

An eye care professional can diagnose myopia and other refractive errors during a comprehensive dilated eye examination. People with this condition often visit their eye care professional with complaints of visual discomfort or blurred vision.

Treatment

How is myopia corrected?

Myopia can be corrected with eyeglasses, contact lenses, or surgery.

Eyeglasses are the simplest and safest way to correct myopia. Your eye care professional can prescribe lenses that will correct the problem and help you to see your best.

Contact lenses work by becoming the first refractive surface for light rays entering the eye, causing a more precise refraction or focus. In many cases, contact lenses may provide clearer vision, wider field of vision, and greater comfort. They are a safe and effective option if fitted and used properly. However, contact lenses may not be the best option for everyone.

If you have certain eye conditions you may not be able to wear contact lenses. Discuss this with your eye care professional.

Refractive surgery aims to permanently change the shape of the cornea, which will improve refractive vision. Surgery can decrease or eliminate dependency on wearing eyeglasses and contact lenses. There are many types of refractive surgeries and surgical options should be discussed with an eye care professional.

Section 10.5

Presbyopia

Excerpted from "Facts about Presbyopia," National Eye
Institute, National Institutes of Health, October 2010.

Presbyopia Defined

What is presbyopia?

Presbyopia is a common type of vision disorder that occurs as you
age. It is often referred to as the aging eye condition. Presbyopia results
in the inability to focus up close, a problem associated with refraction
in the eye.

Can I have presbyopia and another type of refractive error at the same time?

Yes. It is common to have presbyopia and another type of refractive error at the same time. There are several other types of refractive errors: myopia (nearsightedness), hyperopia (farsightedness), and
astigmatism.

An individual may have one type of refractive error in one eye and
a different type of refractive error in the other.

Causes and Risk Factors

How does presbyopia occur?

Presbyopia happens naturally in people as they age. The eye is not
able to focus light directly onto the retina due to the hardening of the
natural lens. Aging also affects muscle fibers around the lens, making
it harder for the eye to focus on up close objects. The ineffective lens
causes light to focus behind the retina, causing poor vision for objects
that are up close.

When you are younger, the lens of the eye is soft and flexible, allowing the tiny muscles inside the eye to easily reshape the lens to focus
on close and distant objects.

Who is at risk for presbyopia?

Anyone over the age of thirty-five is at risk for developing presbyopia. Everyone experiences some loss of focusing power for near objects as they age, but some will notice this more than others.

Symptoms and Detection

What are the signs and symptoms of presbyopia?

Some of the signs and symptoms of myopia include the following:

- Hard time reading small print
- Having to hold reading material farther than arm's distance
- Problems seeing objects that are close to you
- Headaches
- Eyestrain

If you experience any of these symptoms you may want to visit an eye care professional for a comprehensive dilated eye examination. If you wear glasses or contact lenses and still have these issues, a new prescription might be needed.

How is presbyopia diagnosed?

Presbyopia can be found during a comprehensive dilated eye exam. If you notice any changes in your vision, you should visit an eye care professional. Exams are recommended more often after age forty to check for age-related conditions.

Treatment

How is presbyopia corrected?

Eyeglasses are the simplest and safest means of correcting presbyopia. Eyeglasses for presbyopia have higher focusing power in the lower portion of the lens. This allows you to read through the lower portion of the lens and see properly at distance through the upper portion of the lens. It is also possible to purchase reading eyeglasses. These types of glasses do not require a prescription and can help with reading vision.

Chapter 11

Eye Movement and Alignment Disorders

Chapter Contents

Section 11.1

Amblyopia

What is amblyopia?

A common vision problem in children is amblyopia, or "lazy eye." It is so common that it is the reason for more vision loss in children than all other causes put together. Amblyopia is a decrease in the child's vision that can happen even when there is no problem with the structure of the eye. The decrease in vision results when one or both eyes send a blurry image to the brain. The brain then "learns" to only see blurry with that eye, even when glasses are used. Only children can get amblyopia. If it is not treated, it can cause permanent loss of vision.

What kinds of amblyopia are there?

There are several different types and causes of amblyopia: strabismic amblyopia, deprivation amblyopia, and refractive amblyopia. The end result of all forms of amblyopia is reduced vision in the affected eye(s).

What is strabismic amblyopia?

Strabismic amblyopia develops when the eyes are not straight. One eye may turn in, out, up, or down. When this happens, the brain "turns off" the eye that is not straight and the vision subsequently drops in that eye.

What is deprivation amblyopia?

Deprivation amblyopia develops when cataracts or similar conditions "deprive" young children's eyes of visual experience. If not treated very early, these children can have very poor vision. Sometimes this kind of amblyopia can affect both eyes.

What is refractive amblyopia?

Refractive amblyopia happens when there is a large or unequal amount of refractive error (glasses strength) in a child's eyes. Usually the brain will "turn off" the eye that has more farsightedness or more astigmatism. Parents and pediatricians may not think there is a problem because the child's eyes may stay straight. Also, the "good" eye has normal vision. For these reasons, this kind of amblyopia in children may not be found until the child has a vision test. This kind of amblyopia can affect one or both eyes and can be helped if the problem is found early.

Will glasses help a child with amblyopia to see better?

Maybe, but they may not correct it all the way to 20/20. With amblyopia, the brain is "used to" seeing a blurry image and it cannot interpret the clear image that the glasses produce. With time, however, the brain may "relearn" how to see and the vision may increase. Remember, glasses alone do not increase the vision all the way to 20/20, as the brain is used to seeing blurry with that eye. For that reason, the normal eye is treated (with patching or eye drops) to make the amblyopic (weak) eye stronger.

What can be done if my child has equal high amounts of farsightedness and/or astigmatism and is diagnosed with bilateral amblyopia?

Bilateral amblyopia is usually treated with consistent, early glasses and/or contact lenses with follow-up over a long period of time. If asymmetric amblyopia (one eye better than the other) occurs, then patching or eye drops may be added.

When should amblyopia be treated?

Early treatment is always best. If necessary, children with refractive errors (nearsightedness, farsightedness, or astigmatism) can wear glasses or contact lenses when they are as young as one week old. Children with cataracts or other "amblyogenic" conditions are usually treated promptly in order to minimize the development of amblyopia.

How old is too old for amblyopia treatment?

A recent National Institutes of Health (NIH) study confirmed that *some* improvement in vision can be attained with amblyopia therapy initiated in younger teenagers (through age fourteen years). Better treatment success is achieved when treatment starts early, however.

How can I get early treatment for amblyopia?

Some forms of amblyopia, such as that associated with large-deviation strabismus, may be easily detected by parents. Other types of amblyopia (from high refractive error) might cause a child to move very close to objects or squint his or her eyes. Still other forms of amblyopia may *not* be obvious to parents and therefore must be detected by vision screening.

What is vision screening?

Vision screening is strongly recommended by the American Academy of Pediatrics (AAP) over the course of childhood to detect amblyopia early enough to allow successful treatment. Pediatricians check newborns for red reflex to find congenital cataracts. Infants are checked for the ability to fix and follow and whether they have strabismus. Toddlers can have their pupillary red reflexes tested with a direct ophthalmoscope (Brückner test) or by photoscreening, or by remote autorefraction to identify refractive errors that can cause amblyopia. When children can consistently identify objects either by reading or by matching, the acuity of each eye (with the nontested eye patched or covered) is screened to identify amblyopia.

How is amblyopia treated?

One of the most important treatments of amblyopia is correcting the refractive error with consistent use of glasses and/or contact lenses. Other mainstays of amblyopia treatment are to enable as clear an image as possible (for example, by removing a cataract), and forcing the child to use the nondominant eye (via patching or eye drops to blur the better-seeing eye).

When should patching be used for amblyopia treatment?

Patching should only be done if an ophthalmologist recommends it. An ophthalmologist should regularly check how the patch is affecting the child's vision. Although it can be hard to do, patching usually works very well if started early enough and if the parents and child follow the patching instructions carefully. It is important to patch the dominant eye to allow the weak eye to get stronger.

Are there different types of patches?

The classic patch is an adhesive "Band-Aid" which is applied directly to the skin around the eye. These may be available in different sizes for younger and older children. For children wearing glasses, both cloth and semi-transparent stickers (Bangerter foils) may be placed over or onto the spectacles. "Pirate" patches on elastic bands are especially prone to "peeking" and are therefore only occasionally appropriate.

Is there an alternative to patching to treat amblyopia?

Sometimes the stronger (good) eye can be "penalized" or blurred to help the weaker eye get stronger. Blurring the vision in the good eye with drops or with extra power in the glasses will penalize the good eye. This forces the child to use the weaker eye. Ophthalmologists use this treatment instead of patching when the amblyopia is not very bad or when a child is unable to wear the patch as recommended. For mild and moderate degrees of amblyopia, studies have shown that patching or eye drops may be similarly effective. Your pediatric ophthalmologist will help you select the treatment regimen that is best for your child.

Do drops work for all amblyopic children?

Not all children benefit from eye drop treatment for amblyopia. Penalizing eye drops (such as atropine) work less well when the stronger eye is nearsighted.

How many hours per day patching is enough when treating amblyopia?

The mainstay of treating amblyopia is patching of the dominant (good) eye, either full or part time during waking hours. Although classic teaching suggests that the more hours per day patching is performed, the greater the result, recent studies suggest that shorter periods may achieve similar results as longer amounts of patching in patients with moderate amounts of amblyopia.

How long does amblyopia patching therapy take to work?

Although vision improvement frequently occurs within weeks of beginning patching treatment, optimal results often take many months. Once vision has been improved, part-time (maintenance) patching or periodic use of atropine eye drops may be required to keep the vision from slipping or deteriorating. This maintenance treatment may be advisable for several months to years.

During which activities should patching be performed?

The particular activity is not terribly important, compared to the need to keep the patch on during the allotted time. As long as the child is conscious and has his or her eyes open, visual input will be processed by the amblyopic eye. On the other hand, the child may be more cooperative or more open to bargaining if patching is performed during certain, desirable activities (such as watching a preferred television program or video). Some eye doctors believe that the performance of near activities (reading, coloring, hand-held computer games) during treatment may be more stimulating to the brain and produce better or more rapid recovery of vision.

Should patching be performed during school hours?

In many instances, school is an excellent time to patch, taking advantage of a nonparental authority figure. Patching in school hours gives the class an opportunity to learn valuable lessons about accepting differences between children. While in most instances, children may not need to modify their school activities while patching, sometimes adjustments such as sitting in the front row of the classroom will be necessary. If the patient, teacher, and classmates are educated appropriately, school patching need not be a socially stigmatizing experience. On the other hand, frequently a parental or other family figure may be more vigilant in monitoring patching than is possible in the school setting. Parents should be flexible in choosing when to schedule patching.

What if my child refuses to wear the patch?

Many children will resist wearing a patch at first. Successful patching may require persistence and plenty of encouragement from family members, neighbors, teachers, etc. Children will often throw a temper tantrum, but then they eventually learn not to remove the patch. Another way to help is to provide a reward to the child for keeping the patch on for the prescribed time period.

Can surgery be performed to treat amblyopia?

Surgery on the eye muscles is a treatment for strabismus—it can straighten misaligned eyes. By itself, however, surgery does not usually or completely help the amblyopia. Surgery to make the eyes straight can only help enable the eyes to work together as a team. Children with strabismic amblyopia still need close monitoring and treatment for the amblyopia, and this treatment is usually performed before strabismus surgery is considered.

Children who are born with cataracts may need surgery to take out the cataracts. After surgery, the child will usually need vision correction with glasses or contact lenses and patching.

What are appropriate goals of amblyopia treatment?

In all cases, the goal is the best possible vision in each eye. While not every child can be improved to 20/20, most can obtain a substantial improvement in vision. Although there are exceptions, patching does not usually work as well in children who are older than nine years of age.

What happens if amblyopia treatment does not work?

In some cases, treatment for amblyopia may not succeed in substantially improving vision. It is hard to decide to stop treatment, but sometimes it is best for both the child and the family. Children who have amblyopia in one eye and good vision only in their other eye can wear safety glasses and sports goggles to protect the normal eye from injury. As long as the good eye stays healthy, these children function normally in most aspects of society.

Section 11.2

Brown Syndrome

What is Brown syndrome?

Brown syndrome (named after Dr. Harold W. Brown) is also known
as superior oblique tendon sheath syndrome. It is a mechanical problem in which the superior oblique muscle/tendon (on the outside of
the eyeball) does not move freely. This makes looking up and in with
the affected eye difficult. Brown syndrome may be present at birth
(congenital) or begin later. It may be constant or intermittent.

What do the eyes of patients with Brown syndrome look like?

The eyes usually look normal except in side gaze positions. In side
gaze (looking toward the affected side), one eye appears higher than
the other, particularly when looking up. A vertical misalignment is
sometimes noted when looking straight ahead.

Often the higher eye is mistakenly presumed to be the abnormal
eye, but the lower eye is affected. Brown syndrome causes the lower eye
to have trouble looking upward in side gaze. Essentially the affected
eye is "tethered" or held down by the tight superior oblique tendon.

What causes Brown syndrome?

Although the exact cause of Brown syndrome is unknown, it is
clear that there is an abnormality with the tendon that is part of the
superior oblique muscle, with the cartilage structure (trochlea) that
the tendon moves through, or with the combined tendon-trochlea as-
sembly.

These abnormalities may include a reduced elasticity of the superior
oblique muscle and tendon, a thickened tendon, a short and/or tight
sheath, or fibrous adhesions (scarring) of the tendon.

Is Brown syndrome hereditary?

Hereditary cases of Brown syndrome are rare. Most cases arise without a family history (sporadic).

Can Brown syndrome be acquired?

Acquired Brown syndrome is uncommon but may be seen following surgery, after trauma, or in association with inflammatory diseases. Trauma can cause Brown syndrome if a blunt object hits the eye socket in the upper inside corner near the nose. Surgery for the eyelid, frontal sinus, eyeball (retinal detachment), and teeth (dental extraction) have been linked to acquired Brown syndrome. Inflammation of the tendon-trochlea complex (from adult and juvenile rheumatoid arthritis, systemic lupus erythematosus, and sinusitis) can be associated with development of the problem. Sometimes the cause is never identified.

How is Brown syndrome diagnosed?

The eyes are usually straight when looking directly ahead and down. The hallmark sign of Brown syndrome is decreased ability to look upward. In some situations the eyes turn outward (exotropia) when looking up.

Brown syndrome can be associated with an abnormal head position (chin up, face turn, head tilt) for better eye cooperation. The affected eye can get "stuck" after looking up or down for long periods of time. When the eye becomes unstuck, a click is often heard and may be accompanied by pain or discomfort.

Brown syndrome may be more noticeable in children since they often look upward toward adults.

Does Brown syndrome affect one or both eyes?

Ninety percent of patients have only one affected eye, more commonly the right.

Does Brown syndrome cause eye problems besides abnormal eye movements?

Some children with Brown syndrome have poor binocular vision (which can result in poor depth perception), amblyopia, or exotropia.

119

Are there different kinds of Brown syndrome?

Brown syndrome can be classified according to severity. In mild cases there is a reduced ability to look up and in with the affected eye. In moderate cases, there is also a tendency for the eye to move downward as it is turned in. In severe cases there is a tendency for the affected eye to turn downward when the patient looks straight ahead.

Can Brown syndrome improve or resolve without treatment?

Spontaneous resolution sometimes occurs in acquired and intermittent cases. In the congenital form of Brown syndrome, the eye movement problem is usually constant and unlikely to resolve spontaneously.

How is Brown syndrome treated?

Treatment recommendations for Brown syndrome vary according to the cause and severity of the movement disorder. Close observation alone is usually sufficient in mild cases. Visual acuity and the ability to use both eyes at the same time (binocular vision) should be monitored closely in young children. Nonsurgical treatment is often advised for recently acquired, traumatic, and variable cases. Systemic and locally injected corticosteroids have been used to treat inflammatory cases of acquired Brown syndrome. Nonsteroidal anti-inflammatory agents (like ibuprofen) have also been used. Surgical treatment is usually recommended if any of the following are present: eye turns down when looking straight ahead, significant double vision, compromised binocular vision, or pronounced abnormal head position. More than one surgery may be needed for optimal management.

Section 11.3

Nystagmus

What is nystagmus?

Nystagmus is an involuntary, shaking, "to and fro" movement of the eyes.

What are the different types of nystagmus?

Nystagmus is typically classified as congenital or acquired, with multiple subcategories.

Congenital nystagmus onset is typically between six weeks and three months of age. Congenital motor nystagmus tends to be horizontal, bilateral, idiopathic (cause unknown), and is sometimes inherited. Sensory nystagmus also occurs early in life and is secondary to poor vision caused by a variety of eye conditions such as cataract (cloudiness of the eye's lens), strabismus (eye misalignment), and optic nerve hypoplasia.

Acquired nystagmus occurs later and has many etiologies. Acquired nystagmus can be associated with serious medical conditions.

What ocular/medical conditions are associated with nystagmus?

- Cataract
- Strabismus
- Amblyopia
- Optic nerve hypoplasia
- Leber congenital amaurosis
- Aniridia
- Achromatopsia

- Severe refractive error
- Retina coloboma
- Other optic nerve and retina disorders
- Albinism
- Medication use
- Vitamin deficiency
- Fetal alcohol syndrome
- Trauma
- Inner ear (vestibular) problems
- Stroke (most common cause in older people with acquired nystagmus
- Brain tumor (rare cause of acquired nystagmus)

All children and adults with nystagmus should be evaluated by an ophthalmologist (and primary care physician) to determine if any association exists with other conditions.

Is nystagmus inheritable?

Nystagmus can be inheritable, sometimes with a strong family history, and dominant, recessive, and x-linked patterns have been reported. The severity of nystagmus often varies amongst members of an involved family.

How does nystagmus affect a child's visual development? What will the vision be as an adult?

The visual development of a child with nystagmus is quite variable. Some children with nystagmus have a mild reduction in visual acuity (20/50 or better) while others have severe visual disability (20/200 or worse). It is difficult to predict what the visual acuity will be as an adult; however, most individuals with nystagmus have some reduction of visual function.

What does a person with nystagmus actually see?

Children with nystagmus typically see the world similarly to other children, albeit with some blurriness. The world does not appear to "shake." Individuals with adult onset or acquired nystagmus often report the appearance of movement of the seen world (oscillopsia).

Why do people with nystagmus tilt or turn their head?

Nystagmus severity can vary upon direction of gaze; the eyes oscillate more when looking in certain directions. The gaze position of least eye movement is the "null point" and tends to be where vision is best. Tilting or turning the head can thus optimize vision.

Can nystagmus occur in one eye?

Yes, but rarely. Spasmus nutans (triad of nystagmus, head bobbing or nodding, and a head turn or tilt) is often noted to have unilateral nystagmus. However, under close observation the nystagmus is bilateral but highly asymmetric with a high-frequency "shimmering" movement.

Can surgery make nystagmus go away?

Eye muscle surgery (strabismus surgery) may be indicated for some individuals with nystagmus. The goal of surgery in most instances is to help alleviate a significantly abnormal head position or to decrease the amplitude of nystagmus. Surgery can sometimes cause vision improvement but does not fully eliminate nystagmus.

What nonsurgical treatments exist for nystagmus?

Significant refractive error is corrected with glasses or contact lenses. Contact lenses, in some circumstances, can be more visually beneficial than spectacles. Variable success has been noted with medications used to dampen the severity of nystagmus. Unfortunately, the use of these medications is frequently limited by side effects. Botulinum toxin is helpful for some individuals with severe, intractable oscillopsia.

Section 11.4

Strabismus

Crossed eyes, or strabismus as it is medically termed, is a condition in which both eyes do not look at the same place at the same time. It occurs when an eye turns in, out, up, or down and is usually caused by poor eye muscle control or a high amount of farsightedness.

There are six muscles attached to each eye that control how it moves. The muscles receive signals from the brain that direct their movements. Normally, the eyes work together so they both point at the same place. When problems develop with eye movement control, an eye may turn in, out, up, or down. The eye turning may be evident all the time or may appear only at certain times, such as when the person is tired, ill, or has done a lot of reading or close work. In some cases, the same eye may turn each time, while in other cases, the eyes may alternate turning.

Maintaining proper eye alignment is important to avoid seeing double, for good depth perception, and to prevent the development of poor vision in the turned eye. When the eyes are misaligned, the brain receives two different images. At first, this may create double vision and confusion, but over time the brain will learn to ignore the image from the turned eye. If the eye turning becomes constant and is not treated, it can lead to permanent reduction of vision in one eye, a condition called amblyopia or lazy eye.

Some babies' eyes may appear to be misaligned, but are actually both aiming at the same object. This is a condition called pseudostrabismus or false strabismus. The appearance of crossed eyes may be due to extra skin that covers the inner corner of the eyes, or a wide bridge of the nose. Usually, this will change as the child's face begins to grow.

Strabismus usually develops in infants and young children, most often by age three, but older children and adults can also develop the condition. There is a common misconception that a child with strabismus will outgrow the condition. However, this is not true. In fact, strabismus may get worse without treatment. Any child older than four months whose eyes do not appear to be straight all the time should be examined.

Strabismus is classified by the direction the eye turns:

- Inward turning is called esotropia.

- Outward turning is called exotropia.

- Upward turning is called hypertropia.

- Downward turning is called hypotropia.

Other classifications of strabismus include:

- the frequency with which it occurs—either constant or intermittent;

- whether it always involves the same eye—unilateral;

- if the turning eye is sometimes the right eye and other times the left eye—alternating.

Treatment for strabismus may include eyeglasses, prisms, vision therapy, or eye muscle surgery. If detected and treated early, strabismus can often be corrected with excellent results.

What causes strabismus?

Strabismus can be caused by problems with the eye muscles, the nerves that transmit information to the muscles, or the control center in the brain that directs eye movements. It can also develop due to other general health conditions or eye injuries.

Risk factors for developing strabismus include:

- **Family history:** Individuals with parents or siblings who have strabismus are more likely to develop it.

- **Refractive error:** People who have a significant amount of uncorrected farsightedness (hyperopia) may develop strabismus because of the additional amount of eye focusing required to keep objects clear.

- **Medical conditions:** People with conditions such as Down syndrome and cerebral palsy or who have suffered a stroke or head injury are at a higher risk for developing strabismus.

Although there are many types of strabismus that can develop in children or adults, the two most common forms are accommodative esotropia and intermittent exotropia.

Accommodative esotropia often occurs because of uncorrected farsightedness (hyperopia). Because the eye's focusing system is linked to the system that controls where the eyes point, the extra focusing effort needed to keep images clear in farsightedness may cause the eyes to turn inward. Signs and symptoms of accommodative esotropia may include seeing double, closing or covering one eye when doing close work, and tilting or turning of the head.

Intermittent exotropia may develop due to an inability to coordinate both eyes together. The eyes may have a tendency to point beyond the object being viewed. People with intermittent exotropia may experience headaches, difficulty reading, and eyestrain. They also may have a tendency to close one eye when viewing at distance or in bright sunlight.

How is strabismus diagnosed?

Strabismus is diagnosed through a comprehensive eye exam. Testing for strabismus, with special emphasis on how the eyes focus and move, may include:

- **Patient history:** A patient history is obtained to determine any symptoms the patient is experiencing or the parent is observing, and to note the presence of any general health problems, medications taken, or environmental factors that may be contributing to the symptoms.

- **Visual acuity:** Visual acuity measurements are taken to assess the extent to which vision may be affected. As part of the testing, you will be asked to read letters on distance and near reading charts. This test measures visual acuity, which is written as a fraction such as 20/40. When testing distance vision, the top number is the standard distance at which testing is done, twenty feet. The bottom number is the smallest letter size you were able to read at the twenty-foot distance. A person with 20/40 visual acuity would have to get within twenty feet of a letter that should be seen at forty feet in order to see it clearly. "Normal" distance visual acuity is 20/20.

- **Refraction:** A refraction is conducted to determine the appropriate lens power needed to compensate for any refractive error (nearsightedness, farsightedness, or astigmatism). Using an instrument called a phoroptor, your optometrist places a series of lenses in front of your eyes and measures how they focus light using a handheld lighted instrument called a retinoscope. Or the doctor may choose to use an automated instrument that automatically evaluates the refractive power of the eye. The power is then refined by the patient's responses to determine the lenses that allow the clearest vision.

- **Alignment and focusing testing:** How well your eyes focus, move, and work together needs to be assessed. In order to obtain a clear, single image of what is being viewed, the eyes must effectively change focus, move, and work in unison. This testing will look for problems that keep your eyes from focusing effectively or make it difficult to use both eyes together.

- **Examination of eye health:** The structures of the eye are observed to rule out any eye disease that may be contributing to strabismus. The health of the external and internal parts of the eye will be assessed using various testing procedures.

This testing may be done without the use of eye drops to determine how the eyes respond under normal seeing conditions. In some cases, such as for patients who can't respond verbally or when some of the eye's focusing power may be hidden, eye drops may be used. They temporarily keep the eyes from changing focus while testing is done.

Using the information obtained from these tests, along with results of other tests, your optometrist can determine if you have strabismus. Once testing is complete, your optometrist can discuss options for treatment.

How is strabismus treated?

People with strabismus have several treatment options available to improve eye alignment and coordination. They include:

- eyeglasses or contact lenses;

- prism lenses;

- vision therapy;

- eye muscle surgery.

Eyeglasses or contact lenses may be prescribed for patients with uncorrected farsightedness. This may be the only treatment needed for some patients with accommodative esotropia. Once the farsightedness is corrected, the eyes require less focusing effort and may remain straight.

Prism lenses are special lenses that have a prescription for prism power in them. The prisms alter the light entering the eye and assist in reducing the amount of turning the eye has to do to look at objects. Sometimes the prisms are able to fully compensate for and eliminate the eye turning.

127

Vision therapy is a structured program of visual activities prescribed to improve eye coordination and eye focusing abilities. Vision therapy trains the eyes and brain to work together more effectively. These eye exercises help remediate deficiencies in eye movement, eye focusing, and eye teaming and reinforce the eye-brain connection. Treatment may include office-based as well as home training procedures.

Eye muscle surgery can change the length or position of the muscles around the eye in an attempt to better align the eyes. Eye muscle surgery may be able to physically align the eyes so they appear straight. Often a program of vision therapy may also be needed to develop a functional improvement in eye coordination and to keep the eyes from reverting back to their previous condition of misalignment.

Chapter 12

Eyeglasses

Chapter Contents

Section 12.1

How to Read Your Eyeglass Prescription

So, you've just had an eye exam and your optometrist or ophthalmologist has given you an eyeglass prescription. He or she probably mentioned that you are nearsighted or farsighted, or perhaps that you have astigmatism. But what do all those numbers on your eyeglass prescription mean? And what about all those abbreviated terms, such as OD, OS, SPH, and CYL?

This section will help you decipher all parts of your prescription and discuss it knowledgeably with an optician when you're buying eyeglasses.

What OD and OS Mean

The first step to understanding your eyeglass prescription is knowing what "OD" and "OS" mean. They are abbreviations for oculus dexter and oculus sinister, which are Latin terms for right eye and left eye.

Your eyeglass prescription also may have a column labeled "OU." This is the abbreviation for the Latin term oculus uterque, which means "both eyes."

Though the use of these abbreviated Latin terms is traditional for prescriptions written for eyeglasses, contact lenses, and eye medicines, some doctors and clinics have opted to modernize their prescriptions and use RE (right eye) and LE (left eye) instead of OD and OS.

You may have noticed that on your prescription form the information for the right eye (OD) comes before the information for the left eye (OS). Eye doctors write prescriptions this way to avoid making errors, because when they face you, they see your right eye at left (first) and your left eye at right (second).

Other Terms on Your Eyeglass Prescription

Your eyeglass prescription contains other terms and abbreviations as well. These include:

- **Sphere (SPH):** This indicates the amount of lens power, measured in diopters (D), prescribed to correct nearsightedness or farsightedness. If the number appearing under this heading has a minus sign (–), you are nearsighted; if the number has a plus sign (+) or is not preceded by a plus sign or a minus sign, you are farsighted. The term "sphere" means that the correction for nearsightedness or farsightedness is "spherical," or equal in all meridians of the eye.

- **Cylinder (CYL):** This indicates the amount of lens power for astigmatism. If nothing appears in this column, you have no astigmatism. The term "cylinder" means that this lens power added to correct astigmatism is not spherical, but instead is shaped so one meridian has no added curvature, and the meridian perpendicular to this "no added power" meridian contains the maximum power and lens curvature to correct astigmatism. The number in the cylinder column may be preceded with a minus sign (for the correction of nearsighted astigmatism) or a plus sign (for farsighted astigmatism). Cylinder power always follows sphere power in an eyeglass prescription. Meridians of the eye are determined by superimposing a protractor scale on the eye's front surface. The 90-degree meridian is the vertical meridian of the eye, and the 180-degree meridian is the horizontal meridian.

- **Axis:** This describes the lens meridian that contains no cylinder power to correct astigmatism. The axis is defined with a number from 1 to 180. The number 90 corresponds to the vertical meridian of the eye, and the number 180 corresponds to the horizontal meridian. If an eyeglass prescription includes cylinder power, it also must include an axis value, which follows the cyl power and is preceded by an "x" when written freehand. The axis is the lens meridian that is 90 degrees away from the meridian that contains the cylinder power.

- **Add:** This is the added magnifying power applied to the bottom part of multifocal lenses to correct presbyopia. The number appearing in this section of the prescription is always a "plus" power, even if it is not preceded by a plus sign. Generally it will range from +0.75 to +3.00 D and will be the same power for both eyes.

- **Prism:** This is the amount of prismatic power, measured in prism diopters ("p.d." or a superscript triangle when written freehand), prescribed to compensate for eye alignment problems. Only a small percentage of eyeglass prescriptions include prism.

When present, the amount of prism is indicated in either metric or fractional English units (0.5 or ½, for example), and the direction of the prism is indicated by noting the relative position of its "base" or thickest edge. Four abbreviations are used for prism direction: BU = base up; BD = base down; BI = base in (toward the wearer's nose); BO = base out (toward the wearer's ear).

Sphere power, cylinder power, and add power always appear in diopters. They are in decimal form and generally are written in quarter-diopter (0.25 D) increments. Axis values are whole numbers from 1 to 180 and signify only a meridional location, not a power. When prism diopters are indicated in decimal form, typically only one digit appears after the period (e.g., 0.5).

An Example of an Eyeglass Prescription

Confused? Let's use an example to clear things up. (Pun intended.) Here is a sample eyeglass prescription:

OD -2.00 SPH	+2.00 add	0.5 p.d. BD
OS -1.00 -0.50 x 180	+2.00 add	0.5 p.d. BU

In this case, the eye doctor has prescribed -2.00 D sphere for the correction of myopia in the right eye (OD). There is no astigmatism correction for this eye, so no cylinder power or axis is noted. This doctor has elected to add "SPH," to confirm the right eye is being prescribed only spherical power. (Some doctors will add "DS" for "diopters sphere"; others will leave this area blank.)

The left eye (OS) is being prescribed -1.00 D sphere for myopia plus -0.50 D cylinder for the correction of astigmatism. The cyl power has its axis at the 180 meridian, meaning the horizontal (180-degree) meridian of the eye has no added power for astigmatism and the vertical (90-degree) meridian gets the added -0.50 D.

Both eyes are being prescribed an "add power" of +2.00 D for the correction of presbyopia, and this eyeglass prescription includes a prismatic correction of 0.5 prism diopter in each eye. In the right eye, the prism is base down (BD); in the left eye, it's base up (BU).

An Eyeglass Prescription Is Not a Contact Lens Prescription

An eyeglass prescription is for the purchase of eyeglasses only. It does not contain certain information that is crucial to a contact lens prescription and that can be obtained only during a contact lens consultation and fitting.

First of all, not everyone who needs eyeglasses can wear contact lenses successfully. Conditions such as dry eyes or blepharitis can make contact lens wear uncomfortable or unsafe. Even with no preexisting eye conditions, some people have sensitive corneas and simply cannot adapt to contact lenses.

In addition to the information in an eyeglass prescription, a contact lens prescription must specify the base (central) curve of the back surface of the contact lens, the lens diameter, and the specific manufacturer and brand name of the lens.

Also, the power of an eyeglass prescription frequently is modified when determining the best contact lens power. One reason is that eyeglass lenses are worn some distance (usually about twelve millimeters) from the surface of the eye, whereas contact lenses rest directly on the cornea. To provide the same effective power as that prescribed for eyeglasses, the contact lens power may need to be reduced or increased, depending on the degree of your nearsightedness or farsightedness.

An accurate contact lens prescription can be written only after a contact lens fitting has been performed and the prescribing doctor has evaluated your eyes' response to the lenses and to contact lens wear in general.

Your Eyeglass Prescription: It's Yours to Keep

The Federal Trade Commission (FTC) is the U.S. government's consumer protection agency, and in 1980 the FTC's Prescription Release Rule became law. The rule requires eye doctors (both optometrists and ophthalmologists) to give patients a copy of their eyeglass prescription at the end of an eye exam that includes a refraction. The rule is intended to protect the "portability" of your eyeglass prescription, allowing you to use it to buy glasses from the vendor of your choice.

Your eye doctor must give you a copy of the prescription whether or not you ask for it. Eye doctors may not condition the release of your prescription on your agreement to purchase eyeglasses from them, nor may they charge you an extra fee to release your prescription. They also may not disclaim liability for the accuracy of the prescription if you purchase eyeglasses elsewhere.

The FTC enforces the Prescription Release Rule, and eye doctors who violate the rule are subject to a civil penalty of $10,000.

Section 12.2

Types of Eyeglasses

Eyeglasses correct vision problems, such as nearsightedness, farsightedness, astigmatism, and presbyopia, by focusing light more appropriately on the retina.

The type of vision problem that you have determines the shape of the eyeglass lens. For example, a lens that is concave, or curves inward, is used to correct nearsightedness, while a lens that is convex, or curves outward, is used to correct farsightedness. To correct astigmatism, which is caused by distortions in the shape of the cornea, a cylinder-shaped lens is used. Presbyopia requires bifocal or multifocal lenses.

What Are Multifocal Lenses?

People who have more than one vision problem often need glasses with multifocal lenses. Multifocal lenses, bifocals, trifocals, or progressive lenses are lenses that contain two or more vision-correcting prescriptions:

- **Bifocals:** Bifocals are the most common type of multifocal lens. The lens is split into two sections; the upper part is for distance vision and the lower part for near vision. They are usually prescribed for people over the age of forty whose focusing ability has declined because of presbyopia.

- **Trifocals:** Trifocals are simply bifocals with a third section for people who need help seeing objects that are within an arm's reach.

- **Progressive:** Progressive lenses have a continuous gradient (inclined) lens which focuses progressively closer as one looks down through the lens.

What Types of Lenses Are Available?

In the past, eyeglass lenses were made exclusively of glass; today, however, most lenses are made of plastic. Plastic lenses are lighter, do not break as easily as glass lenses, and can be treated with a filter to keep out ultraviolet light, which can be damaging to the eyes. However, glass lenses are more resistant to scratches than plastic ones.

As technology advances so, too, do eyeglass lenses. The following modern lenses are lighter, thinner, and more scratch-resistant than the common plastic and glass lenses:

- **Polycarbonate lenses:** These lenses are impact-resistant and are a good choice for people who regularly participate in sporting activities, work in a job environment in which their glasses may be easily scratched or broken, and for children who may easily drop and scratch their glasses.

- **Photochromic and tinted lenses:** Made from either glass or plastic, these lenses change from clear to tinted when exposed to sunlight. This eliminates the need for prescription sunglasses.

- **High-index plastic lenses:** Designed for people who require strong prescriptions, these lenses are lighter and thinner than the standard, thick lenses that may otherwise be needed.

- **Aspheric lenses:** These lenses are unlike typical lenses, which are spherical in shape. Aspheric lenses are made up of differing degrees of curvature over its surface, which allows the lens to be thinner and flatter than other lenses. This also creates a lens with a much larger usable portion than the standard lens.

If you have questions about which type of lens is right for you, talk to your eye doctor. He or she can help you choose the lenses that are best for you based on your lifestyle and vision needs.

Caring For Your Eyeglasses

Always store your eyeglasses in a clean, dry place away from potential damage. Clean your glasses with water and a non-lint cloth, as necessary, to keep them spot-free and prevent distorted vision.

How Often Should I Change My Glasses?

Generally an eyeglass prescription is good for a year, sometimes longer. Some circumstances may lead to a need for new glasses at a shorter interval. They include:

- increasing nearsightedness in the teen years;

- presbyopia in midlife;

- developing cataracts;

- surgery;

- onset of diabetes.

If your vision is decreasing in one or both eyes, you should check to see if you need new glasses or to be sure that there is no significant disease that may require treatment.

Section 12.3

Sunglasses

Sunglasses: Frequently Asked Questions

If the sun doesn't bother my eyes, do I still need to wear sunglasses?

Yes. The sun has damaging ultraviolet (UV) rays that can cause photokeratitis, pingueculae, and permanent retinal damage.

What exactly are UV rays?

Ultraviolet (UV) rays are located just past the violet portion of the visible light spectrum; sunlight is the main source.

UV light is broken into three different types: UVA, UVB, and UVC:

- UVA has longer wavelengths and passes through glass easily; experts disagree about whether or not UVA damages the eyes.

- UVB rays are the most dangerous, making sunglasses and sunscreen a must; they don't go through glass.

- UVC rays do not reach the Earth because its atmosphere blocks them.

When do UV rays affect my eyes?

Most people think that they're at risk only when they're outside on a sunny day, but UV light can go right through clouds, so it doesn't matter if the sky is overcast. The sun's rays are strongest between 10 a.m. and 2 p.m.

Glare and reflections can give you trouble, so have your sunglasses ready if you'll be around snow, water, or sand, or if you'll be driving (windshields are a big glare source).

The following put you at additional risk: sunlamps, tanning beds and parlors, photosensitizing drugs, and living at high altitudes or near the equator.

Can certain medical problems increase my risk for damage from UV rays?

Yes. People with cataracts (or who have had cataract surgery), macular degeneration, and retinal dystrophies should be extra careful.

What are my options to prevent UV damage to my eyes?

You must wear sunglasses to prevent damage to your eyes. While some contact lenses provide UV protection, they don't cover your whole eye, so you still need sunglasses.

Look for sunglasses that protect you from 99 to 100 percent of both UVA and UVB light. This includes those labeled as "UV 400," which blocks all light rays with wavelengths up to 400 nanometers. (This covers all of UVA and UVB rays.)

Also, you may want to consider wraparound sunglasses to prevent harmful UV rays from entering around the frame.

What are the different kinds of lenses that are available?

With so many lenses available, it's a good idea to ask a professional optician for help when choosing sunglasses. Different tints can help you see better in certain conditions, and a knowledgeable optician can help you choose sunglass tints that are best suited for your needs.

Blue-blockers block blue light and usually have amber lenses. Some evidence indicates blue light is harmful, and could increase risk of eye damage from diseases such as macular degeneration. These lenses are popular among skiers, hunters, boaters, and pilots, who use them to heighten contrast.

Both polarized lenses and anti-reflective coating cut reflected glare. Polarized lenses in particular are popular with those who play water and snow sports. Anti-reflecting coatings reduce glare caused by light reflecting off the back surface of your sunglass lenses.

Mirror-coated lenses limit the amount of light entering your eyes, so you're more comfortable.

Mirror coatings (also called flash coatings) are highly reflective coatings applied to the front surface of sunglass lenses to reduce the amount of light entering the eye. This makes them especially beneficial for activities in very bright conditions, such as snow skiing on a sunny day.

The mirrored sunglasses associated with state troopers are one example of a flash coating. The technology has advanced, however, so that today's choices in mirror coatings include all colors of the rainbow, as well as silver, gold, and copper metallic colors. Hot pink, blue—almost any color is available.

Choosing the color of a mirror coating is a purely cosmetic decision. The color of the mirror coating you choose does not influence your color perception—it's the color of the tinted lens under the coating that determines how mirrored sunglasses affect your color vision.

Gradient lenses are tinted from the top down, so that the top of the lens is darkest. These lenses are good for driving, because they shield your eyes from overhead sunlight and allow more light through the bottom half of the lens so you can see your dashboard clearly.

Double gradient refers to lenses that are also tinted from the bottom up: The top and bottom are darkest and the middle has a lighter tint. Double gradient lenses are a great choice if you want sunglasses that aren't too dark, but shield your eyes well against bright overhead sunlight and light reflecting off sand, water, and other reflective surfaces at your feet.

Photochromic lenses adjust their level of darkness based on the amount of UV light they're exposed to.

What about sunglasses blocking infrared rays?

Infrared rays are located just past the red portion of the visible light spectrum. Though infrared radiation produces heat, most experts agree that the sun's infrared rays do not pose a danger to the eyes.

Which lens color is the best?

Lens color is a personal choice and doesn't affect how well sunglass lenses protect your eyes from UV light. Gray and brown are popular because they distort color perception the least.

Athletes often prefer other tints for their contrast-enhancing properties. For example, yellow lenses are popular with skiers and target shooters because they work well in low light, reduce haze, and increase contrast for a sharper image.

Are impact-resistant lenses necessary?

The U.S. Food and Drug Administration (FDA) requires all sunglass lenses to be impact-resistant. If you play sports or wear sunglasses on the job, you might want to consider ultra-impact-resistant polycarbonate lenses for even greater eye safety.

Do I still need those "UV protective" sunglasses if my lenses are real dark?

Yes! Most people believe that the darkness of the lens is what protects their eyes. The degree of darkness has no effect on UV rays. For adequate protection, you need to buy sunglasses that indicate they block 100 percent of the sun's UV rays.

Are the more expensive sunglasses of better quality?

Not necessarily. While expensive sunglasses usually are high quality, you can also get a good pair for under $20 if you're a careful shopper. Just make sure to check that the lenses provide adequate protection from UV light and are free of distortions.

You can also take them to your eye care professional to have the lenses metered to determine the amount of UV that passes through the lenses. That way you can be sure you are getting the most from your sunglasses.

Children don't need sunglasses, do they?

Children's sunglasses are essential. Children are at particular risk because they're in the sun much more than adults, and their eyes are more sensitive as well. UV damage is cumulative over a person's lifetime, which means you should begin protecting your child's eyes as soon as possible.

Most parents would not allow their children to go outside without shoes, yet many seem unaware of the need to protect their children's eyes.

I wear glasses. What options are available to me?

You can buy prescription sunglasses or glasses with photochromic lenses (which change from clear to dark) from your eye care practitioner. Clip-ons may be a less expensive option, and can be bought at the same time as your regular eyeglasses to perfectly match the frames.

Some eyeglass frames include sun lenses that magnetically attach to the frame. This gives you the convenience of clip-on sunglasses with less risk of scratching your prescription lenses.

Do those sunglasses for specific sports really make a difference?

Yes. Sports eyewear in general tends to be safer than regular sunglasses because the lenses and frames are made of special materials that are unlikely to shatter if struck and can give you the benefits of both sunglasses and protective eyewear.

Also, certain lens colors in performance sunglasses can enhance your vision for certain sports; brown, for example, is popular with golfers because it provides nice contrast on those very green golf courses.

Sunglasses for Kids

Children may not be as interested as adults are in the fashion aspect of sunglasses. But because kids spend much more time outdoors than most adults do, sunglasses that block 100 percent of the sun's harmful ultraviolet (UV) rays are extra important for children.

In fact, many experts believe our eyes get 80 percent of their total lifetime exposure to the sun's UV rays by age eighteen. And since excessive lifetime exposure to UV radiation has been linked to the development of cataracts and other eye problems, it's never too early for kids to begin wearing good-quality sunglasses outdoors.

UV rays aren't the only potential danger from sunlight. Recently, researchers have suggested that long-term exposure to high-energy visible (HEV) light rays, also called "blue light," may also cause eye damage over time. In particular, some believe a high lifetime exposure to HEV light may contribute to the development of macular degeneration later in life.

Children's eyes are more susceptible to UV and HEV radiation than adult eyes because the lenses inside young eyes are less capable of filtering these high-energy rays. This is especially true for young children, so it's wise for kids to start wearing protective sunglasses outdoors as soon as they begin playing in direct sunlight.

Also, be aware that your child's exposure to UV rays increases at high altitudes, in tropical locales, and in highly reflective environments (such as in a snowfield, on the water, or on a sandy beach). Protective sun wear is especially important for kids in these situations.

Choosing Sunglass Lens Colors

The level of UV protection sunglasses provide has nothing to do with the color of the lenses.

As long as your optician certifies that the lenses block 100 percent of the sun's UV rays, the choice of color and tint density is a matter of personal preference.

Most sunglass lenses that block the sun's HEV rays are amber or copper in color. By blocking blue light, these lenses also enhance contrast, a positive feature for outdoor sports and cycling.

Sunglass Styles for Kids

Colorful, adolescent frame styles are still available, but sunglass companies have found a niche in appealing to children's desire to look like their parents or older siblings.

Oval, round, rectangular, cat-eye, and geometric shapes are all popular in cool, sophisticated colors like green, blue, tortoise, and black. Metal frames are very popular, but so are plastic sunglass frames that look like scaled-down versions of trendy adult styles. Also, sporty styles for kids like wraparounds are available in miniature adult editions.

Where to Get Kids' Sunglasses

The best places to find kids' sunglasses are sunglass specialty stores like Sunglass Hut, optical chain stores like Pearle Vision and Lens-Crafters, and your local optician or optical shop.

Some opticians even specialize in children's sunglasses and eyeglasses and have dedicated areas just for kids to play and shop for their frames.

Section 12.4

Fitting Glasses for Children

What type of lenses should be used?

Polycarbonate (shatter proof) lenses which also have built in ultraviolet (UV) protection to block harmful rays from the sun are recommended for children's spectacles.

Which optical shop is best?

Optical shops that frequently work with children are preferable. If frames and lenses are not fit properly, the endeavor of having a child wear glasses may be severely compromised. These optical shops also often have a superior selection of children's frames. Your local independent optical shop will work with your doctor to ensure proper power and continued good fit for your child.

What frame should be chosen?

Glasses must fit well so that they are comfortable and provide clear vision. If uncomfortable, a child may be reluctant to wear spectacles. Children should not be given adult frames to grow into. Every child has a unique face, and frames should be chosen to fit appropriately. One size does not fit all. Remember that your child will spend most waking hours wearing his or her glasses. Quality glasses will not only hold up better, but will be more comfortable for your child. The frame should be adjusted as needed for comfort and alignment on your child's face.

Frames should preferably not touch the cheeks or eyelashes and eyes should be centered in the lenses. The frame and nose pads can be adjusted for optimal fit.

The horizontal line on bifocal lenses should go through the middle or immediately below the pupil.

Glasses for infants and toddlers often come with cable temples. This type of temple wraps around the ear. It is important that the cable not be too tight or the temple length too short.

Do children love glasses as soon as they get them?

Nearsighted (myopic) children often enjoy their glasses immediately. However, far-sighted (hyperopic) and astigmatic children may take several weeks to adjust to wearing spectacles. If after several weeks of attempting to wear the glasses the child does not cooperate, the doctor may prescribe eye drops in an attempt to help the child adjust to the glasses.

How do I care for glasses?

When not being worn, glasses should be placed in a case and should never be placed face down on a surface for fear of scratching the lens. Do not try to adjust the frame, as breakage may occur. Some children wear straps to keep glasses in place.

Chapter 13

Contact Lenses

Chapter Contents

Section 13.1

Types of Contact Lenses

Excerpted from "Types of Contact Lenses,"
U.S. Food and Drug Administration, January 14, 2010.

There are two general categories of contact lenses—soft and rigid gas permeable (RGP). All contact lenses require a valid prescription.

Soft Contact Lenses

Soft contact lenses are made of soft, flexible plastics that allow oxygen to pass through to the cornea. Soft contact lenses may be easier to adjust to and are more comfortable than rigid gas permeable lenses. Newer soft lens materials include silicone-hydrogels to provide more oxygen to your eye while you wear your lenses.

Rigid Gas Permeable (RGP) Contact Lenses

Rigid gas permeable contact lenses (RGPs) are more durable and resistant to deposit buildup, and generally give a clearer, crisper vision. They tend to be less expensive over the life of the lens, since they last longer than soft contact lenses. They are easier to handle and less likely to tear. However, they are not as comfortable initially as soft contacts and it may take a few weeks to get used to wearing RGPs, compared to several days for soft contacts.

Extended-Wear Contact Lenses

Extended-wear contact lenses are available for overnight or continuous wear ranging from one to six nights or up to thirty days. Extended-wear contact lenses are usually soft contact lenses. They are made of flexible plastics that allow oxygen to pass through to the cornea. There are also a very few rigid gas permeable lenses that are designed and approved for overnight wear. Length of continuous wear depends on lens type and your eye care professional's evaluation of your tolerance for overnight wear. It's important for the eyes to have a rest without lenses for at least one night following each scheduled removal.

Disposable (Replacement Schedule) Contact Lenses

The majority of soft contact lens wearers are prescribed some type of frequent replacement schedule. "Disposable," as defined by the U.S. Food and Drug Administration (FDA), means used once and discarded. With a true daily wear disposable schedule, a brand new pair of lenses is used each day.

Some soft contact lenses are referred to as "disposable" by contact lens sellers, but actually, they are for frequent/planned replacement. With extended-wear lenses, the lenses may be worn continuously for the prescribed wearing period (for example, seven days to thirty days) and then thrown away. When you remove your lenses, make sure to clean and disinfect them properly before reinserting.

Specialized Uses of Contact lenses

Conventional contact lenses correct vision in the same way that glasses do, only they are in contact with the eye. Two types of lenses that serve a different purpose are orthokeratology lenses and decorative (plano) lenses.

Orthokeratology (Ortho-K)

Orthokeratology, or Ortho-K, is a lens-fitting procedure that uses specially designed rigid gas permeable (RGP) contact lenses to change the curvature of the cornea to temporarily improve the eye's ability to focus on objects. This procedure is primarily used for the correction of myopia (nearsightedness).

Overnight Ortho-K lenses are the most common type of Ortho-K. There are some Ortho-K lenses that are prescribed only for daytime wear. Overnight Ortho-K lenses are commonly prescribed to be worn while sleeping for at least eight hours each night. They are removed upon awakening and not worn during the day. Some people can go all day without their glasses or contact lenses. Others will find that their vision correction will wear off during the day.

The vision correction effect is temporary. If Ortho-K is discontinued, the corneas will return to their original curvature and the eye to its original amount of nearsightedness. Ortho-K lenses must continue to be worn every night or on some other prescribed maintenance schedule in order to maintain the treatment effect. Your eye care professional will determine the best maintenance schedule for you.

Decorative (Plano) Contact Lenses

Some contact lenses do not correct vision and are intended solely to change the appearance of the eye. These are sometimes called plano, zero-powered, or noncorrective lenses. For example, they can temporarily change a brown-eyed person's eye color to blue, or make a person's eyes look "weird" by portraying Halloween themes. Even though these decorative lenses don't correct vision, they're regulated by the FDA, just like corrective contact lenses. They also carry the same risks to the eye.

The FDA is aware that consumers without valid prescriptions have bought decorative contact lenses from beauty salons, record stores, video stores, flea markets, convenience stores, beach shops, and the internet. Buying contact lenses without a prescription is dangerous!

If you're considering getting decorative contact lenses, you should:

- get an eye exam from a licensed eye care professional;

- get a valid prescription that includes the brand and lens dimensions;

- buy the lenses from an eye care professional or from a vendor who requires that you provide prescription information for the lenses;

- follow directions for cleaning, disinfection, and wearing the lenses, and visit your eye care professional for follow-up eye exams.

Section 13.2

Advantages and Disadvantages of Various Types of Contact Lenses

Reasons to Consider Contact Lenses

- Contact lenses move with your eye, allow a natural field of view, have no frames to obstruct your vision, and greatly reduce distortions.

- They do not fog up, like glasses, nor do they get splattered by mud or rain.

- Contact lenses do not get in the way of your activities.

- Many people feel they look better in contact lenses.

- Contact lenses, compared to eyeglasses, generally offer better sight.

Some Things to Remember about Contact Lenses

- Contact lenses, when compared with glasses, require a longer initial examination and more follow-up visits to maintain eye health, and more time for lens care.

- If you are going to wear your lenses successfully, you will have to clean and store them properly, adhere to lens wearing schedules, and make appointments for follow-up care.

- If you are wearing disposable or planned replacement lenses, you will have to carefully follow the schedule for throwing away used lenses.

[*See* Table 13.1. Advantages and Disadvantages of Various Types of Contact Lenses on the next page.]

Table 13.1. Advantages and Disadvantages of Different Types of Contact Lenses

Lens Types	Advantages	Disadvantages
Rigid gas-permeable (RGP): Made of slightly flexible plastics that allow oxygen to pass through to the eyes.	Excellent vision, short adaptation period, comfortable to wear, correct most vision problems, easy to put on and to care for, durable with a relatively long life, available in tints (for handling purposes) and bifocals.	Require consistent wear to maintain adaptation, can slip off center of eye more easily than other types, debris can easily get under the lenses, requires office visits for follow-up care.
Daily wear soft lenses: Made of soft, flexible plastic that allows oxygen to pass through to the eyes.	Very short adaptation period, more comfortable and more difficult to dislodge than RGP lenses, available in tints and bifocals, great for active lifestyles.	Do not correct all vision problems, vision may not be as sharp as with RGP lenses, require regular office visits for follow-up care, lenses soil easily and must be replaced.
Extended-wear: Available for overnight wear in soft or RGP lenses.	Can usually be worn up to seven days without removal.	Do not correct all vision problems, require regular office visits for follow-up care, increases risk of complication, requires regular monitoring and professional care.
Extended-wear disposable: Soft lenses worn for an extended period of time, from one to six days and then discarded.	Require little or no cleaning, minimal risk of eye infection if wearing instructions are followed, available in tints and bifocals, spare lenses available.	Vision may not be as sharp as RGP lenses, do not correct all vision problems, handling may be more difficult.
Planned replacement: Soft daily wear lenses that are replaced on a planned schedule, most often either every two weeks, monthly, or quarterly.	Require simplified cleaning and disinfection, good for eye health, available in most prescriptions.	Vision may not be as sharp as RGP lenses, do not correct all vision problems, handling may be more difficult.

Section 13.3

Contact Lens Risks

Reprinted from the U.S. Food and
Drug Administration, August 24, 2010.

Wearing contact lenses puts you at risk of several serious conditions, including eye infections and corneal ulcers. These conditions can develop very quickly and can be very serious. In rare cases, these conditions can cause blindness.

You can not determine the seriousness of a problem that develops when you are wearing contact lenses. You have to get help from an eye care professional to determine your problem.

If you experience any symptoms of eye irritation or infection, do the following things:

- Remove your lenses immediately and do not put them back in your eyes.

- Contact your eye care professional right way.

- Don't throw away your lenses. Store them in your case and take them to your eye care professional. He or she may want to use them to determine the cause of your symptoms.

Symptoms of Eye Irritation or Infection

- Discomfort

- Excess tearing or other discharge

- Unusual sensitivity to light

- Itching, burning, or gritty feelings

- Unusual redness

- Blurred vision

- Swelling

- Pain

Serious Hazards of Contact Lenses

Symptoms of eye irritation can indicate a more serious condition. Some of the possible serious hazards of wearing contact lenses are corneal ulcers, eye infections, and even blindness.

Corneal ulcers are open sores in the outer layer of the cornea. They are usually caused by infections. To reduce your chances of infection, you should do the following:

- Rub and rinse your contact lenses as directed by your eye care professional.

- Clean and disinfect your lenses properly according to the labeling instructions.

- Do not "top-off" the solutions in your case. Always discard all of the leftover contact lens solution after each use. Never reuse any lens solution.

- Do not expose your contact lenses to any water: tap, bottled, distilled, lake, or ocean water. Never use nonsterile water (distilled water, tap water, or any homemade saline solution). Tap and distilled water have been associated with Acanthamoeba keratitis, a corneal infection that is resistant to treatment and cure.

- Remove your contact lenses before swimming. There is a risk of eye infection from bacteria in swimming pool water, hot tubs, lakes, and the ocean.

- Replace your contact lens storage case every three to six months.

Other Risks of Contact Lenses

Other risks of contact lenses include the following:

- Pink eye (conjunctivitis)

- Corneal abrasions

- Eye irritation

Section 13.4

Proper Care of Contact Lenses

Taking good care of your contacts is important for keeping healthy eyes. Your optometric physician will teach you about the best way to treat your lenses, but here are a few general rules:

- Every time contact lenses are removed, they must be cleaned, rinsed, and disinfected before wearing again. Some solutions are designed to perform more than one of these functions.

- Always remove, clean, rinse, and disinfect your contacts before wearing again.

- Lenses stored longer than twelve hours may need cleaning, rinsing, and disinfecting again before use. Ask your eye doctor for specific instructions.

Here are the steps for cleaning your lenses:

- Wash your hands, then dry them with a lint-free towel.

- Remove your lenses and clean them. This usually involves putting some solution on the lens while it is in your hand, then taking the index finger of your other hand and gently rubbing your lens in the solution. The cleaning process removes dirt, other debris, and mucous from the lens.

- Rinse your lenses by running a small stream of solution over the lens in your hand.

- Put your lenses in a lens case filled with disinfecting/storage solution. The disinfecting process gets rid of potentially sight-threatening organisms on the lens.

- The next time you wear the lenses, remove them from the case, rinse them, and insert.

Section 13.5

Things to Know about Cosmetic Contacts

Excerpted from "Before You Buy Cosmetic Contact Lenses,"
U.S. Federal Trade Commission, October 2011.

What Are Cosmetic Contacts?

Whether you're planning to cap off a costume with a pair of cat-eye lenses, get the big-eye look of circle lenses, or switch your eye color from blue to violet for the day, cosmetic contacts—contact lenses meant to change the way your eye looks rather than correct your vision—may seem like just another fashion accessory.

But all contact lenses—even purely cosmetic ones—require a prescription. Businesses that sell cosmetic lenses without a prescription are selling them illegally.

Why Get a Prescription?

Lenses need to fit your eye correctly. If they don't, or if they aren't used and cared for properly, they can cause problems like the following:

- Conjunctivitis (pink eye)

- Scratches

- Sores on your cornea

- Blindness

If you're in the market for cosmetic contacts, see an eye care professional for an eye exam and prescription. Don't do business with anyone who doesn't require one.

Chapter 14

Laser-Assisted In Situ Keratomileusis (LASIK) Surgery

Chapter Contents

Section 14.1

LASIK: The Basics

Reprinted from "What Is LASIK?" "When Is LASIK Not for Me?" "What Are the Risks and How Can I Find the Right Doctor for Me?" and "What Should I Expect Before, During, and After Surgery?" U.S. Food and Drug Administration, April 16, 2009.

What Is Laser-Assisted In Situ Keratomileusis (LASIK)?

The Eye and Vision Errors

The cornea is a part of the eye that helps focus light to create an image on the retina. It works in much the same way that the lens of a camera focuses light to create an image on film. The bending and focusing of light is also known as refraction. Usually the shape of the cornea and the eye are not perfect and the image on the retina is out of focus (blurred) or distorted. These imperfections in the focusing power of the eye are called refractive errors. There are three primary types of refractive errors: myopia, hyperopia, and astigmatism. Persons with myopia, or nearsightedness, have difficulty seeing distant objects as clearly as near objects. Persons with hyperopia, or farsightedness, have difficulty seeing near objects as clearly as distant objects. Astigmatism is a distortion of the image on the retina caused by irregularities in the cornea or lens of the eye. Combinations of myopia and astigmatism or hyperopia and astigmatism are common. Glasses or contact lenses are designed to compensate for the eye's imperfections. Surgical procedures aimed at improving the focusing power of the eye are called refractive surgery. In LASIK surgery, precise and controlled removal of corneal tissue by a special laser reshapes the cornea, changing its focusing power.

Other Types of Refractive Surgery

Radial keratotomy, or RK, and photorefractive keratectomy, or PRK, are other refractive surgeries used to reshape the cornea. In RK, a very sharp knife is used to cut slits in the cornea, changing its shape. PRK was the first surgical procedure developed to reshape the cornea, by sculpting, using a laser. Later, LASIK was developed. The same type of laser is used for LASIK and PRK. Often the exact same laser is used for the two types of surgery. The major difference between the two surgeries is the way that the stroma, the middle layer of the cornea, is exposed before it is vaporized with the laser. In PRK, the top layer of the cornea, called the epithelium, is scraped away to expose the stromal layer underneath. In LASIK, a flap is cut in the stromal layer and the flap is folded back.

Another type of refractive surgery is thermokeratoplasty, in which heat is used to reshape the cornea. The source of the heat can be a laser, but it is a different kind of laser than is used for LASIK and PRK. Other refractive devices include corneal ring segments that are inserted into the stroma and special contact lenses that temporarily reshape the cornea (orthokeratology).

When Is LASIK Not For Me?

You are probably *not* a good candidate for refractive surgery if:

- You are not a risk taker. Certain complications are unavoidable in a percentage of patients, and there are no long-term data available for current procedures.

- It will jeopardize your career. Some jobs prohibit certain refractive procedures. Be sure to check with your employer/professional society/military service before undergoing any procedure.

- Cost is an issue. Most medical insurance will not pay for refractive surgery. Although the cost is coming down, it is still significant.

- You required a change in your contact lens or glasses prescription in the past year. This is called refractive instability. Patients who are in their early twenties or younger, whose hormones are fluctuating due to disease such as diabetes, who are pregnant or breastfeeding, or who are taking medications that may cause fluctuations in vision are more likely to have refractive instability and should discuss the possible additional risks with their doctor.

- You have a disease or are on medications that may affect wound healing. Certain conditions, such as autoimmune diseases (e.g., lupus, rheumatoid arthritis), immunodeficiency states (e.g., human immunodeficiency virus [HIV]), and diabetes, and some medications (e.g., retinoic acid and steroids) may prevent proper healing after a refractive procedure.

- You actively participate in contact sports. You participate in boxing, wrestling, martial arts, or other activities in which blows to the face and eyes are a normal occurrence.

- You are not an adult. Currently, no lasers are approved for LASIK on persons under the age of eighteen.

Precautions

The safety and effectiveness of refractive procedures has not been determined in patients with some diseases. Discuss with your doctor if you have a history of any of the following:

- Herpes simplex or Herpes zoster (shingles) involving the eye area

- Glaucoma, glaucoma suspect, or ocular hypertension

- Eye diseases, such as uveitis/iritis (inflammations of the eye)

- Eye injuries or previous eye surgeries

- Keratoconus

Other Risk Factors

Your doctor should screen you for the following conditions or indicators of risk:

- **Blepharitis:** Inflammation of the eyelids with crusting of the eyelashes, that may increase the risk of infection or inflammation of the cornea after LASIK.

- **Large pupils:** Make sure this evaluation is done in a dark room. Although anyone may have large pupils, younger patients and patients on certain medications may be particularly prone to having large pupils under dim lighting conditions. This can cause symptoms such as glare, halos, starbursts, and ghost images (double vision) after surgery. In some patients these symptoms may be debilitating. For example, a patient may no longer be able to drive a car at night or in certain weather conditions, such as fog.

- **Thin corneas:** The cornea is the thin clear covering of the eye that is over the iris, the colored part of the eye. Most refractive procedures change the eye's focusing power by reshaping the cornea (for example, by removing tissue). Performing a refractive procedure on a cornea that is too thin may result in blinding complications.

- **Previous refractive surgery (e.g., RK, PRK, LASIK):** Additional refractive surgery may not be recommended. The decision to have additional refractive surgery must be made in consultation with your doctor after careful consideration of your unique situation.

- **Dry Eyes:** LASIK surgery tends to aggravate this condition.

What Are the Risks and How Can I Find the Right Doctor for Me?

Most patients are very pleased with the results of their refractive surgery. However, like any other medical procedure, there are risks involved. That's why it is important for you to understand the limitations and possible complications of refractive surgery.

Before undergoing a refractive procedure, you should carefully weigh the risks and benefits based on your own personal value system, and try to avoid being influenced by friends that have had the procedure or doctors encouraging you to do so:

- Some patients lose vision. Some patients lose lines of vision on the vision chart that cannot be corrected with glasses, contact lenses, or surgery as a result of treatment.

- Some patients develop debilitating visual symptoms. Some patients develop glare, halos, and/or double vision that can seriously affect nighttime vision. Even with good vision on the vision chart, some patients do not see as well in situations of low contrast, such as at night or in fog, after treatment as compared to before treatment.

- You may be undertreated or overtreated. Only a certain percentage of patients achieve 20/20 vision without glasses or contacts. You may require additional treatment, but additional treatment may not be possible. You may still need glasses or contact lenses after surgery. This may be true even if you required only a very weak prescription before surgery. If you used reading glasses before surgery, you may still need reading glasses after surgery.

- Some patients may develop severe dry eye syndrome. As a result of surgery, your eye may not be able to produce enough tears to keep the eye moist and comfortable. Dry eye not only causes discomfort, but can reduce visual quality due to intermittent blurring and other visual symptoms. This condition may be permanent. Intensive drop therapy and use of plugs or other procedures may be required.

- Results are generally not as good in patients with very large refractive errors of any type. You should discuss your expectations with your doctor and realize that you may still require glasses or contacts after the surgery.

- For some farsighted patients, results may diminish with age. If you are farsighted, the level of improved vision you experience after surgery may decrease with age. This can occur if your manifest refraction (a vision exam with lenses before dilating drops) is very different from your cycloplegic refraction (a vision exam with lenses after dilating drops).

- Long-term data are not available. LASIK is a relatively new technology. The first laser was approved for LASIK eye surgery in 1998. Therefore, the long-term safety and effectiveness of LASIK surgery is not known.

Additional Risks If You Are Considering Monovision or Bilateral Simultaneous Treatment

Monovision: Monovision is one clinical technique used to deal with the correction of presbyopia, the gradual loss of the ability of the eye to change focus for close-up tasks that progresses with age. The intent of monovision is for the presbyopic patient to use one eye for distance viewing and one eye for near viewing. This practice was first applied to fit contact lens wearers and more recently to LASIK and other refractive surgeries. With contact lenses, a presbyopic patient has one eye fit with a contact lens to correct distance vision, and the other eye fit with a contact lens to correct near vision. In the same way, with LASIK, a presbyopic patient has one eye operated on to correct the distance vision, and the other operated on to correct the near vision. In other words, the goal of the surgery is for one eye to have vision worse than 20/20, the commonly referred to goal for LASIK surgical correction of distance vision. Since one eye is corrected for distance viewing and the other eye is corrected for near viewing, the two eyes no longer work together. This results in poorer quality vision and a decrease in depth perception. These effects of monovision are most noticeable in low lighting conditions and when performing tasks requiring very sharp vision. Therefore, you may need to wear glasses or contact lenses to fully correct both eyes for distance or near when performing visually demanding tasks, such as driving at night, operating dangerous equipment, or performing occupational tasks requiring very sharp close vision (e.g., reading small print for long periods of time).

Many patients cannot get used to having one eye blurred at all times. Therefore, if you are considering monovision with LASIK, make sure you go through a trial period with contact lenses to see if you can tolerate monovision before having the surgery performed on your eyes. Find out if you pass your state's driver's license requirements with monovision.

In addition, you should consider how much your presbyopia is expected to increase in the future. Ask your doctor when you should expect the results of your monovision surgery to no longer be enough for you to see nearby objects clearly without the aid of glasses or contacts, or when a second surgery might be required to further correct your near vision.

Bilateral simultaneous treatment: You may choose to have LASIK surgery on both eyes at the same time or to have surgery on one eye at a time. Although the convenience of having surgery on both eyes on the same day is attractive, this practice is riskier than having two separate surgeries.

If you decide to have one eye done at a time, you and your doctor will decide how long to wait before having surgery on the other eye. If both eyes are treated at the same time or before one eye has a chance to fully heal, you and your doctor do not have the advantage of being able to see how the first eye responds to surgery before the second eye is treated.

Another disadvantage to having surgery on both eyes at the same time is that the vision in both eyes may be blurred after surgery until the initial healing process is over, rather than being able to rely on clear vision in at least one eye at all times.

Finding the Right Doctor

If you are considering refractive surgery, make sure you do the following things:

- **Compare:** The levels of risk and benefit vary slightly not only from procedure to procedure, but from device to device, depending on the manufacturer, and from surgeon to surgeon, depending on their level of experience with a particular procedure.

- **Don't base your decision simply on cost and don't settle for the first eye center, doctor, or procedure you investigate:** Remember that the decisions you make about your eyes and refractive surgery will affect you for the rest of your life.

- **Be wary of eye centers that advertise, "20/20 vision or your money back" or "package deals":** There are never any guarantees in medicine.

- **Read:** It is important for you to read the patient handbook provided to your doctor by the manufacturer of the device used to perform the refractive procedure. Your doctor should provide you with this handbook and be willing to discuss his or her outcomes (successes as well as complications) compared to the results of studies outlined in the handbook.

Even the best screened patients under the care of most skilled surgeons can experience serious complications:

- **During surgery:** Malfunction of a device or other error, such as cutting a flap of cornea through and through instead of making a hinge during LASIK surgery, may lead to discontinuation of the procedure or irreversible damage to the eye.

- **After surgery:** Some complications, such as migration of the flap, inflammation, or infection, may require another procedure and/or intensive treatment with drops. Even with aggressive therapy, such complications may lead to temporary loss of vision or even irreversible blindness.

Under the care of an experienced doctor, carefully screened candidates with reasonable expectations and a clear understanding of the risks and alternatives are likely to be happy with the results of their refractive procedure.

Advertising

Be cautious about "slick" advertising and/or deals that sound "too good to be true." Remember, they usually are. There is a lot of competition, resulting in a great deal of advertising and bidding for your business. Do your homework.

What Should I Expect Before, During, and After Surgery?

What to expect before, during, and after surgery will vary from doctor to doctor and patient to patient. This section is a compilation of patient information developed by manufacturers and healthcare professionals, but cannot replace the dialogue you should have with your doctor. Read this information carefully and discuss your expectations with your doctor.

Before Surgery

If you decide to go ahead with LASIK surgery, you will need an initial or baseline evaluation by your eye doctor to determine if you are a good candidate. This is what you need to know to prepare for the exam and what you should expect.

If you wear contact lenses, it is a good idea to stop wearing them before your baseline evaluation and switch to wearing your glasses full-time. Contact lenses change the shape of your cornea for up to several weeks after you have stopped using them, depending on the type of contact lenses you wear. Not leaving your contact lenses out long enough for your cornea to assume its natural shape before surgery can have negative consequences. These consequences include inaccurate measurements and a poor surgical plan, resulting in poor vision after surgery. These measurements, which determine how much corneal tissue to remove, may need to be repeated at least a week after your initial evaluation and before surgery to make sure they have not changed, especially if you wear rigid gas permeable (RGP) or hard lenses. If you wear:

- soft contact lenses, you should stop wearing them two weeks before your initial evaluation;

- toric soft lenses or rigid gas permeable (RGP) lenses, you should stop wearing them at least three weeks before your initial evaluation; or

- hard lenses, you should stop wearing them at least four weeks before your initial evaluation.

You should tell your doctor the following things:

- About your past and present medical and eye conditions

- About all the medications you are taking, including over-the-counter medications and any medications you may be allergic to

Your doctor should perform a thorough eye exam and discuss the following things:

- Whether you are a good candidate

- What the risks, benefits, and alternatives of the surgery are

- What you should expect before, during, and after surgery

- What your responsibilities will be before, during, and after surgery

You should have the opportunity to ask your doctor questions during this discussion. Give yourself plenty of time to think about the risk/benefit discussion, to review any informational literature provided by your doctor, and to have any additional questions answered by your doctor before deciding to go through with surgery and before signing the informed consent form.

You should not feel pressured by your doctor, family, friends, or anyone else to make a decision about having surgery. Carefully consider the pros and cons.

The day before surgery, you should stop using:

- creams;

- lotions;

- makeup;

- perfumes.

These products as well as debris along the eyelashes may increase the risk of infection during and after surgery. Your doctor may ask you to scrub your eyelashes for a period of time before surgery to get rid of residues and debris along the lashes.

Also before surgery, arrange for transportation to and from your surgery and your first follow-up visit. On the day of surgery, your doctor may give you some medicine to make you relax. Because this medicine impairs your ability to drive and because your vision may be blurry, even if you don't drive make sure someone can bring you home after surgery.

During Surgery

The surgery should take less than thirty minutes. You will lie on your back in a reclining chair in an exam room containing the laser system. The laser system includes a large machine with a microscope attached to it and a computer screen.

A numbing drop will be placed in your eye, the area around your eye will be cleaned, and an instrument called a lid speculum will be used to hold your eyelids open.

Your doctor may use a mechanical microkeratome (a blade device) to cut a flap in the cornea.

If a mechanical microkeratome is used, a ring will be placed on your eye and very high pressures will be applied to create suction to the cornea. Your vision will dim while the suction ring is on and you may feel the pressure and experience some discomfort during this part of the procedure. The microkeratome, a cutting instrument, is attached to the suction ring. Your doctor will use the blade of the microkeratome to cut a flap in your cornea. Microkeratome blades are meant to be used only once and then thrown out. The microkeratome and the suction ring are then removed.

Your doctor may use a laser keratome (a laser device), instead of a mechanical microkeratome, to cut a flap on the cornea.

If a laser keratome is used, the cornea is flattened with a clear plastic plate. Your vision will dim and you may feel the pressure and experience some discomfort during this part of the procedure. Laser energy is focused inside the cornea tissue, creating thousands of small bubbles of gas and water that expand and connect to separate the tissue underneath the cornea surface, creating a flap. The plate is then removed.

You will be able to see, but you will experience fluctuating degrees of blurred vision during the rest of the procedure. The doctor will then lift the flap and fold it back on its hinge, and dry the exposed tissue.

The laser will be positioned over your eye and you will be asked to stare at a light. This is not the laser used to remove tissue from the cornea. This light is to help you keep your eye fixed on one spot once the laser comes on. *Note:* If you cannot stare at a fixed object for at least sixty seconds, you may not be a good candidate for this surgery.

When your eye is in the correct position, your doctor will start the laser. At this point in the surgery, you may become aware of new sounds and smells. The pulse of the laser makes a ticking sound. As the laser removes corneal tissue, some people have reported a smell similar to burning hair. A computer controls the amount of laser energy delivered to your eye. Before the start of surgery, your doctor will have programmed the computer to vaporize a particular amount of tissue based on the measurements taken at your initial evaluation. After the pulses of laser energy vaporize the corneal tissue, the flap is put back into position.

A shield should be placed over your eye at the end of the procedure as protection, since no stitches are used to hold the flap in place. It is important for you to wear this shield to prevent you from rubbing your eye and putting pressure on your eye while you sleep, and to protect your eye from accidentally being hit or poked until the flap has healed.

After Surgery

Immediately after the procedure, your eye may burn, itch, or feel like there is something in it. You may experience some discomfort, or in some cases, mild pain and your doctor may suggest you take a mild pain reliever. Both your eyes may tear or water. Your vision will probably be hazy or blurry. You will instinctively want to rub your eye, but don't! Rubbing your eye could dislodge the flap, requiring further treatment. In addition, you may experience sensitivity to light, glare, starbursts or haloes around lights, or the whites of your eye may look red or bloodshot. These symptoms should improve considerably within the first few days after surgery. You should plan on taking a few days off from work until these symptoms subside. You should contact your doctor immediately and not wait for your scheduled visit if you experience severe pain, or if your vision or other symptoms get worse instead of better.

You should see your doctor within the first twenty-four to forty-eight hours after surgery and at regular intervals after that for at least the first six months. At the first postoperative visit, your doctor will remove the eye shield, test your vision, and examine your eye. Your doctor may give you one or more types of eye drops to take at home to help prevent infection and/or inflammation. You may also be advised to use artificial tears to help lubricate the eye. Do not resume wearing a contact lens in the operated eye, even if your vision is blurry.

You should wait one to three days following surgery before beginning any noncontact sports, depending on the amount of activity required, how you feel, and your doctor's instructions.

To help prevent infection, you may need to wait for up to two weeks after surgery or until your doctor advises you otherwise before using lotions, creams, or make-up around the eye. Your doctor may advise you to continue scrubbing your eyelashes for a period of time after surgery. You should also avoid swimming and using hot tubs or whirlpools for one to two months.

Strenuous contact sports such as boxing, football, karate, etc., should not be attempted for at least four weeks after surgery. It is important to protect your eyes from anything that might get in them and from being hit or bumped.

During the first few months after surgery, your vision may fluctuate:

- It may take up to three to six months for your vision to stabilize after surgery.

- Glare, haloes, difficulty driving at night, and other visual symptoms may also persist during this stabilization period. If further correction or enhancement is necessary, you should wait until your eye measurements are consistent for two consecutive visits at least three months apart before re-operation.

- It is important to realize that although distance vision may improve after re-operation, it is unlikely that other visual symptoms such as glare or haloes will improve.

- It is also important to note that no laser company has presented enough evidence for the U.S. Food and Drug Administration (FDA) to make conclusions about the safety or effectiveness of enhancement surgery.

Contact your eye doctor immediately if you develop any new, unusual, or worsening symptoms at any point after surgery. Such symptoms could signal a problem that, if not treated early enough, may lead to a loss of vision.

Section 14.2

Wavefront-Guided LASIK

"Custom LASIK or Wavefront LASIK: Individualized Vision," reprinted with permission from www.AllAboutVision.com. © 2011 Access Media Group LLC. All rights reserved.

Custom laser-assisted in situ keratomileusis (LASIK) surgery, also known as wavefront LASIK or wavefront-guided LASIK, uses three-dimensional (3-D) measurements of how your eye processes images to guide the laser in reshaping the front part of the eye (cornea).

With a wavefront measurement system, some extremely precise, individualized vision correction outcomes may be achieved that would be impossible with traditional LASIK surgery, contact lenses, or eyeglasses.

You should be qualified under U.S. Food and Drug Association (FDA) guidelines before custom wavefront LASIK is considered for your eye condition. Depending on the custom laser system used and other factors such as appropriate thickness of your cornea, you might be considered a candidate if you have mild to moderately high degrees of common vision defects such as myopia, hyperopia, and astigmatism.

With custom LASIK, your eye's ability to focus light rays is measured, and a 3-D map used in wavefront technology is created that demonstrates irregularities in the way your eye processes images. Information contained in the map guides the laser in customizing the treatment to reshape your eye's corneal surface so that these irregularities can be corrected.

Standard prescriptions for glasses, contacts, or traditional LASIK procedures can correct ordinary vision defects such as myopia, hyperopia, and astigmatism. But other irregularities associated with the eye's optical system could not be addressed until the advent of wavefront and related technology used in custom LASIK.

Potential Benefits of Wavefront-Guided Custom LASIK

Wavefront technology is groundbreaking because it has the potential to improve not only how much you can see, visual acuity measured by the standard 20/20 eye chart, but also how well you can see, in terms of contrast sensitivity and fine detail.

This translates into a reduced risk of post-LASIK complications, such as glare, halos, and difficulty with night vision.

How much you see depends on vision defects known as lower-order aberrations associated with common refractive errors, including myopia, hyperopia, and astigmatism, which traditional LASIK can treat.

How well you see can depend on presence of the type and numbers of visual distortions known as higher-order aberrations, which are optical defects other than common refractive errors.

Higher-order aberrations can create problems such as decreased contrast sensitivity or night vision, glare, shadows, and halos. However, higher-order aberrations do not always affect vision. Unlike traditional LASIK, custom LASIK treats both lower- and higher-order aberrations.

Custom LASIK's advantage lies in the area of quality of vision:

- Greater chance of achieving 20/20 vision

- Greater chance of achieving better than 20/20 vision

- Reduced chance of losing best-corrected vision

- Reduced chance of losing visual quality or contrast sensitivity

- Reduced chance of night-vision disturbances and glare

Potential also exists for custom LASIK to treat people who have lost best-corrected vision from any past refractive surgery: LASIK, photorefractive keratotomy (PRK), radial keratotomy (RK), etc.

Wavefront LASIK creates a highly individualized laser correction of your eye's surface, guided by precise analysis of vision errors that occur as light rays travel through your eye. "Sometimes patients complain about vision quality problems, such as not being able to see in dim or low light. This is referred to as poor contrast sensitivity," said Roger Steinert, MD, vice chair of clinical ophthalmology and professor at University of California Irvine.

"Prior to the advent of wavefront measurements, there wasn't anything we could do to measure or treat higher-order aberrations," Steinert said. "With this technology breakthrough, we can now measure these disorders, show the patient what's going on in their eye, link that information to the laser, and actually correct higher-order aberrations that diminish contrast sensitivity. Wavefront technology enables the surgeon to improve overall vision quality better than in the past."

Not all refractive surgeons agree that wavefront-guided LASIK can treat higher-order aberrations. In fact, studies show that both wavefront LASIK and conventional LASIK can sometimes cause these aberrations because of artificial changes made to the natural shape of the eye's surface.

However, wavefront-guided LASIK may be less likely to induce higher-order aberrations than conventional LASIK, according to discussion in the April 2005 issue of *Ophthalmology Times*.

Most refractive surgeons now use wavefront-guided LASIK in their practices, according to recent surveys such as those conducted by the American Society of Cataract and Refractive Surgery (ASCRS).

Wavefront-Guided LASIK and Contrast Sensitivity

While visual outcomes as noted on familiar eye charts can be similar for wavefront-guided and conventional LASIK, research has linked wavefront-guided procedures to better results in areas such as improved contrast sensitivity.

A study reported in June 2009[1] found that 84 percent of 324 eyes that underwent wavefront-guided LASIK procedures for myopia with or without astigmatism achieved 20/20 uncorrected vision or better. In specific tests measuring contrast sensitivity and night vision, significant improvement was noted. Custom LASIK was found to induce certain types of aberrations, which did not appear to affect good visual outcomes.

In certain cases, outcomes such as improved night vision with use of wavefront-guided LASIK appear to surpass results that can be achieved with conventional LASIK.

In August 2004, the U.S. Navy announced that patients at its refractive surgery center were achieving better distance vision and night vision after custom LASIK than after traditional LASIK.

In a small study, 88 percent of contrast sensitivity measurements improved after wavefront-guided LASIK, while only 40 percent improved after regular LASIK. This was one month after surgery.

Uncorrected visual acuity of 20/20 or better was achieved by similar numbers, however: 72 percent of the wavefront group and 70 percent of the regular LASIK group. The study was published in the March 2004 issue of *Ophthalmology*, the clinical journal of the American Academy of Ophthalmology.

How Custom LASIK Works

The process for determining a custom LASIK treatment begins with the use of a wavefront device to transmit a safe ray of light into your eye. The light is then reflected back off the retina, out through the pupil, and into the device, where the reflected wave of light is received and arranged into a unique pattern that captures your lower- and higher-order aberrations.

All of these visual irregularities are then displayed as a 3-D map, referred to as a wavefront map. This information is then electronically transferred to the laser (in wavefront-guided systems), and computer-matched to the eye's position, enabling the surgeon to customize the LASIK procedure laser treatment (or "ablation") to your unique visual requirements.

Getting Wavefront-Guided Custom LASIK

Numbers of LASIK procedures in general grew significantly in 2004 and 2005, with many leading LASIK surgeons reporting in publications such as *EyeWorld* (published by ASCRS) that most eligible patients were opting for more expensive custom LASIK.

However, deteriorating economic conditions in the United States and elsewhere during 2008 and 2009 caused demand for custom LASIK and similar elective vision correction procedures to plunge.

About 1.4 million LASIK procedures were performed annually in the U.S. in 2005, 2006, and 2007, according to a report filed in April 2009 by TLC Vision Corp., which operates laser surgery centers nationwide.

The company report cites research from a leading industry analyst (MarketScope).

The report says the number of LASIK procedures dropped to 1 million in 2008. About 760,000 procedures were performed in the U.S. in 2009, representing almost a 50 percent decline from previous years.

Custom LASIK costs usually are significantly more than traditional LASIK, partly because surgeons pay a higher royalty fee to the device manufacturer for each procedure.

Research is continuing into expanding the degree of vision errors (such as high myopia) that can be corrected with custom LASIK. Investigations also are underway for use of custom LASIK to create multifocal corrections in a procedure known as PresbyLASIK, which would enable older eyes that have developed presbyopia to see at near, middle, and distant ranges at the same time.

Investigators have reported early promising results of wavefront LASIK, combined with automated topographical measurements of the eye's surface during a procedure, to help reduce surgically induced aberrations and astigmatism. Early studies also indicate that night vision might be further improved with this approach.[2]

Like conventional LASIK, custom LASIK won't cure all vision-related problems, so it's important to discuss its applications with your eye doctor or surgeon to determine if you are a good candidate.

Notes

1. Wavefront-guided LASIK for myopia: effect on visual acuity, contrast sensitivity, and higher order aberrations. *Journal of Refractive Surgery.* June 2009.

2. Abstract: What does true integration of topographic and refractive wavefront parameters in excimer laser surgery involve. NewVision Clinics, Melbourne, Victoria, Australia. Presentation for 2009 European Society of Cataract and Refractive Surgery (ESCRS) conference.

Chapter 15

Photorefractive Keratectomy (PRK) Eye Surgery

Photorefractive keratectomy, or PRK, is a type of laser eye surgery used to correct mild to moderate nearsightedness, farsightedness, and/or astigmatism.

All laser vision correction surgeries work by reshaping the cornea, or clear front part of the eye, so that light traveling through it is properly focused onto the retina located in the back of the eye. There are a number of different surgical techniques used to reshape the cornea. During PRK, an eye surgeon uses a laser to reshape the cornea. This laser, which delivers a cool pulsing beam of ultraviolet light, is used on the surface of the cornea, not underneath a flap on the cornea, as in LASIK.

What are the advantages of PRK?

PRK is highly accurate in correcting many cases of nearsightedness. Approximately 90 percent of PRK patients have 20/20 vision without glasses or contact lenses one year after the surgery; 95 to 98 percent have 20/40 or better without glasses or contacts.

PRK is thought to leave the cornea stronger after surgery. It is preferable to LASIK in cases of thin corneal thickness or with patients who desire to pursue boxing as a recreational activity.

What are the disadvantages of PRK?

Disadvantages of PRK include:

- Mild discomfort, including minor eye irritation and watering, for one to three days following the procedure.

- It is expensive, typically costing as much as LASIK (around $2,500 per eye).

- Somewhat longer time to best uncorrected vision (best vision is vision attained using glasses or contacts). Typically, patients are 80 percent at one month after surgery, and 95 to 100 percent by three months after surgery. LASIK, in contrast, corrects vision much faster.

- The outcome is not completely predictable and some patients may still require glasses.

When both eyes are treated, some patients should be cautioned to consider taking off from work for approximately one week, during which time the eye irritation and vision improve to a more acceptable level.

What are the potential side effects of PRK?

Many PRK patients experience some discomfort in the first twenty-four to forty-eight hours after surgery, and almost all experience sensitivity to light. Within the first six months after surgery, other potential side effects may include:

- Loss of best vision achieved with glasses.

- Seeing a minor glare. This can be permanent, depending on a patient's pupil size in dim light.

- Mild halos around images.

Other potential side effects include delayed surface healing or mild corneal haze or irregularity that could affect the best vision achieved with glasses. Usually, the quality of vision long-term is as good as, if not better, than that achieved with LASIK.

How do I prepare for PRK surgery?

Before your PRK surgery, you will meet with a doctor and a coordinator who will discuss with you what you should expect during and after the surgery. During this session, your medical history will be evaluated, and you will have your eyes tested. Likely tests will include measuring corneal thickness, refraction, and pupil dilation. Your surgeon will answer any further questions you may have. Afterwards, you can schedule an appointment for the PRK procedure.

If you wear rigid gas-permeable contact lenses, you should not wear them starting three weeks before the date of your surgery. Other types of contact lenses shouldn't be worn for at least three days prior to surgery. Be sure to bring your glasses so your prescription can be reviewed.

On the day of your surgery, eat a light meal before coming and take all of your prescribed medications. Do not wear eye makeup or have any bulky accessories in your hair that will interfere with positioning your head under the laser. If you are not feeling well that morning, call the doctor's office to determine whether the procedure needs to be postponed.

What happens during the PRK procedure?

The PRK procedure is done under local anesthesia and takes a maximum of about ten minutes to do both eyes. During PRK, an eye surgeon uses a laser to reshape the cornea. This laser, which delivers a cool pulsing beam of ultraviolet light, is used on the surface of the cornea, not underneath the cornea as in LASIK.

What should I expect after PRK surgery?

Most of the time, a bandage contact lens will be applied immediately after the procedure. This contact lens is usually worn for the first three to four days to allow the surface of the eye to heal. You should expect to visit your eye doctor at least a few times during the first six months after surgery, with the first visit being one to three days after surgery. Once the surface of the eye is healed, the bandage contact lens is removed.

Your vision may fluctuate between clear and blurry for the first few weeks following surgery and you may need to wear glasses for night driving or reading until your vision stabilizes. Your eyes will be dry even though they do not feel that way. Your doctor will give you prescription eye drops to prevent infection and keep your eyes moist. These drops may cause a slight burn or momentary blurring of your vision upon using them. Do not use any drops not approved by your ophthalmologist.

Your vision will gradually improve, and usually will be good enough to allow you to drive a car within two to three weeks following surgery.

Keep in mind, however, that your best vision may not be obtained for up to six weeks to six months following surgery.

Will I still need reading glasses to correct presbyopia after I have had PRK?

Presbyopia happens in all patients over the age of forty and can be corrected with reading glasses or with laser refractive surgery doing something called monovision, where, using contact lenses, the non-dominant eye is corrected for reading and the dominant eye is corrected for distance. PRK is not used to correct presbyopia.

Chapter 16

Laser Epithelial Keratomileusis (LASEK) Surgery

LASEK (laser epithelial keratomileusis) is a newer variation of photorefractive keratotomy (PRK), a procedure in which laser energy is applied directly to the eye's outer surface for reshaping and vision correction.

To understand how LASEK works, you first must know the fundamental differences between laser-assisted in situ keratomileusis (LASIK), PRK, and LASEK:

- With LASIK, a thin flap is cut into the eye's surface and then lifted. Laser energy is applied to the eye for reshaping, and the flap is replaced to serve as a type of natural bandage for quicker healing.

- An eye surgeon using PRK does not cut a thin flap into the eye's surface, as occurs with LASIK. Instead, laser energy is applied directly to the eye's surface. The ultra thin, outer layer of the eye (epithelium) is removed completely by laser energy during a PRK procedure, and eventually grows back.

- A LASEK procedure involves preserving the extremely thin epithelial layer by lifting it from the eye's surface before laser energy is applied for reshaping. After the LASEK procedure, the epithelium is replaced on the eye's surface.

"LASEK Eye Surgery: How It Works," reprinted with permission from www .AllAboutVision.com. © 2011 Access Media Group LLC. All rights reserved.

In LASIK, the thicker flap is created with a microkeratome cutting tool or a special laser. With LASEK, the ultra thin flap is created with a special cutting tool known as a trephine.

LASEK is used mostly for people with corneas that are too thin or too steep for LASIK, when it may be difficult to create a thicker LASIK flap. LASEK was developed to reduce the chance of complications that occur when the flap created during LASIK does not have the ideal thickness or diameter.

According to a survey of members of the American Society of Cataract and Refractive Surgery (ASCRS), the popularity of LASEK is growing among refractive eye surgeons, as it is with epi-LASIK—another variation of the procedure. Epi-LASIK uses a plastic blade, called an epithelial separator, to detach part of the epithelial layer from the eye.

However, eyes undergoing LASEK procedures generally heal more slowly and result in more complaints of discomfort than with LASIK. For this reason, some surgeons prefer to perform PRK rather than LASEK or epi-LASIK because they find no advantage in the latter procedures.

In fact, a 2008 study published in the *Journal of Refractive Surgery* indicated that people undergoing PRK tended to have less pain and healed slightly faster than people who had undergone a surgical technique called butterfly LASEK. "Butterfly" refers to the shape and type of thin flap lifted in LASIK, which is thought to increase comfort and healing time.

The LASEK Procedure

During LASEK, your surgeon uses local anesthesia. Then he or she cuts the epithelium, or outer layer of the cornea, with a fine blade (trephine). Then the surgeon covers the eye with a diluted alcohol solution for approximately thirty seconds, which loosens the edges of the epithelium.

After sponging the alcohol solution from the eye, the surgeon uses a tiny hoe to lift the edge of the epithelial flap and gently fold it back out of the way.

Then the same excimer laser used for LASIK or PRK sculpts the corneal tissue underneath. Afterward, a type of spatula is used to place the epithelial flap back on the eye.

In a new variation of LASEK, the same plastic blade (epithelial separator) used in epi-LASIK creates the thin epithelial flap. But because alcohol is applied during the procedure as it is in straight LASEK, the procedure is called epi-LASEK with an "E" instead of an "I."

After LASEK

In many ways, LASEK vision recovery is slower than LASIK recovery, but there are some differences. According to doctors who perform LASEK, the flap edge heals in about a day, though patients usually wear a bandage contact lens for approximately four days to protect the eye.

Your eye may feel irritated during the first day or two afterward. Also, with LASEK compared with LASIK, it often takes longer to recover good vision—up to four to seven days—but this can vary from one person to the next. You also may experience more pain with LASEK compared with LASIK.

Talking to Your Doctor

If you are considering LASIK, but your doctor says you need LASEK, ask why. It's not for everyone, but many surgeons who perform LASEK consider it a better option for some patients who will probably not do very well with LASIK.

Also, in some studies LASEK has been associated with faster recovery of sensation or nerve function in the eye's surface (cornea) compared with LASIK. It also may cause dry eye less frequently than LASIK.

However, keep in mind that a 2007 study published in the *Journal of Cataract and Refractive Surgery* concluded that the outcome of LASEK depends on the surgeon's experience.

Therefore, it's always a good idea to ask how many procedures your surgeon has performed.

Chapter 17

Phakic Intraocular Lenses

What Are Phakic Lenses?

Phakic intraocular lenses, or phakic lenses, are lenses made of plastic or silicone that are implanted into the eye permanently to reduce a person's need for glasses or contact lenses. Phakic refers to the fact that the lens is implanted into the eye without removing the eye's natural lens. During phakic lens implantation surgery, a small incision is made in the front of the eye. The phakic lens is inserted through the incision and placed just in front of or just behind the iris.

What do they treat?

Phakic lenses are used to correct refractive errors, errors in the eye's focusing power. All phakic lenses approved by the U.S. Food and Drug Administration (FDA) are for the correction of nearsightedness (myopia).

People who are nearsighted have more difficulty seeing distant objects than near objects. For these people, the images of distant objects come to focus in front of the retina instead of on the retina.

Ideally, phakic lenses cause light entering the eye to be focused on the retina, providing clear distance vision without the aid of glasses or contact lenses.

Excerpted from the following documents from the U.S. Food and Drug Administration: "What Are Phakic Lenses?" November 24, 2010; "Are Phakic Lenses for You?" November 24, 2010; "What Are the Risks?" April 16, 2009; "Before, During, and After Surgery," June 26, 2009; and "Questions for Your Doctor," April 30, 2009.

Can they be removed?

Phakic lenses are intended to be permanent. While the lenses can be surgically removed, return to your previous level of vision or condition of your eye cannot be guaranteed.

What is the difference between phakic intraocular lenses and intraocular lenses following cataract surgery?

Phakic intraocular lenses are implanted in the eye without removing the natural lens. This is in contrast to intraocular lenses that are implanted into eyes after the eye's cloudy natural lens (cataract) has been removed during cataract surgery.

Are Phakic Lenses For You?

You are probably *not* a good candidate for phakic lenses if any of the following are true:

- You are not an adult. There are no phakic lenses approved by the FDA for persons under the age of twenty-one.

- You are not a risk taker. Certain complications are unavoidable in a percentage of patients, and there are no long-term data available for phakic lenses.

- You required a change in your contact lens or glasses prescription in the last six to twelve months in order to obtain the best possible vision for you. This is called refractive instability. Patients who are in their early twenties or younger, whose hormones are fluctuating due to disease such as diabetes, who are pregnant or breastfeeding, or who are taking medications that may cause fluctuations in vision are more likely to have refractive instability and should discuss the possible additional risks with their doctor.

- You may jeopardize your career. Some jobs prohibit certain refractive procedures. Be sure to check with your employer/professional society/military service before undergoing any procedure.

- Cost is an issue. Most medical insurance will not pay for refractive surgery.

- You have a disease or are on medications that may affect wound healing. Certain conditions, such as autoimmune diseases (e.g., lupus, rheumatoid arthritis), immunodeficiency states (e.g., human immunodeficiency virus [HIV]), and diabetes, and some medications (e.g., retinoic acid and steroids) may prevent proper healing after intraocular surgery.

- You have a low endothelial cell count or abnormal endothelial cells. If the cells that pump the fluid out of your cornea, the endothelial cells, are low in number relative to your age, or if your endothelial cells are abnormal, you have a higher risk of developing a cloudy cornea and requiring a corneal transplant.

- You actively participate in sports with a high risk of eye trauma. Your eye may be more susceptible to damage should you receive a blow to the face or eye, such as a blow to the head during boxing or being hit in the eye by a ball during baseball. Your eye may be more susceptible to rupture or retinal detachment, and the phakic lens may dislocate.

- You only have one eye with potentially good vision. If you only have one eye with good vision with glasses or contact lenses, due to disease, irreparable damage, or amblyopia (eye with poor vision since childhood that cannot be corrected with glasses or contact lenses), you and your doctor should consider the risk of possible damage and/or loss of vision to your better eye as a result of phakic lens implantation.

- You have large pupils. If your pupil dilates in low lighting conditions to a size that is larger than the size of the lens, you have a higher risk of experiencing visual disturbances after surgery that may affect your ability to function comfortably or normally under such conditions (e.g., while driving at night).

- You have a shallow anterior chamber. If the space between the cornea and the iris, the anterior chamber, is narrow, you have a higher risk of developing complications, such as greater endothelial cell loss, due to implantation of the phakic lens.

- You have an abnormal iris. If your pupil is irregularly shaped, you have a higher risk of developing visual disturbances.

- You have had uveitis. If you have had inflammation in your eye, you may have a recurrence or worsening of your disease and/or may develop additional complications, such as glaucoma, as a result of surgery.

- You have had problems with the posterior part of your eye. If you have had any problems in the back part of your eye or are at risk for such problems, for example, proliferative diabetic retinopathy (growth of abnormal vessels in the back of the eye due to diabetes) or retinal detachment, you may not be a good candidate for phakic lens implantation. The phakic lens may not allow your eye doctor to get a clear view of the back part of your eye, preventing or delaying detection of a new or worsening problem, and/or the phakic lens may prevent or make treatment of a problem in the back of your eye more difficult.

The safety and effectiveness of phakic lenses have *not* been studied in patients with certain conditions. If any of the following apply to you, make sure you discuss them with your doctor:

- You have glaucoma (damage to the nerve of the eye resulting in loss of peripheral and then central vision due to too high pressure inside the eye), ocular hypertension (high eye pressure), or glaucoma suspect (some indications, but not clear, that patient has glaucoma). You may have a higher risk of developing or worsening of glaucoma as a result of phakic lens implantation.

- You have pseudoexfoliation syndrome (abnormal deposits of material in the eye visible on the structures in the front part of the eye, such as on the front of the natural lens and the back of the cornea). This syndrome is associated with glaucoma and weakness of the structures holding the natural lens in place (the zonules). You may have a higher risk of surgical complications and/or complications after surgery if you have this syndrome.

- You have had an eye injury or previous eye surgery.

- Your need for visual correction is outside the range for which the phakic lens has been approved. Ask your eye doctor if the phakic lens that he or she recommends for you has been approved to treat your refractive error and/or check FDA-approved phakic lenses for the approved refractive range.

- You are over the age of forty-five years old. Some phakic lenses have not been studied in patients over the age of forty-five.

What Are the Risks?

Implanting a phakic lens involves a surgical procedure. As in any other medical procedure, there are risks involved. That's why it is important for you to understand the limitations and risks of phakic intraocular lens implant surgery.

Before undergoing surgery for implantation of a phakic intraocular lens, you should carefully weigh the risks and benefits and try to avoid being influenced by other people encouraging you to do it.

Risks

- You may lose vision. Some patients lose vision as a result of phakic lens implant surgery that cannot be corrected with glasses, contact lenses, or another surgery. The amount of vision loss may be severe.

- You may develop debilitating visual symptoms. Some patients develop glare, halos, double vision, and/or decreased vision in situations of low-level lighting that can cause difficulty with performing tasks, such as driving, particularly at night or under foggy conditions.

- You may need additional eye surgery to reposition, replace, or remove the phakic lens implant. These surgeries may be necessary for your safety or to improve your visual function. If the lens power is not right, then a phakic lens exchange may be needed. You may also have to have the lens repositioned, removed, or replaced, if the lens does not stay in the right place, is not the right size, and/or causes debilitating visual symptoms. Every additional surgical procedure has its own risks.

- You may be undertreated or overtreated. Many treated patients do not achieve 20/20 vision after surgery. The power of the implanted phakic lens may be too strong or too weak. This is because of the difficulties with determining exactly what power lens you need. This means that you will probably still need glasses or contact lenses to perform at least some tasks. For example, you may need glasses for reading, even if you did not need them before surgery. This also means that you may need a second surgery to replace the lens with another, if the power of the originally implanted lens was too far from what you needed.

- You may develop increased intraocular pressure. You may experience increased pressure inside the eye after surgery, which may require surgery or medication to control. You may need long-term treatment with glaucoma medications. If the pressure is too high for too long, you may lose vision.

- Your cornea may become cloudy. The endothelial cells of your cornea are a thin layer of cells responsible for pumping fluid out of the cornea to keep it clear. If the endothelial cells become too few in number, the endothelial cell pump will fail and the cornea will become cloudy, resulting in loss of vision. You start with a certain number of cells at birth, and this number continuously decreases as you age, since these cells are not replenished. Normally, you die from old age before the number of endothelial cells becomes so low that your cornea becomes cloudy. Some lens designs have shown that their implantation causes endothelial cells to be lost at a faster rate than normal. If the number of endothelial cells drops too low and your cornea becomes cloudy, you will lose vision and you may require a corneal transplant in order to see more clearly.

- You may develop a cataract. You may get a cataract, clouding of the natural lens. The amount of time for a cataract to develop can vary greatly. If your cataract develops and progresses enough to significantly decrease your vision, you may require cataract surgery. Your doctor will then have to remove both your natural and your phakic lenses.

- You may develop a retinal detachment. The retina is the tissue that lines the inside of the back of your eyeball. It contains the light-sensing cells that collect and send images to your brain, much like the film in a camera. The risk of the retina becoming detached from the back of your eye increases after intraocular surgery. It is not known at this time how much your risk of retinal detachment will increase as a result of phakic intraocular lens implantation surgery.

- You may experience infection, bleeding, or severe inflammation (pain, redness, and decreased vision). These are rare complications that can sometimes lead to permanent loss of vision or loss of the eye.

- Long-term data are not available. Phakic lenses are a new technology and have only recently been approved by the FDA. Therefore, there may be other risks to having phakic lenses implanted that we don't yet know about.

Before, During, and After Surgery

What should I expect before surgery?

Initial visit: Before deciding to have phakic intraocular lens implantation surgery, you will need an initial examination to make sure your eye is healthy and suitable for surgery. Your doctor will take a complete history about your medical and eye health and perform a thorough examination of both eyes, which will include measurements of your pupils, anterior chamber depth (the distance between your cornea and iris), and endothelial cell counts (the number of cells on the back of your cornea).

If you wear contact lenses, your doctor may ask you to stop wearing them before your initial examination (from the day of to a few weeks before), so that your refraction (measure of how much your eye bends light) and central keratometry readings (measure of how much the cornea curves) are more accurate.

At this time, you should tell your doctor if you:

- take any medications, including over-the-counter medications, vitamins, and other supplements;
- have any allergies;
- have had any eye conditions;
- have undergone any previous eye surgery; or
- have had any medical conditions.

Deciding to have surgery: To help you decide whether phakic lenses are right for you, talk to your doctor about your expectations and whether there are elements of your medical history, eye history, or eye examination that might increase your risk or prevent you from having the outcome you expect. Before you sign an informed consent document (a form giving permission to your doctor to operate on your eye), you should discuss with your doctor the following things:

- Whether you are a good candidate
- What the risks, benefits, and alternatives of the surgery are
- What you should expect before, during, and after surgery
- What your responsibilities will be before, during, and after surgery

You should have the opportunity to ask your doctor questions during this discussion. Ask your doctor for the patient labeling of the lens that he or she recommends for you. Give yourself plenty of time to think about the risk/benefit discussion, to review any informational literature provided by your doctor, and to have any additional questions answered by your doctor before deciding to go through with surgery and before signing the informed consent document. You should not feel pressured by anyone to make a decision about having surgery.

How should I prepare for surgery?

Within weeks of surgery: About one to two weeks before surgery, your eye doctor may schedule you for a laser iridotomy to prepare your eye for implantation of the phakic lens. Before the procedure, your eye doctor may put drops in your eye to make the pupil small and to numb the eye. While you are seated, you doctor will rest a large lens on your eye. He or she will then make a small hole (or holes) in the extreme outer edge of the iris (the colored part of your eye) with a laser. This hole (holes) are to prevent fluid buildup and pressure in the back chamber of your eye after phakic lens implantation surgery. This procedure is usually performed in an office or clinic setting, not in an operating room, and usually takes only a few minutes.

After the iridotomy procedure, the doctor may have you wait around awhile before checking your eye pressure and letting you go home. The procedure should not prevent you from driving home, but you should check with your eye doctor when you schedule your appointment. You will be given a prescription for steroid drops to put in your eye at home for several days to reduce inflammation from the iridotomy procedure. It is important that you follow all instructions your doctor gives you after the iridotomy procedure.

Possible complications of laser iridotomy include the following:

- iritis (inflammation in the front part of the eye)

- increase in eye pressure (usually within one to four hours after the procedure)

- cataract (clouding of the natural lens) from the laser

- hyphema (bleeding into the anterior chamber of the eye, behind the cornea and in front of the iris, that can cause high pressure inside the eye)

- injury to the cornea from the laser that can result in clouding of the cornea

- incomplete opening of the hole all the way through the iris

- closure of the new opening

- rarely, retinal burns

Your doctor may ask you to stop wearing contact lenses before your surgery (anywhere from the day of the surgery to a few weeks before). Before your surgery, your eye doctor may ask you to temporarily stop taking certain medications that increase the risk of bleeding during surgery. How long before surgery you may need to stop these medications depends upon which medications you are using and the conditions they are treating. You and your eye doctor may need to discuss stopping certain medications with the doctor who prescribed them, since you may need some of these medications to prevent life-threatening events.

Within days of surgery: Your doctor may give you prescriptions for antibiotic drops to prevent infection and/or anti-inflammatory drops to prevent inflammation to put in your eye for a few days before surgery.

Arrange for transportation to and from surgery and to your follow-up doctor's appointment the day after surgery, since you will be unable to drive. Your doctor will let you know when it is safe for you to drive again.

Your eye doctor will probably tell you not to eat or drink anything after midnight the night before your surgery.

What should I expect during surgery?

The day of surgery: Just before surgery, drops will be put in your eye. You will have to lie down for the surgery and remain still. If you cannot lie down flat on your back, you may not be a good candidate for this surgery. Usually, patients are not put to sleep for this type of surgery, but you may be given a sedative or other medication to make you relax and an intravenous (i.v.) line may be started. Your doctor may inject medication around the eye to numb the eye. The doctor also may give you an injection around the eye to also prevent you from being able to move your eye or see out of your eye. You will have to ask your doctor to find out exactly which of these types of anesthesia will be used in your case. Your eye and the surrounding area will be cleaned and an instrument called a lid speculum will be used to hold your eyelids open.

The doctor will make an incision in your cornea, sclera (the white part of your eye), or limbus (where the cornea meets the sclera). He or she will place a lubricant into your eye to help protect the back of the cornea (the endothelial cells) during the insertion of the phakic lens. The doctor will insert the phakic lens through the incision in the eye into the anterior chamber, behind the cornea and in front of the iris. Depending upon the type of phakic lens, the doctor will either attach the lens to the front of the iris in the anterior chamber of the eye or move it through the pupil into position behind the iris and in front of the lens in the posterior chamber of the eye. The doctor will remove the lubricant and may close the incision with tiny stitches, depending

189

upon the type of incision. Your doctor will place some eye drops or ointment in your eye and cover your eye with a patch and/or a shield. The surgery will probably take around thirty minutes.

After the surgery is over, you may be brought to a recovery room for a couple of hours before you will be allowed to go home. You will be given prescriptions for antibiotic and anti-inflammatory drops to use at home as directed. You will be given an implant identification card, which you should keep as a permanent record of the lens that was implanted in your eye. Make sure you show this card to anyone who takes care of your eyes in the future. You will be asked to go home and take it easy for the rest of the day.

What should I expect after surgery?

Immediately after surgery: After the surgical procedure, you may be sensitive to light and have a feeling that something is in your eye. You may experience minor discomfort after the procedure. Your doctor may prescribe pain medication to make you more comfortable during the first few days after the surgery. You should contact your eye doctor immediately if you have severe pain.

You should see your eye doctor the day after surgery. Your doctor will remove the patch and/or shield and will check your vision and the condition of your eye. Your doctor will instruct you on how to use the eye drops that you were prescribed for after the surgery. You will need to take these drops for up to a few weeks after surgery to decrease inflammation and help prevent infection. Your doctor may instruct you to continue wearing the shield all day and all night or just at night. You should wear the shield until your doctor tells you that you no longer have to do so. The shield is meant to prevent you from rubbing your eye or putting pressure on your eye while you sleep and to protect your eye from accidentally being hit or poked while it is healing.

As you recover: Your vision will probably be somewhat hazy or blurry for the first several days after surgery. Your vision should start to improve after the first several days, but may continue to fluctuate for the next several weeks. It usually takes about two to four weeks for the vision to stabilize. Do *not* rub your eyes, especially for the first three to five days. You may also experience sensitivity to light, glare, starbursts or halos around lights, or the whites of your eye may look red or bloodshot. These symptoms should decrease as your eye recovers over the next several weeks.

You should contact your doctor immediately if you develop severe pain or if your vision or other symptoms get worse instead of better.

Follow all postoperative instructions given to you by your surgeon and surgical center.

Remember to do the following things:

- Wash your hands before putting drops in your eye.

- Use the prescribed medications to help minimize the risk of infection and inflammation. Serious infection or inflammation can result in loss of vision.

- Try not to get water in your eyes until your doctor says it is okay to do so.

- Try not to bend from the waist to pick up objects on the floor, as this can cause undue pressure to your eyes. Do not lift any heavy objects.

- Do not engage in any strenuous activity until your doctor says it is okay to do so. It will take about eight weeks for your eye to heal.

Long-term: Your doctor will instruct you to return for additional follow-up visits to monitor your progress. Initially, these visits will be closer together (a few days to a few weeks apart) and then they will be spread out (several weeks to several months apart). It is important to go to all of these appointments, even if you think you are doing well, so that the doctor can check for complications that you may not be aware of.

Because you will have a permanent implant in your eye with long-term risks, and especially since all these risks are not known at this time, you will need to be followed by an eye doctor on a regular basis for the rest of your life. Endothelial cell counts will have to be performed on a regular basis. You and your doctor should maintain records of these measurements, so as to be able to estimate the rate of cell loss. It is especially important for you to have your endothelial cells counted before you and your eye doctor consider any other intraocular procedures, such as cataract surgery, that will decrease the endothelial cell count even further.

Annual eye exams are usually recommended. However, if you have any problems with your vision or your eyes, such as flashing lights, floating spots, or blank spots in your vision (symptoms of a retinal detachment), you should see an eye doctor right away and inform him or her that you have a phakic lens implant. When participating in sports or other activities during which you might injure your eye, like home improvement work, always wear protective eyewear, such as safety goggles.

Questions for Your Doctor

Use the following checklist to help you guide your discussion with your doctor about phakic lenses.

Know what makes you a poor candidate:

- Do I have any conditions that would increase my risks?

- Are the size of my pupils under low lighting conditions bigger than the size of the lens? If so, what are my additional risks?

- Is my anterior chamber shallow? If so, what are my additional risks?

Know all the benefits, risks, and alternatives:

- What are the benefits of the phakic lens for my amount of near-sightedness?

- What are the risks of having the phakic lens implanted?

- What is my risk of needing a corneal transplant in the future, if I have the phakic lens implanted, based on my age and my endothelial cell count?

- What could happen if I get hit in the eye or head after phakic lens implantation that might be different from what could happen if I did not have the lens implanted? Are my chances greater for a more severe injury after phakic lens implantation?

- Can the phakic lens be removed? What are the risks of removing the phakic lens?

- What other options are available for correcting my nearsightedness?

Know preoperative, operative, and postoperative expectations:

- Will I need to limit my activities after treatment? If so, for how long?

- What quality of vision can I expect in the first week, first few months, and a year after surgery?

- What is the possibility that the phakic lens will not completely correct my vision or that my prescription might be worse than before surgery? What options for additional treatment will be available to me, if needed?

- How likely is it that I will need to wear glasses or contact lenses immediately after surgery and as I grow older?

- Should I have the phakic lens implanted in both eyes?

- What vision problems might I experience if I have the phakic lens implanted in only one eye?

- How long will I have to wait before having surgery on my other eye?

Know what the costs are:

- How much will the surgery and follow-up cost? Will my health insurance cover this surgery?

- Will there be additional costs if I need additional procedures because the phakic lens implanted in my eye is too strong or too weak or because I have astigmatism? What is the likelihood of this happening?

Part Three

Understanding and Treating Disorders of the Cornea, Conjunctiva, Sclera, Iris, and Pupil

Chapter 18

The Cornea
and Corneal Disease:
An Overview

What is the cornea?

The cornea is the eye's outermost layer. It is the clear, dome-shaped surface that covers the front of the eye.

Structure of the cornea: Although the cornea is clear and seems to lack substance, it is actually a highly organized group of cells and proteins. Unlike most tissues in the body, the cornea contains no blood vessels to nourish or protect it against infection. Instead, the cornea receives its nourishment from the tears and aqueous humor that fills the chamber behind it. The cornea must remain transparent to refract light properly, and the presence of even the tiniest blood vessels can interfere with this process. To see well, all layers of the cornea must be free of any cloudy or opaque areas.

The corneal tissue is arranged in five basic layers, each having an important function. These five layers are as follows:

- *Epithelium:* The epithelium is the cornea's outermost region, comprising about 10 percent of the tissue's thickness. The epithelium functions primarily to: (1) Block the passage of foreign material, such as dust, water, and bacteria, into the eye and other layers of the cornea; and (2) Provide a smooth surface that absorbs oxygen and cell nutrients from tears, then distributes these nutrients to the rest of the cornea. The epithelium is filled with thousands of

Excerpted from "Facts about the Cornea and Corneal Disease," National Eye Institute, National Institutes of Health, March 2010.

tiny nerve endings that make the cornea extremely sensitive to pain when rubbed or scratched. The part of the epithelium that serves as the foundation on which the epithelial cells anchor and organize themselves is called the basement membrane.

- *Bowman Layer:* Lying directly below the basement membrane of the epithelium is a transparent sheet of tissue known as Bowman layer. It is composed of strong layered protein fibers called collagen. Once injured, Bowman layer can form a scar as it heals. If these scars are large and centrally located, some vision loss can occur.

- *Stroma:* Beneath Bowman layer is the stroma, which comprises about 90 percent of the cornea's thickness. It consists primarily of water (78 percent) and collagen (16 percent), and does not contain any blood vessels. Collagen gives the cornea its strength, elasticity, and form. The collagen's unique shape, arrangement, and spacing are essential in producing the cornea's light-conducting transparency.

- *Descemet Membrane:* Under the stroma is Descemet membrane, a thin but strong sheet of tissue that serves as a protective barrier against infection and injuries. Descemet membrane is composed of collagen fibers (different from those of the stroma) and is made by the endothelial cells that lie below it. Descemet membrane is regenerated readily after injury.

- *Endothelium:* The endothelium is the extremely thin, innermost layer of the cornea. Endothelial cells are essential in keeping the cornea clear. Normally, fluid leaks slowly from inside the eye into the middle corneal layer (stroma). The endothelium's primary task is to pump this excess fluid out of the stroma. Without this pumping action, the stroma would swell with water, become hazy, and ultimately opaque. In a healthy eye, a perfect balance is maintained between the fluid moving into the cornea and fluid being pumped out of the cornea. Once endothelium cells are destroyed by disease or trauma, they are lost forever. If too many endothelial cells are destroyed, corneal edema and blindness ensue, with corneal transplantation the only available therapy.

Refractive errors: About 120 million people in the United States wear eyeglasses or contact lenses to correct nearsightedness, farsightedness, or astigmatism. These vision disorders—called refractive errors—affect the cornea and are the most common of all vision problems in this country.

Refractive errors occur when the curve of the cornea is irregularly shaped (too steep or too flat). When the cornea is of normal shape and curvature, it bends, or refracts, light on the retina with precision. However, when the curve of the cornea is irregularly shaped, the cornea bends light imperfectly on the retina. This affects good vision. The refractive process is similar to the way a camera takes a picture. The cornea and lens in your eye act as the camera lens. The retina is similar to the film. If the image is not focused properly, the film (or retina) receives a blurry image. The image that your retina "sees" then goes to your brain, which tells you what the image is.

When the cornea is curved too much, or if the eye is too long, far-away objects will appear blurry because they are focused in front of the retina. This is called myopia, or nearsightedness. Myopia affects over 25 percent of all adult Americans.

Hyperopia, or farsightedness, is the opposite of myopia. Distant objects are clear, and close-up objects appear blurry. With hyperopia, images focus on a point beyond the retina. Hyperopia results from an eye that is too short.

Astigmatism is a condition in which the uneven curvature of the cornea blurs and distorts both distant and near objects. A normal cornea is round, with even curves from side to side and top to bottom. With astigmatism, the cornea is shaped more like the back of a spoon, curved more in one direction than in another. This causes light rays to have more than one focal point and focus on two separate areas of the retina, distorting the visual image. Two-thirds of Americans with myopia also have astigmatism.

Refractive errors are usually corrected by eyeglasses or contact lenses. Although these are safe and effective methods for treating refractive errors, refractive surgeries are becoming an increasingly popular option.

What is the function of the cornea?

Because the cornea is as smooth and clear as glass but is strong and durable, it helps the eye in two ways:

- It helps to shield the rest of the eye from germs, dust, and other harmful matter. The cornea shares this protective task with the eyelids, the eye socket, tears, and the sclera, or white part of the eye.

- The cornea acts as the eye's outermost lens. It functions like a window that controls and focuses the entry of light into the eye. The cornea contributes between 65 and 75 percent of the eye's total focusing power.

The cornea also serves as a filter, screening out some of the most damaging ultraviolet (UV) wavelengths in sunlight. Without this protection, the lens and the retina would be highly susceptible to injury from UV radiation.

How does the cornea respond to injury?

The cornea copes very well with minor injuries or abrasions. If the highly sensitive cornea is scratched, healthy cells slide over quickly and patch the injury before infection occurs and vision is affected. If the scratch penetrates the cornea more deeply, however, the healing process will take longer, at times resulting in greater pain, blurred vision, tearing, redness, and extreme sensitivity to light. These symptoms require professional treatment. Deeper scratches can also cause corneal scarring, resulting in a haze on the cornea that can greatly impair vision. In this case, a corneal transplant may be needed.

What are some diseases and disorders affecting the cornea?

Allergies: Allergies affecting the eye are fairly common. The most common allergies are those related to pollen, particularly when the weather is warm and dry. Symptoms can include redness, itching, tearing, burning, stinging, and watery discharge, although they are not usually severe enough to require medical attention. Antihistamine decongestant eye drops can effectively reduce these symptoms, as do rain and cooler weather, which decrease the amount of pollen in the air.

An increasing number of eye allergy cases are related to medications and contact lens wear. Also, animal hair and certain cosmetics, such as mascara, face creams, and eyebrow pencil, can cause allergies that affect the eye. Touching or rubbing eyes after handling nail polish, soaps, or chemicals may cause an allergic reaction. Some people have sensitivity to lip gloss and eye makeup. Allergy symptoms are temporary and can be eliminated by not having contact with the offending cosmetic or detergent.

Conjunctivitis (pink eye): This term describes a group of diseases that cause swelling, itching, burning, and redness of the conjunctiva, the protective membrane that lines the eyelids and covers exposed areas of the sclera, or white of the eye. Conjunctivitis can spread from one person to another and affects millions of Americans at any given time. Conjunctivitis can be caused by a bacterial or viral infection, allergy, environmental irritants, a contact lens product, eye drops, or eye ointments.

At its onset, conjunctivitis is usually painless and does not adversely affect vision. The infection will clear in most cases without requiring medical care. But for some forms of conjunctivitis, treatment will be needed. If treatment is delayed, the infection may worsen and cause corneal inflammation and a loss of vision.

Corneal infections: Sometimes the cornea is damaged after a foreign object has penetrated the tissue, such as from a poke in the eye. At other times, bacteria or fungi from a contaminated contact lens can pass into the cornea. Situations like these can cause painful inflammation and corneal infections called keratitis. These infections can reduce visual clarity, produce corneal discharges, and perhaps erode the cornea. Corneal infections can also lead to corneal scarring, which can impair vision and may require a corneal transplant.

As a general rule, the deeper the corneal infection, the more severe the symptoms and complications. It should be noted that corneal infections, although relatively infrequent, are the most serious complication of contact lens wear.

Minor corneal infections are commonly treated with anti-bacterial eye drops. If the problem is severe, it may require more intensive antibiotic or anti-fungal treatment to eliminate the infection, as well as steroid eye drops to reduce inflammation. Frequent visits to an eye care professional may be necessary for several months to eliminate the problem.

Dry eye: The continuous production and drainage of tears is important to the eye's health. Tears keep the eye moist, help wounds heal, and protect against eye infection. In people with dry eye, the eye produces fewer or less quality tears and is unable to keep its surface lubricated and comfortable.

The main symptom of dry eye is usually a scratchy or sandy feeling as if something is in the eye. Other symptoms may include stinging or burning of the eye; episodes of excess tearing that follow periods of very dry sensation; a stringy discharge from the eye; and pain and redness of the eye. Sometimes people with dry eye experience heaviness of the eyelids or blurred, changing, or decreased vision, although loss of vision is uncommon.

Dry eye is more common in women, especially after menopause. Surprisingly, some people with dry eye may have tears that run down their cheeks. This is because the eye may be producing less of the lipid and mucin layers of the tear film, which help keep tears in the eye. When this happens, tears do not stay in the eye long enough to thoroughly moisten it.

Dry eye can occur in climates with dry air, as well as with the use of some drugs, including antihistamines, nasal decongestants, tranquilizers, and anti-depressant drugs. People with dry eye should let their healthcare providers know all the medications they are taking, since some of them may intensify dry eye symptoms.

People with connective tissue diseases, such as rheumatoid arthritis, can also develop dry eye. It is important to note that dry eye is sometimes a symptom of Sjögren syndrome, a disease that attacks the body's lubricating glands, such as the tear and salivary glands. A complete physical examination may diagnose any underlying diseases.

Artificial tears, which lubricate the eye, are the principal treatment for dry eye. They are available over the counter as eye drops. Sterile ointments are sometimes used at night to help prevent the eye from drying. Using humidifiers, wearing wrap-around glasses when outside, and avoiding outside windy and dry conditions may bring relief. For people with severe cases of dry eye, temporary or permanent closure of the tear drain (small openings at the inner corner of the eyelids where tears drain from the eye) may be helpful.

Fuchs dystrophy: Fuchs dystrophy is a slowly progressing disease that usually affects both eyes and is slightly more common in women than in men. Although doctors can often see early signs of Fuchs dystrophy in people in their thirties and forties, the disease rarely affects vision until people reach their fifties and sixties.

Fuchs dystrophy occurs when endothelial cells gradually deteriorate without any apparent reason. As more endothelial cells are lost over the years, the endothelium becomes less efficient at pumping water out of the stroma. This causes the cornea to swell and distort vision. Eventually, the epithelium also takes on water, resulting in pain and severe visual impairment.

Epithelial swelling damages vision by changing the cornea's normal curvature and causing a sight-impairing haze to appear in the tissue. Epithelial swelling will also produce tiny blisters on the corneal surface. When these blisters burst, they are extremely painful.

At first, a person with Fuchs dystrophy will awaken with blurred vision that will gradually clear during the day. This occurs because the cornea is normally thicker in the morning; it retains fluids during sleep that evaporate in the tear film while we are awake. As the disease worsens, this swelling will remain constant and reduce vision throughout the day.

When treating the disease, doctors will try first to reduce the swelling with drops, ointments, or soft contact lenses. They also may instruct a person to use a hair dryer, held at arm's length or directed across the face, to dry out the epithelial blisters. This can be done two or three times a day.

When the disease interferes with daily activities, a person may need to consider having a corneal transplant to restore sight. The short-term success rate of corneal transplantation is quite good for people with Fuchs dystrophy. However, some studies suggest that the long-term survival of the new cornea can be a problem.

Corneal dystrophies: A corneal dystrophy is a condition in which one or more parts of the cornea lose their normal clarity due to a buildup of cloudy material. There are over twenty corneal dystrophies that affect all parts of the cornea. These diseases share many traits:

- They are usually inherited.

- They affect the right and left eyes equally.

- They are not caused by outside factors, such as injury or diet.

- Most progress gradually.

- Most usually begin in one of the five corneal layers and may later spread to nearby layers.

- Most do not affect other parts of the body, nor are they related to diseases affecting other parts of the eye or body.

- Most can occur in otherwise totally healthy people, male or female.

Corneal dystrophies affect vision in widely differing ways. Some cause severe visual impairment, while a few cause no vision problems and are discovered during a routine eye examination. Other dystrophies may cause repeated episodes of pain without leading to permanent loss of vision.

Some of the most common corneal dystrophies include Fuchs dystrophy, keratoconus, lattice dystrophy, and map-dot-fingerprint dystrophy.

Herpes zoster (shingles): This infection is produced by the varicella-zoster virus, the same virus that causes chickenpox. After an initial outbreak of chickenpox (often during childhood), the virus remains inactive within the nerve cells of the central nervous system. But in some people, the varicella-zoster virus will reactivate at another time in their lives. When this occurs, the virus travels down long nerve fibers and infects some part of the body, producing a blistering rash (shingles), fever, painful inflammations of the affected nerve fibers, and a general feeling of sluggishness.

Varicella-zoster virus may travel to the head and neck, perhaps involving an eye, part of the nose, cheek, and forehead. In about 40 percent of those with shingles in these areas, the virus infects the cornea. Doctors will often prescribe oral anti-viral treatment to reduce the risk of the virus infecting cells deep within the tissue, which could inflame and scar the cornea. The disease may also cause decreased corneal sensitivity, meaning that foreign matter, such as eyelashes, in the eye are not felt as keenly. For many, this decreased sensitivity will be permanent.

Be aware that corneal problems may arise months after the shingles are gone. For this reason, it is important that people who have had facial shingles schedule follow-up eye examinations.

Iridocorneal endothelial syndrome: More common in women and usually diagnosed between ages thirty and fifty, iridocorneal endothelial (ICE) syndrome has three main features: (1) Visible changes in the iris, the colored part of the eye that regulates the amount of light entering the eye; (2) Swelling of the cornea; and (3) The development of glaucoma, a disease that can cause severe vision loss when normal fluid inside the eye cannot drain properly. ICE is usually present in only one eye.

ICE syndrome is actually a grouping of three closely linked conditions: iris nevus (or Cogan-Reese) syndrome; Chandler syndrome; and essential (progressive) iris atrophy (hence the acronym ICE). The most common feature of this group of diseases is the movement of endothelial cells off the cornea onto the iris. This loss of cells from the cornea often leads to corneal swelling, distortion of the iris, and variable degrees of distortion of the pupil, the adjustable opening at the center of the iris that allows varying amounts of light to enter the eye. This cell movement also plugs the fluid outflow channels of the eye, causing glaucoma.

The cause of this disease is unknown. While we do not yet know how to keep ICE syndrome from progressing, the glaucoma associated with the disease can be treated with medication, and a corneal transplant can treat the corneal swelling.

Keratoconus: This disorder—a progressive thinning of the cornea—is the most common corneal dystrophy in the United States, affecting one in every two thousand Americans. It is more prevalent in teenagers and adults in their twenties. Keratoconus arises when the middle of the cornea thins and gradually bulges outward, forming a rounded cone shape. This abnormal curvature changes the cornea's refractive power, producing moderate to severe distortion (astigmatism) and blurriness (nearsightedness) of vision. Keratoconus may also cause swelling and a sight-impairing scarring of the tissue.

Studies indicate that keratoconus stems from one of several possible causes:

- An inherited corneal abnormality. About 7 percent of those with the condition have a family history of keratoconus.

- An eye injury, i.e., excessive eye rubbing or wearing hard contact lenses for many years.

- Certain eye diseases, such as retinitis pigmentosa, retinopathy of prematurity, and vernal keratoconjunctivitis.

- Systemic diseases, such as Leber congenital amaurosis, Ehlers-Danlos syndrome, Down syndrome, and osteogenesis imperfecta.

Keratoconus usually affects both eyes. At first, people can correct their vision with eyeglasses. But as the astigmatism worsens, they must rely on specially fitted contact lenses to reduce the distortion and provide better vision. Although finding a comfortable contact lens can be an extremely frustrating and difficult process, it is crucial because a poorly fitting lens could further damage the cornea and make wearing a contact lens intolerable.

In most cases, the cornea will stabilize after a few years without ever causing severe vision problems. But in about 10 to 20 percent of people with keratoconus, the cornea will eventually become too scarred or will not tolerate a contact lens. If either of these problems occur, a corneal transplant may be needed. This operation is successful in more than 90 percent of those with advanced keratoconus. Several studies have also reported that 80 percent or more of these patients have 20/40 vision or better after the operation.

The National Eye Institute is conducting a natural history study—called the Collaborative Longitudinal Evaluation of Keratoconus Study—to identify factors that influence the severity and progression of keratoconus.

Lattice dystrophy: Lattice dystrophy gets its name from an accumulation of amyloid deposits, or abnormal protein fibers, throughout the middle and anterior stroma. During an eye examination, the doctor sees these deposits in the stroma as clear, comma-shaped overlapping dots and branching filaments, creating a lattice effect. Over time, the lattice lines will grow opaque and involve more of the stroma. They will also gradually converge, giving the cornea a cloudiness that may also reduce vision.

In some people, these abnormal protein fibers can accumulate under the cornea's outer layer—the epithelium. This can cause erosion of the epithelium. This condition is known as recurrent epithelial erosion. These erosions: (1) Alter the cornea's normal curvature, resulting in temporary vision problems; and (2) Expose the nerves that line the cornea, causing severe pain. Even the involuntary act of blinking can be painful.

To ease this pain, a doctor may prescribe eye drops and ointments to reduce the friction on the eroded cornea. In some cases, an eye patch may be used to immobilize the eyelids. With effective care, these erosions usually heal within three days, although occasional sensations of pain may occur for the next six to eight weeks.

By about age forty, some people with lattice dystrophy will have scarring under the epithelium, resulting in a haze on the cornea that can greatly obscure vision. In this case, a corneal transplant may be needed. Although people with lattice dystrophy have an excellent chance for a successful transplant, the disease may also arise in the donor cornea in as little as three years. In one study, about half of the transplant patients with lattice dystrophy had a recurrence of the disease from between two to twenty-six years after the operation. Of these, 15 percent required a second corneal transplant. Early lattice and recurrent lattice arising in the donor cornea responds well to treatment with the excimer laser.

Although lattice dystrophy can occur at any time in life, the condition usually arises in children between the ages of two and seven.

Map-dot-fingerprint dystrophy: This dystrophy occurs when the epithelium's basement membrane develops abnormally (the basement membrane serves as the foundation on which the epithelial cells, which absorb nutrients from tears, anchor and organize themselves). When the basement membrane develops abnormally, the epithelial cells cannot properly adhere to it. This, in turn, causes recurrent epithelial erosions, in which the epithelium's outermost layer rises slightly, exposing a small gap between the outermost layer and the rest of the cornea.

Epithelial erosions can be a chronic problem. They may alter the cornea's normal curvature, causing periodic blurred vision. They may also expose the nerve endings that line the tissue, resulting in moderate to severe pain lasting as long as several days. Generally, the pain will be worse on awakening in the morning. Other symptoms include sensitivity to light, excessive tearing, and foreign body sensation in the eye.

Map-dot-fingerprint dystrophy, which tends to occur in both eyes, usually affects adults between the ages of forty and seventy, although it can develop earlier in life. Also known as epithelial basement membrane dystrophy, map-dot-fingerprint dystrophy gets its name from the unusual appearance of the cornea during an eye examination. Most often, the affected epithelium will have a map-like appearance, i.e., large, slightly gray outlines that look like a continent on a map. There may also be clusters of opaque dots underneath or close to the map-like patches. Less frequently, the irregular basement membrane will form concentric lines in the central cornea that resemble small fingerprints.

Typically, map-dot-fingerprint dystrophy will flare up occasionally for a few years and then go away on its own, with no lasting loss of vision. Most people never know that they have map-dot-fingerprint dystrophy, since they do not have any pain or vision loss. However, if treatment is needed, doctors will try to control the pain associated with the epithelial erosions. They may patch the eye to immobilize it, or prescribe lubricating eye drops and ointments. With treatment, these erosions usually heal within three days, although periodic flashes of pain may occur for several weeks thereafter. Other treatments include anterior corneal punctures to allow better adherence of cells; corneal scraping to remove eroded areas of the cornea and allow regeneration of healthy epithelial tissue; and use of the excimer laser to remove surface irregularities.

Ocular herpes: Herpes of the eye, or ocular herpes, is a recurrent viral infection that is caused by the herpes simplex virus and is the most common infectious cause of corneal blindness in the United States. Previous studies show that once people develop ocular herpes, they have up to a 50 percent chance of having a recurrence. This second flare-up could come weeks or even years after the initial occurrence.

Ocular herpes can produce a painful sore on the eyelid or surface of the eye and cause inflammation of the cornea. Prompt treatment with anti-viral drugs helps to stop the herpes virus from multiplying and destroying epithelial cells. However, the infection may spread deeper into the cornea and develop into a more severe infection called stromal keratitis, which causes the body's immune system to attack and destroy stromal cells. Stromal keratitis is more difficult to treat than less severe ocular herpes infections. Recurrent episodes of stromal keratitis can cause scarring of the cornea, which can lead to loss of vision and possibly blindness.

Like other herpetic infections, herpes of the eye can be controlled. An estimated four hundred thousand Americans have had some form of ocular herpes. Each year, nearly fifty thousand new and recurring cases are diagnosed in the United States, with the more serious stromal keratitis accounting for about 25 percent. In one large study, researchers found that recurrence rate of ocular herpes was 10 percent within one year, 23 percent within two years, and 63 percent within twenty years. Some factors believed to be associated with recurrence include fever, stress, sunlight, and eye injury.

The National Eye Institute supported the Herpetic Eye Disease Study, a group of clinical trials that studied various treatments for severe ocular herpes.

Pterygium: A pterygium is a pinkish, triangular-shaped tissue growth on the cornea. Some pterygia grow slowly throughout a person's life, while others stop growing after a certain point. A pterygium rarely grows so large that it begins to cover the pupil of the eye.

Pterygia are more common in sunny climates and in the twenty to forty age group. Scientists do not know what causes pterygia to develop. However, since people who have pterygia usually have spent a significant time outdoors, many doctors believe ultraviolet (UV) light from the sun may be a factor. In areas where sunlight is strong, wearing protective eyeglasses, sunglasses, or hats with brims is suggested. While some studies report a higher prevalence of pterygia in men than in women, this may reflect different rates of exposure to UV light.

Because a pterygium is visible, many people want to have it removed for cosmetic reasons. It is usually not too noticeable unless it becomes red and swollen from dust or air pollutants. Surgery to remove a pterygium is not recommended unless it affects vision. If a pterygium is surgically removed, it may grow back, particularly if the patient is less than forty years of age. Lubricants can reduce the redness and provide relief from the chronic irritation.

Stevens-Johnson syndrome: Stevens-Johnson syndrome (SJS), also called erythema multiforme major, is a disorder of the skin that can also affect the eyes. SJS is characterized by painful, blistery lesions on the skin and the mucous membranes (the thin, moist tissues that line body cavities) of the mouth, throat, genital region, and eyelids. SJS can cause serious eye problems, such as severe conjunctivitis; iritis, an inflammation inside the eye; corneal blisters and erosions; and corneal holes. In some cases, the ocular complications from SJS can be disabling and lead to severe vision loss.

Scientists are not certain why SJS develops. The most commonly cited cause of SJS is an adverse allergic drug reaction. Almost any drug—but most particularly sulfa drugs—can cause SJS. The allergic reaction to the drug may not occur until seven to fourteen days after first using it. SJS can also be preceded by a viral infection, such as herpes or the mumps, and its accompanying fever, sore throat, and sluggishness. Treatment for the eye may include artificial tears, antibiotics, or corticosteroids. About one-third of all patients diagnosed with SJS have recurrences of the disease.

SJS occurs twice as often in men as women, and most cases appear in children and young adults under thirty, although it can develop in people at any age.

What is a corneal transplant? Is it safe?

A corneal transplant involves replacing a diseased or scarred cornea with a new one. When the cornea becomes cloudy, light cannot penetrate the eye to reach the light-sensitive retina. Poor vision or blindness may result.

In corneal transplant surgery, the surgeon removes the central portion of the cloudy cornea and replaces it with a clear cornea, usually donated through an eye bank. A trephine, an instrument like a cookie cutter, is used to remove the cloudy cornea. The surgeon places the new cornea in the opening and sews it with a very fine thread. The thread stays in for months or even years until the eye heals properly (removing the thread is quite simple and can easily be done in an ophthalmologist's office). Following surgery, eye drops to help promote healing will be needed for several months.

Corneal transplants are very common in the United States; about forty thousand are performed each year. The chances of success of this operation have risen dramatically because of technological advances, such as less irritating sutures, or threads, which are often finer than a human hair; and the surgical microscope. Corneal transplantation has restored sight to many, who a generation ago would have been blinded permanently by corneal injury, infection, or inherited corneal disease or degeneration.

What problems can develop from a corneal transplant?

Even with a fairly high success rate, some problems can develop, such as rejection of the new cornea. Warning signs for rejection are decreased vision, increased redness of the eye, increased pain, and increased sensitivity to light. If any of these last for more than six hours, you should immediately call your ophthalmologist. Rejection can be successfully treated if medication is administered at the first sign of symptoms.

A study supported by the National Eye Institute (NEI) suggests that matching the blood type, but not tissue type, of the recipient with that of the cornea donor may improve the success rate of corneal transplants in people at high risk for graft failure. Approximately 20 percent of corneal transplant patients—between six thousand and eight thousand a year—reject their donor corneas. The NEI-supported study, called the Collaborative Corneal Transplantation Study, found that high-risk patients may reduce the likelihood of corneal rejection if their blood types match those of the cornea donors. The study also concluded that intensive steroid treatment after transplant surgery improves the chances for a successful transplant.

Are there alternatives to a corneal transplant?

Phototherapeutic keratectomy (PTK) is one of the latest advances in eye care for the treatment of corneal dystrophies, corneal scars, and certain corneal infections. Only a short time ago, people with these disorders would most likely have needed a corneal transplant. By combining the precision of the excimer laser with the control of a computer, doctors can vaporize microscopically thin layers of diseased corneal tissue and etch away the surface irregularities associated with many corneal dystrophies and scars. Surrounding areas suffer relatively little trauma. New tissue can then grow over the now-smooth surface. Recovery from the procedure takes a matter of days, rather than months, as with a transplant. The return of vision can occur rapidly, especially if the cause of the problem is confined to the top layer of the cornea. Studies have shown close to an 85 percent success rate in corneal repair using PTK for well-selected patients.

The excimer laser: One of the technologies developed to treat corneal disease is the excimer laser. This device emits pulses of ultraviolet light—a laser beam—to etch away surface irregularities of corneal tissue. Because of the laser's precision, damage to healthy, adjoining tissue is reduced or eliminated.

The PTK procedure is especially useful for people with inherited disorders, whose scars or other corneal opacities limit vision by blocking the way images form on the retina. PTK has been approved by the U.S. Food and Drug Administration.

Current corneal research: Vision research funded by the National Eye Institute (NEI) is leading to progress in understanding and treating corneal disease.

For example, scientists are learning how transplanting corneal cells from a patient's healthy eye to the diseased eye can treat certain conditions that previously caused blindness. Vision researchers continue to investigate ways to enhance corneal healing and eliminate the corneal scarring that can threaten sight. Also, understanding how genes produce and maintain a healthy cornea will help in treating corneal disease.

Genetic studies in families afflicted with corneal dystrophies have yielded new insight into thirteen different corneal dystrophies, including keratoconus. To identify factors that influence the severity and progression of keratoconus, the NEI is conducting a natural history study—called the Collaborative Longitudinal Evaluation of Keratoconus (CLEK) study—that is following more than 1,200 patients with the disease. Scientists are looking for answers to how rapidly their keratoconus will progress, how bad their vision will become, and whether they will need corneal surgery to treat it. Results from the CLEK study will enable eye care practitioners to better manage this complex disease.

The NEI also supported the Herpetic Eye Disease Study (HEDS), a group of clinical trials that studied various treatments for severe ocular herpes. HEDS researchers reported that oral acyclovir reduced by 41 percent the chance that ocular herpes, a recurrent disease, would return. The study clearly showed that acyclovir therapy can benefit people with all forms of ocular herpes. Current HEDS research is examining the role of psychological stress and other factors as triggers of ocular herpes recurrences.

Chapter 19

Cataract

Chapter Contents

Section 19.1

Facts about Cataract

Excerpted from "Facts about Cataract,"
National Eye Institute, National Institutes of Health,
September 2009.

Cataract Defined

What is a cataract?

A cataract is a clouding of the lens in the eye that affects vision. Most cataracts are related to aging. Cataracts are very common in older people. By age eighty, more than half of all Americans either have a cataract or have had cataract surgery.

A cataract can occur in either or both eyes. It cannot spread from one eye to the other.

Are there other types of cataract?

Yes. Although most cataracts are related to aging, there are other types of cataract:

- **Secondary cataract:** Cataracts can form after surgery for other eye problems, such as glaucoma. Cataracts also can develop in people who have other health problems, such as diabetes. Cataracts are sometimes linked to steroid use.

- **Traumatic cataract:** Cataracts can develop after an eye injury, sometimes years later.

- **Congenital cataract:** Some babies are born with cataracts or develop them in childhood, often in both eyes. These cataracts may be so small that they do not affect vision. If they do, the lenses may need to be removed.

- **Radiation cataract:** Cataracts can develop after exposure to some types of radiation.

Causes and Risk Factors

What causes cataracts?

The lens lies behind the iris and the pupil. It works much like a camera lens. It focuses light onto the retina at the back of the eye, where an image is recorded. The lens also adjusts the eye's focus, letting us see things clearly both up close and far away. The lens is made of mostly water and protein. The protein is arranged in a precise way that keeps the lens clear and lets light pass through it.

But as we age, some of the protein may clump together and start to cloud a small area of the lens. This is a cataract. Over time, the cataract may grow larger and cloud more of the lens, making it harder to see.

Researchers suspect that there are several causes of cataract, such as smoking and diabetes. Or, it may be that the protein in the lens just changes from the wear and tear it takes over the years.

How can cataracts affect my vision?

Age-related cataracts can affect your vision in two ways:

- Clumps of protein reduce the sharpness of the image reaching the retina. The lens consists mostly of water and protein. When the protein clumps up, it clouds the lens and reduces the light that reaches the retina. The clouding may become severe enough to cause blurred vision. Most age-related cataracts develop from protein clumpings. When a cataract is small, the cloudiness affects only a small part of the lens. You may not notice any changes in your vision. Cataracts tend to "grow" slowly, so vision gets worse gradually. Over time, the cloudy area in the lens may get larger, and the cataract may increase in size. Seeing may become more difficult. Your vision may get duller or blurrier.

- The clear lens slowly changes to a yellowish/brownish color, adding a brownish tint to vision. As the clear lens slowly colors with age, your vision gradually may acquire a brownish shade. At first, the amount of tinting may be small and may not cause a vision problem. Over time, increased tinting may make it more difficult to read and perform other routine activities. This gradual change in the amount of tinting does not affect the sharpness of the image transmitted to the retina. If you have advanced lens discoloration, you may not be able to identify blues and purples. You may be wearing what you believe to be a pair of black socks, only to find out from friends that you are wearing purple socks.

Who is at risk for cataract?

The risk of cataract increases as you get older. Other risk factors for cataract include the following:

- Certain diseases such as diabetes.
- Personal behavior such as smoking and alcohol use.
- The environment, such as prolonged exposure to sunlight.

Symptoms and Detection

What are the symptoms of a cataract?

The most common symptoms of a cataract are as follows:

- Cloudy or blurry vision.
- Colors seem faded.
- Glare. Headlights, lamps, or sunlight may appear too bright. A halo may appear around lights.
- Poor night vision.
- Double vision or multiple images in one eye. (This symptom may clear as the cataract gets larger.)
- Frequent prescription changes in your eyeglasses or contact lenses.

These symptoms also can be a sign of other eye problems. If you have any of these symptoms, check with your eye care professional.

How is a cataract detected?

Cataract is detected through a comprehensive eye exam that includes the following:

- **Visual acuity test:** This eye chart test measures how well you see at various distances.
- **Dilated eye exam:** Drops are placed in your eyes to widen, or dilate, the pupils. Your eye care professional uses a special magnifying lens to examine your retina and optic nerve for signs of damage and other eye problems. After the exam, your close-up vision may remain blurred for several hours.
- **Tonometry:** An instrument measures the pressure inside the eye. Numbing drops may be applied to your eye for this test.

Your eye care professional also may do other tests to learn more about the structure and health of your eye.

Treatment

How is a cataract treated?

The symptoms of early cataract may be improved with new eyeglasses, brighter lighting, anti-glare sunglasses, or magnifying lenses. If these measures do not help, surgery is the only effective treatment. Surgery involves removing the cloudy lens and replacing it with an artificial lens.

A cataract needs to be removed only when vision loss interferes with your everyday activities, such as driving, reading, or watching TV. You and your eye care professional can make this decision together. Once you understand the benefits and risks of surgery, you can make an informed decision about whether cataract surgery is right for you. In most cases, delaying cataract surgery will not cause long-term damage to your eye or make the surgery more difficult. You do not have to rush into surgery.

Sometimes a cataract should be removed even if it does not cause problems with your vision. For example, a cataract should be removed if it prevents examination or treatment of another eye problem, such as age-related macular degeneration or diabetic retinopathy. If your eye care professional finds a cataract, you may not need cataract surgery for several years. In fact, you might never need cataract surgery. By having your vision tested regularly, you and your eye care professional can discuss if and when you might need treatment.

If you choose surgery, your eye care professional may refer you to a specialist to remove the cataract.

If you have cataracts in both eyes that require surgery, the surgery will be performed on each eye at separate times, usually four to eight weeks apart.

Many people who need cataract surgery also have other eye conditions, such as age-related macular degeneration or glaucoma. If you have other eye conditions in addition to cataract, talk with your doctor. Learn about the risks, benefits, alternatives, and expected results of cataract surgery.

What are the different types of cataract surgery?

There are two types of cataract surgery. Your doctor can explain the differences and help determine which is better for you:

- **Phacoemulsification, or phaco:** A small incision is made on the side of the cornea, the clear, dome-shaped surface that covers the front of the eye. Your doctor inserts a tiny probe into the eye. This device emits ultrasound waves that soften and break up the lens so that it can be removed by suction. Most cataract surgery today is done by phacoemulsification, also called "small incision cataract surgery."

- **Extracapsular surgery:** Your doctor makes a longer incision on the side of the cornea and removes the cloudy core of the lens in one piece. The rest of the lens is removed by suction.

After the natural lens has been removed, it often is replaced by an artificial lens, called an intraocular lens (IOL). An IOL is a clear, plastic lens that requires no care and becomes a permanent part of your eye. Light is focused clearly by the IOL onto the retina, improving your vision. You will not feel or see the new lens.

Some people cannot have an IOL. They may have another eye disease or have problems during surgery. For these patients, a soft contact lens, or glasses that provide high magnification, may be suggested.

What are the risks of cataract surgery?

As with any surgery, cataract surgery poses risks, such as infection and bleeding. Before cataract surgery, your doctor may ask you to temporarily stop taking certain medications that increase the risk of bleeding during surgery. After surgery, you must keep your eye clean, wash your hands before touching your eye, and use the prescribed medications to help minimize the risk of infection. Serious infection can result in loss of vision.

Cataract surgery slightly increases your risk of retinal detachment. Other eye disorders, such as high myopia (nearsightedness), can further increase your risk of retinal detachment after cataract surgery. One sign of a retinal detachment is a sudden increase in flashes or floaters. Floaters are little "cobwebs" or specks that seem to float about in your field of vision. If you notice a sudden increase in floaters or flashes, see an eye care professional immediately. A retinal detachment is a medical emergency. If necessary, go to an emergency service or hospital. Your eye must be examined by an eye surgeon as soon as possible. A retinal detachment causes no pain. Early treatment for retinal detachment often can prevent permanent loss of vision. The sooner you get treatment, the more likely you will regain good vision. Even if you are treated promptly, some vision may be lost.

Talk to your eye care professional about these risks. Make sure cataract surgery is right for you.

Is cataract surgery effective?

Cataract removal is one of the most common operations performed in the United States. It also is one of the safest and most effective types of surgery. In about 90 percent of cases, people who have cataract surgery have better vision afterward.

What happens before surgery?

A week or two before surgery, your doctor will do some tests. These tests may include measuring the curve of the cornea and the size and shape of your eye. This information helps your doctor choose the right type of IOL.

You may be asked not to eat or drink anything twelve hours before your surgery.

What happens during surgery?

At the hospital or eye clinic, drops will be put into your eye to dilate the pupil. The area around your eye will be washed and cleansed.

The operation usually lasts less than one hour and is almost painless. Many people choose to stay awake during surgery. Others may need to be put to sleep for a short time.

If you are awake, you will have an anesthetic to numb the nerves in and around your eye.

After the operation, a patch may be placed over your eye. You will rest for a while. Your medical team will watch for any problems, such as bleeding. Most people who have cataract surgery can go home the same day. You will need someone to drive you home.

What happens after surgery?

Itching and mild discomfort are normal after cataract surgery. Some fluid discharge is also common. Your eye may be sensitive to light and touch. If you have discomfort, your doctor can suggest treatment. After one or two days, moderate discomfort should disappear.

For a few days after surgery, your doctor may ask you to use eye drops to help healing and decrease the risk of infection. Ask your doctor about how to use your eye drops, how often to use them, and what effects they can have. You will need to wear an eye shield or eyeglasses to help protect your eye. Avoid rubbing or pressing on your eye.

When you are home, try not to bend from the waist to pick up objects on the floor. Do not lift any heavy objects. You can walk, climb stairs, and do light household chores.

In most cases, healing will be complete within eight weeks. Your doctor will schedule exams to check on your progress.

Can problems develop after surgery?

Problems after surgery are rare, but they can occur. These problems can include infection, bleeding, inflammation (pain, redness, swelling), loss of vision, double vision, and high or low eye pressure. With prompt medical attention, these problems can usually be treated successfully.

Sometimes the eye tissue that encloses the IOL becomes cloudy and may blur your vision. This condition is called an after-cataract. An after-cataract can develop months or years after cataract surgery.

An after-cataract is treated with a laser. Your doctor uses a laser to make a tiny hole in the eye tissue behind the lens to let light pass through. This outpatient procedure is called an yttrium aluminum garnet (YAG) laser capsulotomy. It is painless and rarely results in increased eye pressure or other eye problems. As a precaution, your doctor may give you eye drops to lower your eye pressure before or after the procedure.

When will my vision be normal again?

You can return quickly to many everyday activities, but your vision may be blurry. The healing eye needs time to adjust so that it can focus properly with the other eye, especially if the other eye has a cataract. Ask your doctor when you can resume driving.

If you received an IOL, you may notice that colors are very bright. The IOL is clear, unlike your natural lens that may have had a yellowish/brownish tint. Within a few months after receiving an IOL, you will become used to improved color vision. Also, when your eye heals, you may need new glasses or contact lenses.

What can I do if I already have lost some vision from cataract?

If you have lost some sight from cataract or cataract surgery, ask your eye care professional about low vision services and devices that may help you make the most of your remaining vision. Ask for a referral to a specialist in low vision. Many community organizations and agencies offer information about low vision counseling, training, and other special services for people with visual impairments. A nearby school of medicine or optometry may provide low vision services.

Section 19.2

New Cataract Early Detection Technique

"From Outer Space to the Eye Clinic: New Cataract Early Detection Technique," National Eye Institute National Institutes of Health, January 8, 2009.

A compact fiber-optic probe developed for the space program has now proven valuable for patients in the clinic as the first noninvasive early detection device for cataracts, the leading cause of vision loss worldwide.

Researchers from the National Eye Institute (NEI), part of the National Institutes of Health, and the National Aeronautics and Space Administration (NASA) collaborated to develop a simple, safe eye test for measuring a protein related to cataract formation. If subtle protein changes can be detected before a cataract develops, people may be able to reduce their cataract risk by making simple lifestyle changes, such as decreasing sun exposure, quitting smoking, stopping certain medications, and controlling diabetes.

"By the time the eye's lens appears cloudy from a cataract, it is too late to reverse or medically treat this process," said Manuel B. Datiles III, M.D., NEI medical officer and lead author of the clinical study. "This technology can detect the earliest damage to lens proteins, triggering an early warning for cataract formation and blindness."

The new device is based on a laser light technique called dynamic light scattering (DLS). It was initially developed to analyze the growth of protein crystals in a zero-gravity space environment. NASA's Rafat R. Ansari, Ph.D., senior scientist at the John H. Glenn Research Center and co-author of the study, brought the technology's possible clinical applications to the attention of NEI vision researchers when he learned that his father's cataracts were caused by changes in lens proteins.

Several proteins are involved in cataract formation, but one known as alpha-crystallin serves as the eye's own anti-cataract molecule. Alpha-crystallin binds to other proteins when they become damaged, thus preventing them from bunching together to form a cataract. However, humans are born with a fixed amount of alpha-crystallin, so if the supply becomes depleted due to radiation exposure, smoking, diabetes, or other causes, a cataract can result.

"We have shown that this noninvasive technology that was developed for the space program can now be used to look at the early signs of protein damage due to oxidative stress, a key process involved in many medical conditions, including age-related cataract and diabetes, as well as neurodegenerative diseases such as Alzheimer and Parkinson," said NASA's Dr. Ansari. "By understanding the role of protein changes in cataract formation, we can use the lens not just to look at eye disease, but also as a window into the whole body."

The recent NEI-NASA clinical trial, reported in the December 2008 *Archives of Ophthalmology*, looked at 380 eyes of people aged seven to eighty-six who had lenses ranging from clear to severe cloudiness from cataract. Researchers used the DLS device to shine a low-power laser light through the lenses. They had previously determined alpha-crystallin's light-scattering ability, which was then used to detect and measure the amount of alpha-crystallin in the lenses.

They found that as cloudiness increased, alpha-crystallin in the lenses decreased. Alpha-crystallin amounts also decreased as the participants' ages increased, even when the lenses were still transparent. These age-related, pre-cataract changes would remain undetected by currently available imaging tools.

"This research is a prime example of two government agencies sharing scientific information for the benefit of the American people," said NEI director Paul A. Sieving, M.D., Ph.D. "At an individual level, this device could be used to study the effectiveness of anti-cataract therapies or the tendency of certain medications to cause cataract formation."

The DLS technique will now assist vision scientists in looking at long-term lens changes due to aging, smoking, diabetes, LASIK surgery, eye drops for treating glaucoma, and surgical removal of the vitreous gel within the eye, a procedure known to cause cataracts within six months to one year. It may also help in the early diagnosis of Alzheimer disease, in which an abnormal protein may be found in the lens. In addition, NASA researchers will continue to use the device to look at the impact of long-term space travel on the visual system.

"During a three-year mission to Mars, astronauts will experience increased exposure to space radiation that can cause cataracts and other problems," Dr. Ansari explained. "In the absence of proper countermeasures, this may pose a risk for NASA. This technology could help us understand the mechanism for cataract formation so we can work to develop effective countermeasures to mitigate the risk and prevent it in astronauts."

Section 19.3

Reducing Risk of Cataract

Cataracts is a complex disease with many probable contributing factors even within a single individual. Identifying those factors and doing our best to control them may reduce our risk of developing the disease. That said, let's outline the known risk factors for cataracts and discuss how each of us can lower our risk.

Risk Factors

As with high blood pressure, asthma, arthritis, and most other chronic health conditions, some risk factors for cataracts are beyond our control. But specific behavioral and lifestyle choices we make, such as not smoking, do minimize our risk.

Nonmodifiable Risk Factors

Genetic variation: Nature is thought to have a hand in whether we develop cataracts. Studies of identical twins show that the genetic lotto determines perhaps half of our risk for cataracts. Environmental factors—that is, the modifiable risk factors outlined below—account for the rest.

Advancing age: As we age, the risk of cataract development inevitably increases. While we can't turn back the calendar pages, we can change how we age. A small but intriguing study found that elderly adults who reach age ninety with their mental faculties intact are less likely to have cataracts than their peers who show signs of mental decline.

The researchers propose that lack of cataract development might be a marker, or indicator, that a person has aged well in general. This idea seems to have been confirmed by an Australian study reporting that those with cataracts have a higher rate of hearing loss and by other studies that have noted increased mortality among those with cataracts. Make no mistake—having cataracts doesn't cause mortality. It simply may be a red flag that indicates more widespread tissue damage in the body.

Ethnicity: Some evidence suggests that our ethnic ancestry influences the likelihood of developing cataracts. In fact, cataracts is the leading cause of treatable vision loss among black Americans age forty and over, and it's the number one cause of low vision among Americans of Latino, African, and European descent.

Female gender: For reasons that remain murky, women are more likely than men to develop certain types of cataracts. According to the National Eye Institute, women also have greater difficulty getting the care they need due to lack of access transportation and other problems that affect women disproportionately.

Modifiable or Partially Modifiable Risk Factors

Excessive sunlight exposure: A higher level of exposure to ultraviolet radiation from the sun's rays is thought to make cataract development more likely. One published case report, for example, concludes that working at altitudes above the protective ozone layer puts airline pilots at increased risk of cataracts. Newer studies have not confirmed such an association, and research is under way to prove or disprove the link.

Having diabetes: According to the American Diabetes Association, people with diabetes are 60 percent more likely than those without diabetes to develop cataracts. The condition tends to have an earlier onset and to progress more rapidly than in people with cataracts who do not have diabetes. People with diabetes are also at higher risk for treatment-related complications.

The National Institutes of Health (NIH) tracks statistics on the number of Americans with cataracts. The average prevalence for people age sixty-five and over is 118 people with cataracts per 1,000 population. However, the rate for those without diabetes is 107 per 1,000, while the rate among those with diabetes jumps to 182 per 1,000. The risk of onset and progression of cataracts correlates with the duration and severity of diabetes.

Poor nutrition: Although further study is needed, vision researchers believe that a diet high in saturated fat and refined carbohydrates may be linked to the development of cataracts. They're also investigating the possibility that low blood calcium levels may contribute to cataract development. A recent study shows that nutrient deficiencies are especially likely to contribute to the development of nuclear cataracts—that is, a cataract in the center, or nucleus, of the eye. This kind of cataract is especially detrimental to vision and is the most common form of the disease.

Another study reports that a high intake of vitamin E and the antioxidants lutein and zeaxanthin, found in dark leafy greens like spinach and kale, is associated with a significantly decreased risk of cataracts.

Smoking: Although scientists don't understand exactly how smoking promotes the cataract formation, there is a clear correlation between the two. The relationship is dose related, so heavy smokers have a higher risk than those who smoke less. Researchers are beginning to investigate whether environmental tobacco smoke (secondhand smoke) is a risk factor as well.

Alcohol abuse: A higher incidence of cataracts has been found among people who chronically abuse alcohol. Having more than one drink per day also increases the risk of complications associated with cataract surgery.

Researchers have proposed several other factors that may increase the risk of cataracts, such as a family history of the disease, myopia (nearsightedness), obesity, and high blood pressure.

Risk Reduction

As you reviewed the list of modifiable risk factors for cataracts, did you notice a theme? Hard living is hazardous to your health. Moderation is the key. Here are some guidelines to keep in mind:

- **Limit your sunlight exposure:** The long-held belief that exposure to ultraviolet radiation contributes to the development of cataracts has been called into question by recent research. Until more studies can be carried out, it's best to limit your exposure to bright sunlight and to wear sunglasses with UV-filtering lenses or a hat with a brim when you must be in the sun.

- **Tightly control your blood sugar if you have diabetes:** In addition to following general recommendations for a healthy, active lifestyle, tightly controlling your blood sugar will reduce your risk of the onset and progression of cataracts.

- **Follow a healthy diet:** New research shows that a diet containing adequate amounts of protein, vitamin A, thiamin (vitamin B1), riboflavin (vitamin B2), and niacin (vitamin B3) may help protect your eyes against development of nuclear cataracts. The B vitamins are found in whole, unprocessed foods such as beans, potatoes, meat, turkey, molasses, and bananas. Unfiltered beer is an unexpectedly rich source of B vitamins because it contains brewer's yeast, which has a high content of B1, B2, B3, and other B vitamins. Even so, you should drink beer and other alcoholic beverages only in moderation.

- **Stop smoking or don't start:** Smoking is so closely linked with eventual cataract development that the surgeon general's warning label on cigarette packages now includes cataracts. (So many diseases are caused by smoking, though, that they can't all be printed on a single package, so the list rotates.) The good news is that the threat of cataracts and other grim diseases recedes when you quit smoking. The risk continues to drop the longer you remain smoke-free.

- **Use alcohol only in moderation:** You should limit your intake to no more than one drink a day for women or no more than two drinks a day for men.

Section 19.4

Cataract Surgery

"Guide to Cataract Surgery," © 2011 Prevent Blindness America
(www.preventblindness.org). Reprinted with permission.

According to Prevent Blindness America's Vision Problems in the U.S. report, nearly 20.5 million Americans age forty and older have cataracts. By age eighty, more than half of all Americans will have a cataract. Every year in the United States, more than one million cataract surgeries are performed. Cataract surgeries are performed without complication in 95 percent of cases.

Why Do Cataracts Form?

Cataracts are probably caused by changes related to aging. Throughout our lives, our bodies replace old cells with new ones. As we grow older, the old cells in our eye's lens build up and block light as it tries to pass through. The end result is cloudy vision.

Besides getting older, other factors may cause cataracts to form. Eye infections, some medicines (such as steroids), injuries, or exposure to intense heat or radiation may cause cataracts. Too much exposure to nonvisible sunlight (called UV or ultraviolet light) and various diseases, such as diabetes or metabolic disorders, may also contribute to cataracts forming.

What Are the Types of Cataracts?

- **Age-related:** Ninety-five percent of cataracts are age-related, usually after age forty.

- **Congenital:** These are present at birth, usually caused by infection or inflammation during pregnancy; possibly inherited.

- **Traumatic:** Lens damage from a hard blow, cut, puncture, intense heat, or chemical burn may cause cataracts.

- **Secondary:** Some medicines, eye disease, eye infection, or diseases such as diabetes cause these cataracts.

How Can the Eye Doctor Tell If I Have a Cataract?

Everyone who gets a cataract experiences it differently. But a person with a cataract commonly experiences cloudy or blurry vision. Lights may cause a glare, seem too dim, or seem too bright. It may be hard to read or drive, especially at night. If you have a cataract, you may see halos around lights, such as car headlights, that make it hard to focus clearly. Colors may not seem as bright as they used to be. Or you may have to change your eyeglass prescription often.

To find out if you have cataracts, your eye doctor will want to:

- find out your general medical history;
- find out your specific eye history, including problems and symptoms;
- test your vision (visual acuity);
- test your side vision (peripheral vision);
- test your eye movement;
- test you for glaucoma (by measuring the eye's internal pressure);
- do a microscopic exam of the front of the eye (using something called a slit lamp) to assess the density of the cataract and how it interferes with light passing through the lens;
- widen (dilate) the pupils of your eyes to examine the retina, the optic nerve (which carries visual messages from the retina to the brain), and the macula (responsible for the best part of central vision);
- test you to see how glare affects your vision.

Should I Have Cataract Surgery?

You must decide whether to have cataract surgery. Cataracts will not cause large vision changes for some people. A cataract at the outer edge of your lens, for example, may hardly affect your vision. A cataract at the center of your lens, however, may greatly affect your sight. Only you can decide if a change in your vision keeps you from doing all the things you want or need to do.

Note: If a cataract keeps your eye doctor from viewing the inside of your eye, he or she may suggest surgery.

When Can I Avoid Cataract Surgery?

Prevent Blindness America recommends that individuals do not have cataract surgery if:

- cataracts have not affected your lifestyle or kept you from doing all the things you want and need to do;

- your vision will not improve with surgery because of other eye problems;

- glasses or contact lenses can provide satisfactory vision;

- you are not well enough/fit enough for the surgery;

- you do not want surgery.

What Kind of Lens Will Replace My Cataract Lens?

When the eye surgeon removes the lens with the cataract, you will need something to replace it, so that you can focus and see clearly. You have three choices to replace your own lens:

- Intraocular lenses (IOLs)

- Contact lenses

- Cataract glasses

Intraocular Lenses

Intraocular lenses (IOLs) replace your cataract, or cloudy lens. If you have certain eye diseases or problems which prevent safe placement of an IOL, you will need either contact lenses or cataract glasses in order to see clearly after surgery.

IOLs have become the most popular choice for replacing lenses with cataracts. Unlike contact lenses, these lenses are implanted inside the eye and are meant to be permanent. They do not require replacement or cleaning. The eye surgeon implants the IOL in about the same place as your natural lens, so that it results in the most natural vision.

IOLs are the best option to replace your own lenses. However if you have certain other eye diseases or problems, you may not be able to have lens implants. You and your eye doctor will need to discuss whether any restrictions apply.

Contact Lenses

If you are unable to have an IOL implant, you may opt to wear contact lenses after cataract surgery. By wearing a contact lens on your operated eye, you will be able to see about as well as you did before the cataract developed. These lenses cannot cure all your vision problems. You may still need glasses for close-up work.

There are two types of contact lenses: daily-wear and extended-wear. You must remove daily-wear contact lenses before you go to sleep. You can wear extended-wear contact lenses for longer periods of time. Extended-wear contact lenses are usually prescribed for people who would have trouble inserting and removing daily wear contacts (for example, people with severe arthritis).

Cataract Glasses

Cataract glasses may be an option if you cannot have an IOL implant or if you cannot wear contact lenses. Cataract glasses are also safe and relatively inexpensive, but they may take some getting used to after surgery. The lenses in cataract glasses are different from regular eyeglasses, so you will see things in a different way. Objects will look larger (by about 25 percent) and may seem to appear suddenly in your side vision (peripheral field of vision). Vertical lines may appear curved, and it may be hard to judge distances.

If you have cataracts in both eyes but only have surgery in one eye, your eyes won't be able to work together when you wear cataract glasses after surgery. The glasses lens for your operated eye makes things appear larger while your other eye will view images as they truly are. Your brain won't be able to put the two images together for normal (binocular) vision. You will have this condition, called monocular aphakia (one eye without a lens), until after your second cataract operation.

Choosing an Eye Surgeon

Once you decide to have cataract surgery, you'll need to choose an eye surgeon to perform the operation. Some things to keep in mind are the surgeon's experience and skill, how easy it is to talk to him or her and have your questions answered, and your previous experience with this eye doctor, if any.

Referrals may help you choose an eye surgeon. Ask friends who have had cataract surgery or contact a university with a medical school or a hospital for names and references.

If an eye doctor has recommended surgery, you may want to get a second opinion. Make an appointment to see an eye doctor who does not work with, and was not referred by, your regular doctor. You do not have to tell this doctor that someone else has already recommended surgery—let this doctor come to his or her own conclusions about whether you need cataract surgery.

Here are some points you may want to bring up with your doctor. Check the questions you'd like your eye doctor to answer during your next appointment or conversation:

- Do I really need surgery? What will I gain by having it?

- What are the risks?

- What is surgery like? Will it hurt? What will I see?

- Will any other problems like glaucoma or diabetes affect my cataracts or my surgery?

- How long will I need to recover from the surgery?

- Will I need glasses after surgery? If I wear contacts, can I wear them again after surgery?

- Are there some things I won't be able to do after surgery? If so, for how long?

- Will someone have to take care of me after surgery? If so, for how long?

- Will the medicines I take for other illnesses interfere with surgery or my recovery?

- How experienced is the doctor? Is he or she board certified?

- Is a payment plan available?

Getting Ready for Surgery

On the day of your surgery, or a few days ahead of time, you may need to see your primary care doctor for a few tests. Because you will be given some form of anesthesia, your doctor will probably ask you not to eat or drink anything after midnight the day before your surgery. If you take medicines or have diabetes, ask your doctor whether different guidelines apply.

Removing the cataract and inserting an intraocular lens usually takes the surgeon ten to fifteen minutes. The entire process, from arriving at the hospital or surgical center to going home, takes about half a day. Less than 1 percent of surgeries require an overnight hospital stay.

On the day of your surgery, you will be given some eye drops to widen (dilate) your pupils. You may also be given a mild sedative to help you relax. A healthcare worker will take you into the operating room where an anesthesiologist or nurse anesthetist will give you a local or an intravenous anesthetic. He or she will monitor your condition.

You will not feel the surgery because the topical anesthetic numbs your eye during the operation. You may see some lights or vague shapes, but that is all.

Your surgeon will use a special microscope, which magnifies and illuminates the area of the procedure as he or she removes your cataract.

You may not remember much about the operation after it is over. You may feel a little drowsy afterward, but as the sedative wears off, you will be encouraged to walk around a bit. Your doctor will monitor your condition for a while, explain how to care for your eye at home, and schedule a follow-up appointment.

Once you're fully recovered, you will be allowed to go home. It is a good idea to have a friend or relative drive you. You may feel tired after surgery, so try to relax the rest of the day.

At home, you should not experience much discomfort. Some people describe the feeling as having an eyelash or a cinder in their eye— slightly uncomfortable but not painful. You will apply eye drops or ointment as your doctor prescribes, and you will learn to rely on your untreated eye during this time.

Three Kinds of Cataract Removal

During the cataract operation, your surgeon will first remove the clouded lens. (If you are able to have a lens implant, your doctor will perform this procedure right after removing your cataract lens.) There are three methods for removing the clouded lens:

- Phacoemulsification

- Extracapsular

- Intracapsular

Phacoemulsification

The most common procedure, phacoemulsification requires a smaller incision in the cornea or, less commonly, the sclera. The surgeon uses sound waves (an ultrasonic device) to break the lens into small pieces, and then suctions the tiny pieces out through the same incision.

Next, the doctor will insert the lens into place. Again, the capsular bag will remain to strengthen the eye and to preserve normal architecture. Most IOLs are foldable, so they can be inserted through the same small incision. The lens usually unfolds slowly once it is placed into the capsular bag. The incision can be closed with either one stitch, or usually none at all.

Phacoemulsification, with its smaller incision, offers the fastest healing and recovery time, produces little discomfort, and reduces the chance of uneven focus (astigmatism) or distorted vision.

Extracapsular and Intracapsular

Less common are the extracapsular and intracapsular procedures. An extracapsular cataract extraction may be needed if your lens is too hard to phacoemalsify. The extracapsular procedure removes only the inside of the lens but leaves the capsular bag that holds the lens in place. Leaving the capsular bag adds to the structural strength of the eye and promotes easier healing.

During the intracapsular procedure, your eye surgeon removes the lens and the entire capsular bag that holds it. Your doctor will make an incision in the sclera, use a special tool to freeze the lens, and then remove it through the incision. He or she may then implant the IOL in front of the iris, where its loops hold it in place. Another option is to suture the IOL to the wall of the eye. This latter option enables the IOL to be placed behind the iris.

Cost of Surgery

Basic charges you can expect for cataract surgery include fees for the hospital/surgical center, the doctor, the anesthesiologist, basic tests before surgery, medicine after surgery, and follow-up visits with your doctor. Ask your doctor to estimate each of the costs. You may also need new glasses or contact lenses after surgery.

If you have private health insurance or Medicare, it will usually pay for a part of most costs. Try to find out what your health insurance will cover before the surgery. Extra insurance (secondary supplemental insurance) also may cover 80 percent of the amounts not covered by your primary insurance. You may have to pay 20 percent of the balance. Ask your doctor about his or her billing and payment methods. Newer "bifocal" IOLs are not usually covered by insurance.

Some hospitals and surgical centers may be able to help you with financial planning. This may include putting together a payment plan or filing claims to your insurance company. Filling out insurance forms can be hard—so be sure to ask questions ahead of time.

Possible Complications from Surgery

Less than 5 percent of patients experience complications from cataract surgery, but you should discuss possible problems with your doctor.

Here are three areas of complications:

- Problems during surgery, called operative complications, such as severe bleeding, happen to less than 1 percent of patients. Up to 2 percent of patients lose the gel-like substance that fills the inside of the eye (vitreous humor) during surgery. Complication rates may be higher if you have certain medical or ocular diseases.

- Problems soon after surgery, called early postoperative complications, can include leaking from the wound, bleeding, or infections.

- Problems after healing, called late postoperative complications, include retinal detachment (this requires surgery to correct but happens in about one out of every one hundred patients), swelling of the cornea, or swelling of the retina (called cystoid macular edema). Infection is a rare complication. This happens in fewer than one in every one thousand patients, but it may cause severe vision loss.

Remember, the risk of severe problems or blindness from cataract surgery is very low. Still, it may ease your mind to talk about your concerns with your doctor before surgery.

Sometimes after the extracapsular or phacoemulsification procedure, the capsular bag that remains in your eye can become cloudy. This is called an after cataract or posterior capsular opacification. If this happens, your doctor may suggest laser surgery to make a tiny hole through the cloudy lens capsule. This hole will let you see clearly again.

Your Recovery

After surgery, most of the healing takes place in the first few days. But it may take up to one month for your eye to fully heal. For the first week or two, or as your doctor recommends, you should minimize vigorous physical activity. You should restrict any lifting or deep bending, which causes increased eye pressure. If you experience severe pain, loss of vision, or a sudden increase in redness or swelling of your operated eye, call your eye doctor right away.

Other Do's and Don'ts

- Do use your medication as directed.
- Do sit down and lift your feet to put on your shoes.
- Do try to sleep on your back or on the unoperated side.

- Do have someone else drive while your eye is healing.
- Do wear sunglasses in bright light.
- Do keep follow-up appointments with your doctor.
- Do keep moderately active.
- Don't rub or press your eye.
- Don't bend over to pick things up; kneel instead.
- Don't get soap, shampoo, or other irritants in your eye.

Take Care of Your Eye

Here are some pointers that can help you recover more quickly.

Applying Eye Medications

Use the eye drops or ointment that your doctor prescribed to help your eye heal. This medicine protects against infection and helps decrease swelling.

How to Apply Eye Drops or Ointment

Tilt your head back. Pull your lower eyelid down to create a "cup" that holds the drops or ointment. Put in the prescribed amount of medicine and close your eye to distribute it evenly. If you have trouble doing this, ask a friend or relative for help. Start with a fresh bottle of medicine after surgery so germs don't get transferred.

Eye Shields

Your doctor may want you to use an eye shield at night to protect your eye while you sleep.

Follow-Up Care

Your doctor will suggest a schedule for follow-up visits. The first one will be the day after your surgery. It is important to keep these appointments to find out whether your eye is healing well. These visits will also let you ask your doctor any questions you have about medicine or your activities (such as heavy lifting or exercising).

Chapter 20

Other Corneal Disorders

Section 20.1

Bullous Keratopathy

Bullous keratopathy is a condition in which the cornea becomes permanently swollen. This occurs because the inner layer of the cornea, the endothelium, has been damaged and is not pumping fluid properly. The cause of the endothelial damage could be from trauma, glaucoma, or inflammation after eye surgery. Endothelial keratoplasty (EK) is the recommended treatment for bullous keratopathy.

Certain intraocular lens implant designs can damage the cornea. Sometimes it is helpful to replace a lens implant with a newer design when a transplant is being performed to prevent damage to the transplant.

The causes of bullous keratopathy have changed over the last two decades. Twenty years ago, the most common reason for bullous keratopathy was complications from cataract surgery with or without problems from intraocular lenses. Over the past twenty years, cataract surgery techniques and intraocular lens implants have improved dramatically. Now, corneal problems are less common after cataract surgery. Currently, one of the most common reasons for developing bullous keratopathy, or secondary corneal decompensation, is from problems related to glaucoma surgery.

Glaucoma surgery can lead to corneal failure because of direct damage to the cornea either during surgery or in the immediate postoperative period. Often this is from the cornea coming into contact with the other structures in the eye like the iris or lens. Another association between glaucoma and bullous keratopathy is that sometimes the cornea can decompensate after a laser treatment is performed to treat acute angle closure glaucoma. In acute angle closure glaucoma, the iris blocks the normal flow of eye fluid from the area where it is produced behind the iris to the trabecular meshwork in front of the iris, where the fluid drains from the eye. The treatment for acute angle closure glaucoma is to make a hole in the peripheral iris so the fluid can bypass the areas of blockage. Typically if a drainage hole is made in the iris before acute angle closure happens, it does not cause corneal problems. However, when the drainage hole (called an iridotomy) has to be made after the eye is inflamed from the onset of acute angle closure, there can be secondary decompensation of the cornea either immediately or even years later. This is particularly a problem in Asian eyes, where the space between the iris and cornea is often smaller. Being farsighted (hyperopia) can be a risk factor for this type of glaucoma.

Section 20.2

Cogan Dystrophy (Map-Dot-Fingerprint Dystrophy)

"Cogan's Dystrophy (Map-Dot-Fingerprint Dystrophy)," © 2011 St. Luke's Cataract and Laser Institute (www.stlukeseye.com). All rights reserved. Reprinted with permission.

Overview

Cogan dystrophy is a disease that affects the cornea. It is commonly called map-dot-fingerprint dystrophy because of microscopic dot and fingerprint-like patterns that form within the layers of the cornea.

The cornea is comprised of five layers. Cogan affects the superficial cornea layer called the epithelium. The epithelium's bottom or basement layer of cells becomes thickened and uneven. This weakens the bond between the cells and sometimes causes the epithelium to become loosened and slough off in areas. This problem is called corneal erosion.

Even though this disease is commonly known as a dystrophy (a term that describes genetic diseases), Cogan is not necessarily an inherited problem. It often affects both eyes and is typically diagnosed after the age of thirty. Cogan usually becomes progressively worse with age.

Signs and Symptoms

Some patients with Cogan dystrophy have no symptoms at all. The symptoms among patients may vary widely in severity and include:

- light sensitivity;

- glare;

- fluctuating vision;

- blurred vision;

- irregular astigmatism (uneven corneal surface);

- mild to extreme irritation and discomfort that is worse in the morning.

Detection and Diagnosis

The doctor examines the layers of the cornea with a slit lamp microscope. In some cases, corneal topography may be needed to evaluate and monitor astigmatism resulting from the disease.

Treatment

The treatment for Cogan is dependent on the severity of the problem. The first step is to lubricate the cornea with artificial tears to keep the surface smooth and comfortable. Lubricating ointments are recommended at bedtime so the eyes are more comfortable in the morning. Salt solution drops or ointments such as sodium chloride are often prescribed to reduce swelling and improve vision. Gas-permeable contacts are occasionally fit for patients with irregular astigmatism to create a smooth, even corneal surface and improve vision.

For patients with recurrent corneal erosion, soft, bandage contact lenses may be used to keep the eye comfortable and allow the cornea to heal. In some cases, laser treatment may beneficial. The surgeon removes the epithelium with an excimer laser, creating a regular, smooth surface. The epithelium quickly regenerates, usually within a matter of days, forming a better bond with the underlying cell layer.

Section 20.3

Corneal Abrasions

What is the cornea?

The cornea is the clear front window of the eye. It covers the colored portion of the eye, much like a watch crystal covers the face of a watch. The cornea is composed of five layers. The outermost layer is called the epithelium.

What is a corneal abrasion?

A corneal abrasion is an injury to the epithelium. Abrasions are painful. Common causes of corneal abrasions include problems from contact lenses, fingernails, paper cuts, tree or bush limbs, or rubbing of the eye. There are some eye conditions, such as dry eye, that may make injury more likely.

The corneal surface usually heals within a day or two, but the eye may be very uncomfortable while it is healing. Tearing, light sensitivity, and the feeling that something is in the eye—"foreign body sensation"—will accompany even a small abrasion.

How are abrasions treated?

A common treatment is to patch the scratched eye, thus preventing the blinking eyelid from moving over the healing area. Another common treatment is repeated application of ointment to the eye, which forms a soothing layer between the inner eyelid and the abrasion. Antibiotics are often used because of the small risk of infection. Sometimes a drop is used to dilate the pupil to help with pain associated with light sensitivity.

Even after the surface has healed, the cornea may still be sensitive to wind and dust. Often, additional lubrication is helpful, both during the day and at bedtime, until the sensitivity has disappeared. Some other diseases, such as dry eye or diabetes, may slow healing.

What is a corneal erosion?

A corneal erosion is a spontaneous breakdown of the epithelium, sometimes at the site of an earlier abrasion. The symptoms are similar to a corneal abrasion: foreign body sensation, tearing, and light sensitivity. These symptoms may vary, are often unpredictable, and may occur upon awakening. An erosion may occur when the eyes are dry or irritated.

How are corneal erosions treated?

Several treatments are used to alleviate the discomfort of erosions and to speed healing:

- lubricating drops and ointments;
- drops or ointments containing salt;
- a special contact lens used to bandage the cornea;
- micro-puncture of the epithelium;
- removal of the damaged epithelium.

Recurrent corneal erosions can be stubborn and frustrating. Your eye doctor may be able to identify other contributing factors. Your attention to extra lubrication for the cornea is often the key to ending the erosion cycle.

Section 20.4

Corneal Ulcers and Infections

Excerpted from "Corneal Ulcers and Infections,"
© 2011 A.D.A.M., Inc. Reprinted with permission.

The cornea is the clear (transparent) tissue at the front of the eye. A corneal ulcer is an erosion or open sore in the outer layer of the cornea. It is often caused by infection.

Causes

Corneal ulcers are most commonly caused by an infection with bacteria, viruses, fungi, or a parasite:

- Acanthamoeba keratitis occurs in contact lens users, especially in people who make their own homemade cleaning solutions.

- Fungal keratitis can occur after a corneal injury involving plant material, or in people with a suppressed immune system.

- Herpes simplex keratitis is a serious viral infection. It may cause repeated attacks that are triggered by stress, exposure to sunlight, or any condition that impairs the immune system.

Corneal ulcers or infections may also be caused by:

- eyelids that do not close all the way, such as with Bell palsy;

- foreign bodies in the eye;

- scratches (abrasions) on the eye surface;

- severely dry eyes;

- severe allergic eye disease;

- various inflammatory disorders.

Contact lens wear, especially soft contact lenses worn overnight, may cause a corneal ulcer.

Symptoms

Symptoms of infection or ulcers of the cornea include:

- blurry or hazy vision;
- eye that appears red or bloodshot;
- itching and discharge;
- sensitivity to light (photophobia);
- very painful and watery eyes;
- white patch on the cornea (with herpes).

Exams and Tests

- Examination of scrapings from the ulcer
- Fluorescein stain of the cornea
- Keratometry (measurement of the corneal curvature)
- Pupillary reflex response
- Refraction test
- Slit-lamp examination
- Tests for dry eye
- Visual acuity

Blood tests to check for inflammatory disorders may also be needed.

Treatment

Treatment for corneal ulcers and infections depends on the cause. Treatment should be started as soon as possible to prevent scarring of the cornea.

If the exact cause is not known, patients may start treatment with antibiotic drops that work against many kinds of bacteria.

Once the exact cause is known, drops that treat bacteria, herpes, other viruses, or a fungus are prescribed.

Corticosteroid eye drops may be used to reduce swelling and inflammation in certain conditions.

Your doctor may also recommend that you:

- avoid eye makeup;
- don't wear contact lenses at all, or don't wear them at night;

- take pain medications;
- wear an eye patch to keep light out and help with symptoms;
- wear protective glasses.

Severe ulcers may need to be treated with corneal transplantation.

Outlook (Prognosis)

Many people recover completely from corneal ulcers or infections, or they have only a minor change in vision.

However, a corneal ulcer or infection can cause long-term damage to the cornea and lead to a noticeable worsening of vision.

Possible Complications

Untreated corneal ulcers and infections may lead to:

- loss of the eye (rare);
- severe vision loss;
- scars on the cornea.

When to Contact a Medical Professional

Call your healthcare provider if:

- you have symptoms of corneal ulcers or an infection;
- you have been diagnosed with this condition and your symptoms become worse after treatment.

Prevention

Prompt, early attention by an ophthalmologist for an eye infection may prevent ulcers from forming. Wash hands and pay very close attention to cleanliness while handling contact lenses. Avoid wearing contact lenses overnight.

Alternative Names

Bacterial keratitis; fungal keratitis; acanthamoeba keratitis; herpes simplex keratitis

Section 20.5

Keratoconus

What Is Keratoconus?

Keratoconus, often abbreviated to "KC," is a non-inflammatory eye condition in which the normally round dome-shaped cornea progressively thins, causing a cone-like bulge to develop. This results in significant visual impairment.

Who Gets Keratoconus?

The actual incidence of KC is not known. It is not a common eye disease, but it is by no means rare. It has been estimated to occur in one out of every two thousand persons in the general population. Keratoconus is generally first diagnosed in young people at puberty or in their late teens. It is found in all parts of the United States and the rest of the world. It has no known significant geographic, cultural, or social pattern.

What Happens?

The cornea is the clear window of the eye and is responsible for refracting most of the light coming into the eye. Therefore, abnormalities of the cornea severely affect the way we see the world, making simple tasks, like driving, watching TV, or reading a book, difficult.

In its earliest stages, keratoconus causes slight blurring and distortion of vision and increased sensitivity to light. These symptoms usually first appear in the late teens and early twenties. Keratoconus may progress for ten to twenty years and then slow or stabilize. Each eye may be affected differently.

What Can Be Done about It?

In the early stages, eyeglasses or soft contact lenses may be used to correct the mild nearsightedness and astigmatism caused in the early stages of keratoconus. As the disorder progresses and the cornea continues to thin and change shape, rigid gas permeable (RGP) contact lenses are generally prescribed to correct vision more adequately. The contact lenses must be carefully fitted, and frequent checkups and lens changes may be needed to achieve and maintain good vision. Intacs, intracorneal rings, are sometimes used to improve contact lens fit.

Corneal cross-linking is a new treatment option under investigation to halt the progression of keratoconus.

In severe cases, a corneal transplant may be needed due to scarring, extreme thinning, or contact lens intolerance. This is a surgical procedure that replaces the keratoconus cornea with healthy donor tissue.

What Causes Keratoconus?

The exact cause of keratoconus is unknown. There are many theories based on research and its association with other conditions. However, no one theory explains it all and it may be caused by a combination of things.

It is believed that genetics, the environment, and the endocrine system all play a role in keratoconus.

Genetic

One scientific view is that keratoconus is developmental (i.e., genetic) in origin because in some cases there does appear to be a familial association. From the presently available information there is less than a one in ten chance that a blood relative of a keratoconic patient will have keratoconus. The majority of patients with keratoconus do not have other family members with the disease. Some studies show that keratoconus corneas lack important anchoring fibrils that structurally stabilize the anterior cornea. This increased flexibility allows that cornea to "bulge forward" into a cone-shaped appearance.

Environmental

Eye rubbing: Keratoconus corneas are more easily damaged by minor trauma such as eye rubbing. Poorly fit contact lenses (that rub against the irregularity of the KC cornea) have been suggested as a possible cause of keratoconus; this has not been proven and remains questionable.

Allergies: Many who have keratoconus report vigorous eye rubbing and also have allergies (which cause eye itching and irritation, leading to eye rubbing), however the link to allergic disease also remains unclear. A higher percentage of keratoconic patients have atopic disease than the general population. Disorders such as hay fever, eczema, asthma, and food allergies are all considered atopic diseases. Those with KC are advised to avoid eye rubbing as much as possible.

Oxidative stress: Some studies indicate an abnormal processing of the superoxide radicals in the keratoconus cornea and an involvement of oxidative stress in the pathogenesis of this disease. Keratoconus corneas lack the ability to self-repair routine damage easily repaired by normal corneas. Like any tissues in the body, the cornea creates harmful byproducts of cell metabolism called free radicals. Normal corneas, like any other body tissue, have a defense system in place to neutralize these free radicals so they don't damage the collagen, the structural part of the cornea, weakening it and causing the cornea to thin and bulge. The keratoconus corneas do not posses the ability to eliminate the free radicals, so they stay in the tissue and can cause structural damage.

Hormonal: Another hypothesis is that the endocrine system may be involved because keratoconus is generally first detected at puberty and progresses during pregnancy. This theory is still controversial and has not been proven.

Symptoms and Diagnosis

The earliest signs of keratoconus are usually blurring of vision and the need for frequent changes in eyeglass prescription, or blurred vision that cannot be corrected with glasses.

Symptoms of keratoconus generally begin in late teenage years or early twenties, but can start at any time. Other symptoms include:

- difficultly driving at night;
- halos and ghosting, especially at night;
- eye strain;
- headaches and general eye pain;
- eye irritation, excessive eye rubbing.

Keratoconus, especially in the early stages, can be difficult to diagnose, and all of the above symptoms could be associated with other eye problems. Simply recognizing symptoms does not by itself diagnose keratoconus. Keratoconus requires a diagnosis from a competent eye doctor who is trained in not only recognizing the symptoms but also observing signs of keratoconus through direct measurement as well as inspection of the cornea at a microscopic level using a slit lamp.

Always consult your medical doctor to confirm a diagnosis of keratoconus.

Diagnosis

Keratoconus can usually be diagnosed with a slit-lamp examination. The classic signs of keratoconus that the doctor will see when examining your eyes include:

- corneal thinning;
- Fleischer ring (an iron-colored ring surrounding the cone);
- Vogt striae (stress lines caused by corneal thinning);
- apical scarring (scarring at the apex of the cone).

The doctor will also measure the curvature of the cornea. This is done by:

- Keratometry, an instrument that shines a pattern of light onto the cornea. The shape of the reflection of the pattern tells the doctor how the eye is curved.
- Corneal topography, a computerized instrument that makes three-dimensional "maps" of the cornea.

Corneal topography has facilitated the diagnosis of keratoconus, helping establish the diagnosis earlier, follow progression more accurately, and differentiate keratoconus from other conditions.

Treatment Options Overview

Treatment options for keratoconus focus on correcting the distorted vision caused by the thinning and bulging of the cornea.

Eyeglasses or soft contact lenses may be used to correct the mild nearsightedness and astigmatism caused by keratoconus in its earliest stage, however at some point a rigid gas permeable (RGP) contact lens will correct KC vision better.

Rigid gas permeable contact lenses (abbreviated to RGP or GP) will correct vision as KC progresses. The rigid lens material enables the lens to vault over the cornea, replacing the cornea's irregular shape with a smooth, uniform refracting surface to improve vision.

Intacs plastic rings are inserted into the mid layer of the cornea to flatten it, changing the shape and location of the cone.

Corneal cross-linking (CXL) is a new treatment option in U.S. Food and Drug Administration (FDA) clinical trials in the United States. The goal of this procedure is to is to stop progression of the keratoconus.

Corneal transplant surgery is necessary in very advanced keratoconus due to scarring, extreme thinning, or contact lens intolerance.

Section 20.6

Pterygium

What is a pterygium?

Pterygium means "wing" and refers to a winglike growth that spreads over the cornea. Pterygia are more common in the tropics and are associated with early exposure to the sun (especially during childhood and teen years).

A pterygium may be confused with a pinguecula, a benign degeneration of the conjunctiva that does not extend over the cornea. A pinguecula is a yellowish patch or bump on the surface of the eye in a similar location. A pinguecula does not progressively grow. Both are caused by damage due to exposure to ultraviolet (UV) light (sun).

What is the cause of a pterygium?

The most likely cause is damage to the conjunctiva by the sun's ultraviolet rays. Pterygia usually grow over the edge of the cornea nearest the nose. Pterygia are not spread from person to person.

What are the effects of a pterygium?

Pterygia are usually small and have no harmful effects. They sometimes cause redness, burning, itching, and/or an unacceptable appearance. Larger pterygia can cause blurred vision by altering the shape of the cornea, producing astigmatism. Some pterygia grow over the center of the cornea, causing loss of vision.

How can a pterygium be treated?

Artificial tears usually relieve irritation and burning caused by pterygia. Anti-allergy drops or even anti-inflammatory drops may be used for more significant symptoms. If vision is affected or if the pterygia become large, surgical excision may be indicated. Methods to decrease recurrence rate include grafting of conjunctiva tissue from another part of the eye, anti-metabolite drugs, or even radiation. Regrowth of the pterygium is a common late complication.

How can a pterygium be prevented?

Prevention starts in childhood. Hats with brims are important to protect children's eyes. Sunglasses with UV protection are encouraged for children.

Chapter 21

Corneal Transplant

Chapter Contents

Section 21.1

All About Corneal Transplant

The cornea is the clear layer on the front of the eye. A corneal transplant is surgery to replace the cornea with tissue from a donor. It is one of the most common transplants done.

Description

You will probably be awake during the transplant. Local anesthesia (numbing medicine) will be injected around your eye to block pain and temporarily prevent eye muscle movement. You may receive a sedative to help you relax.

The tissue for your corneal transplant will come from a person (donor) who has recently died and who previously agreed to donate their tissue. The donated cornea is processed and tested by a local eye bank to make sure it is safe for use in your surgery.

The most common type of corneal transplant is called "penetrating keratoplasty." During this procedure, your surgeon will remove a small round piece of your cornea. Then your surgeon will sew the donated cornea into the opening of your eye.

Newer techniques may be used for some patients. During these, only the inner or outer layers of the cornea are replaced, rather than all the layers.

Why the Procedure Is Performed

Corneal transplantation is recommended for people who have:

- vision problems caused by thinning of the cornea, usually due to keratoconus;

- scarring of the cornea from severe infections or injuries;

- vision loss caused by cloudiness of the cornea, usually due to Fuchs dystrophy.

Risks

Sometimes, the body rejects the transplanted tissue. This occurs in a small number of patients and can often be controlled with steroid eye drops. The risk of rejection decreases over time but never disappears completely.

Other risks for a corneal transplant are:

- bleeding;
- infection of the eye;
- glaucoma (high pressure in the eye that can cause vision loss);
- swelling of the front of the eye.

The risks for any anesthesia are:

- allergic reactions to medicines;
- breathing problems.

Before the Procedure

Tell your doctor about any medical conditions you may have. Also tell your doctor what medicines you are taking, even drugs, supplements, and herbs you bought without a prescription.

You may need to limit medicines that make it hard for your blood to clot for ten days before the surgery. Some of these are aspirin, ibuprofen (Advil, Motrin), and warfarin (Coumadin).

You may take your other daily medicines the morning of your surgery. But check with your doctor if you take diuretics (water pills) or insulin or pills for diabetes.

You will need to stop eating and drinking most fluids after midnight the night before your surgery. You can have water, apple juice, and plain coffee or tea (without cream or sugar) up to two hours before surgery. Do not drink alcohol twenty-four hours before or after surgery.

On the day of your surgery, wear loose, comfortable clothing. Do not wear any jewelry. Do not put creams, lotions, or makeup on your face or around your eyes.

You will need to have someone drive you home after your surgery.

Note: These are general guidelines. Your surgeon may have specific requirements or instructions.

After the Procedure

You will go home on the same day as your surgery. Your doctor will give you an eye patch to wear for about one to four days.

Your doctor will prescribe eye drops to help your eye heal and prevent infection and rejection.

Your doctor will remove the stitches at a follow-up visit;. Some stitches may remain in place for as long as a year.

Outlook (Prognosis)

Full recovery of eyesight may take up to a year. Most patients who have successful corneal transplants will enjoy good vision for many years. But, if you have other eye problems, those problems may still reduce your eyesight.

Often glasses or contact lenses may be needed to achieve the best vision. Laser vision correction may be an option if there is nearsightedness, farsightedness, or astigmatism present after the transplant has fully healed.

Newer cornea transplant techniques usually have faster recovery times and fewer complications.

Alternative Names

Keratoplasty; penetrating keratoplasty

References

Blackmon S, Semchyshyn T, Kim, T. Penetrating and lamellar keratoplasty. In: Tasman W, Jaeger EA, eds. *Duane's Ophthalmology. 15th ed.* Philadelphia, Pa: Lippincott Williams & Wilkins; 2009:chap 26.

Section 21.2

Caring for Your Eyes after Corneal Transplant

Your transplant must be taken care of in order to be successful. The following are general guidelines on the care of your eye after transplant surgery:

- Always wear a pair of glasses or a shield over your eye for two months after surgery. This protects your eye from being hit or bumped.

- Always wear the shield while sleeping.

- Never rub or push on your eye.

- Do not get water in your eye for two weeks.

- Bring whatever eye medicine you are using to each appointment.

- Unless told otherwise, you may do any physical activity except lifting anything over twenty pounds for two months.

- Contact your doctor's office or your doctor immediately if:
  - you develop severe pain;
  - your vision gets worse or blurry;
  - your eye becomes red;
  - your eye develops any infection.

- If any of these symptoms develop, even if it's on a weekend, call.

- It is very important that you take your eye medicines as directed and that you do not miss or run out of your eye drops or ointments.

Chapter 22

Disorders of the Conjunctiva, Sclera, and Pupil

Chapter Contents

Section 22.1

Conjunctivitis

Conjunctivitis is an inflammation or infection of the conjunctiva, the thin transparent layer of tissue that lines the inner surface of the eyelid and covers the white part of the eye. Conjunctivitis, often called "pink eye," is a common eye disease, especially in children. It may affect one or both eyes. Some forms of conjunctivitis can be highly contagious and easily spread in schools and at home. While conjunctivitis is usually a minor eye infection, sometimes it can develop into a more serious problem.

Conjunctivitis may be caused by a viral or bacterial infection. It can also occur due to an allergic reaction to irritants in the air like pollen and smoke, chlorine in swimming pools, and ingredients in cosmetics or other products that come in contact with the eyes. Sexually transmitted diseases like chlamydia and gonorrhea are less common causes of conjunctivitis.

People with conjunctivitis may experience the following symptoms:

- A gritty feeling in one or both eyes

- Itching or burning sensation in one or both eyes

- Excessive tearing

- Discharge coming from one or both eyes

- Swollen eyelids

- Pink discoloration to the whites of one or both eyes

- Increased sensitivity to light

What Causes Conjunctivitis?

The cause of conjunctivitis varies depending on the offending agent. There are three main categories of conjunctivitis: allergic, infectious, and chemical.

Allergic Conjunctivitis

- Allergic conjunctivitis occurs more commonly among people who already have seasonal allergies. At some point they come into contact with a substance that triggers an allergic reaction in their eyes.

- Giant papillary conjunctivitis is a type of allergic conjunctivitis caused by the chronic presence of a foreign body in the eye. This condition occurs predominantly with people who wear hard or rigid contact lenses, wear soft contact lenses that are not replaced frequently, have an exposed suture on the surface or the eye, or have a glass eye.

Infectious Conjunctivitis

- Bacterial conjunctivitis is an infection most often caused by staphylococcal or streptococcal bacteria from your own skin or respiratory system. Infection can also occur by transmittal from insects, physical contact with other people, poor hygiene (touching the eye with unclean hands), or by use of contaminated eye makeup and facial lotions.

- Viral conjunctivitis is most commonly caused by contagious viruses associated with the common cold. The primary means of contracting this is through exposure to coughing or sneezing by persons with upper respiratory tract infections. It can also occur as the virus spreads along the body's own mucous membranes connecting lungs, throat, nose, tear ducts, and conjunctiva.

- Ophthalmia neonatorum is a severe form of bacterial conjunctivitis that occurs in newborn babies. This is a serious condition that could lead to permanent eye damage unless it is treated immediately. Ophthalmia neonatorum occurs when an infant is exposed to chlamydia or gonorrhea while passing through the birth canal.

Chemical Conjunctivitis

Chemical conjunctivitis can be caused by irritants like air pollution, chlorine in swimming pools, and exposure to noxious chemicals.

How Is Conjunctivitis Diagnosed?

Conjunctivitis can be diagnosed through a comprehensive eye examination. Testing, with special emphasis on evaluation of the conjunctiva and surrounding tissues, may include:

- Patient history to determine the symptoms the patient is experiencing, when the symptoms began, and the presence of any general health or environmental conditions that may be contributing to the problem.

- Visual acuity measurements to determine the extent to which vision may be affected.

- Evaluation of the conjunctiva and external eye tissue using bright light and magnification.

- Evaluation of the inner structures of the eye to ensure that no other tissues are affected by the condition.

- Supplemental testing may include taking cultures or smears of conjunctival tissue, particularly in cases of chronic conjunctivitis or when the condition is not responding to treatment.

Using the information obtained from these tests, your optometrist can determine if you have conjunctivitis and advise you on treatment options.

How Is Conjunctivitis Treated?

Treatment of conjunctivitis is directed at three main goals:

1. To increase patient comfort.

2. To reduce or lessen the course of the infection or inflammation.

3. To prevent the spread of the infection in contagious forms of conjunctivitis.

The appropriate treatment for conjunctivitis depends on its cause:

- **Allergic conjunctivitis:** The first step should be to remove or avoid the irritant, if possible. Cool compresses and artificial tears sometimes relieve discomfort in mild cases. In more severe cases, nonsteroidal anti-inflammatory medications and antihistamines may be prescribed. Cases of persistent allergic conjunctivitis may also require topical steroid eye drops.

- **Bacterial conjunctivitis:** This type of conjunctivitis is usually treated with antibiotic eye drops or ointments. Improvement can occur after three or four days of treatment, but the entire course of antibiotics needs to be used to prevent recurrence.

- **Viral conjunctivitis:** There are no available drops or ointments to eradicate the virus for this type of conjunctivitis. Antibiotics will not cure a viral infection. Like a common cold, the virus just has to run its course, which may take up to two or three weeks in some cases. The symptoms can often be relieved with cool compresses and artificial tear solutions. For the worst cases, topical steroid drops may be prescribed to reduce the discomfort from inflammation, but do not shorten the course of the infection. Some doctors may perform an ophthalmic iodine eye wash in the office in hopes of shortening the course of the infection. This newer treatment has not been well studied yet, therefore no conclusive evidence of the success exists.

- **Chemical conjunctivitis:** Treatment for chemical conjunctivitis requires careful flushing of the eyes with saline and may require topical steroids. The more acute chemical injuries are medical emergencies, particularly alkali burns, which can lead to severe scarring, intraocular damage, or even loss of the eye.

Contact Lens Wearers

Contact lens wearers may need to discontinue wearing their lenses while the condition is active. Your doctor can advise you on the need for temporary restrictions on contact lens wear.

If the conjunctivitis developed due to wearing contact lenses, your eye doctor may recommend that you switch to a different type of contact lens or disinfection solution. Your optometrist might need to alter your contact lens prescription to a type of lens that you replace more frequently to prevent the conjunctivitis from recurring.

Self-Care

Practicing good hygiene is the best way to control the spread of conjunctivitis. Once an infection has been diagnosed, follow these steps:

- Don't touch your eyes with your hands.
- Wash your hands thoroughly and frequently.
- Change your towel and washcloth daily, and don't share them with others.
- Discard eye cosmetics, particularly mascara.
- Don't use anyone else's eye cosmetics or personal eye care items.
- Follow your eye doctor's instructions on proper contact lens care.

You can soothe the discomfort of viral or bacterial conjunctivitis by applying warm compresses to your affected eye or eyes. To make a compress, soak a clean cloth in warm water and wring it out before applying it gently to your closed eyelids.

For allergic conjunctivitis, avoid rubbing your eyes. Instead of warm compresses, use cool compresses to soothe your eyes. Over-the-counter eye drops are available. Antihistamine eye drops should help to alleviate the symptoms, and lubricating eye drops help to rinse the allergen off of the surface of the eye.

See your doctor of optometry when you experience conjunctivitis to help diagnose the cause and the proper course of action.

Section 22.2

Dry Eye

Excerpted from "Facts about Dry Eye," National Eye Institute, National Institutes of Health, August 2009.

Dry Eye Defined

What is dry eye?

Dry eye occurs when the eye does not produce tears properly, or when the tears are not of the correct consistency and evaporate too quickly.

In addition, inflammation of the surface of the eye may occur along with dry eye. If left untreated, this condition can lead to pain, ulcers, or scars on the cornea, and some loss of vision. However, permanent loss of vision from dry eye is uncommon.

What are the types of dry eye?

- Aqueous tear-deficient dry eye is a disorder in which the lacrimal glands fail to produce enough of the watery component of tears to maintain a healthy eye surface.

- Evaporative dry eye may result from inflammation of the meibomian glands, also located in the eyelids. These glands make the lipid or oily part of tears that slows evaporation and keeps the tears stable.

Dry eye can be associated with the following things:

- Inflammation of the surface of the eye, the lacrimal gland, or the conjunctiva
- Any disease process that alters the components of the tears
- An increase in the surface of the eye, as in thyroid disease when the eye protrudes forward
- Cosmetic surgery, if the eyelids are opened too widely

Frequently Asked Questions About Dry Eye

What are tears, and how do they relate to dry eye?

Tears, made by the lacrimal gland, are necessary for overall eye health and clear vision. Tears bathe the surface of the eye, keeping it moist, and wash away dust and debris. They also help protect the eye from bacterial and other types of infections.

Tears are composed of three major components: an outer, oily, lipid layer produced by the meibomian glands; a middle, watery, lacrimal layer produced by the lacrimal glands; and an inner, mucous or mucin layer produced by goblet cells located within a thin transparent layer over the white part of the eye and covering the inner surface of the eyelids. Tears are made of proteins (including growth factors), electrolytes, and vitamins that are critical to maintaining the health of the eye surface and to preventing infection.

Tears are constantly produced to bathe, nourish, and protect the eye surface. They are also produced in response to emergencies, such as a particle of dust in the eye, an infection or irritation of the eye, or an onset of strong emotions. When the lacrimal glands fail to produce sufficient tears, dry eye can result.

Any disease process that alters the components of tears can make them unhealthy and result in dry eye.

Symptoms

What are the symptoms of dry eye?

Dry eye symptoms may include any of the following:

- Stinging or burning of the eye

- A sandy or gritty feeling as if something is in the eye
- Episodes of excess tears following very dry eye periods
- A stringy discharge from the eye
- Pain and redness of the eye
- Episodes of blurred vision
- Heavy eyelids
- Inability to cry when emotionally stressed
- Uncomfortable contact lenses
- Decreased tolerance of reading, working on the computer, or any activity that requires sustained visual attention
- Eye fatigue

Note: If symptoms of dry eye persist, consult an eye care professional to get an accurate diagnosis of the condition and begin treatment to avoid permanent damage.

Causes and Risk Factors

What are the causes of dry eye?

Dry eye can be a temporary or chronic condition:

- Dry eye can be a side effect of some medications, including antihistamines, nasal decongestants, tranquilizers, certain blood pressure medicines, Parkinson medications, birth control pills, and antidepressants.
- Skin disease on or around the eyelids can result in dry eye.
- Diseases of the glands in the eyelids, such as meibomian gland dysfunction, can cause dry eye.
- Dry eye can occur in women who are pregnant.
- Women who are on hormone replacement therapy may experience dry eye symptoms.
- Dry eye can also develop after the refractive surgery known as LASIK. These symptoms generally last three to six months, but may last longer in some cases.
- Dry eye can result from chemical and thermal burns that scar the membrane lining the eyelids and covering the eye.

- Allergies can be associated with dry eye.

- Infrequent blinking, associated with staring at computer or video screens, may also lead to dry eye symptoms.

- Both excessive and insufficient dosages of vitamins can contribute to dry eye.

- Homeopathic remedies may have an adverse impact on a dry eye condition.

- Loss of sensation in the cornea from long-term contact lens wear can lead to dry eye.

- Dry eye can be associated with immune system disorders such as Sjögren syndrome, lupus, and rheumatoid arthritis. Sjögren leads to inflammation and dryness of the mouth, eyes, and other mucous membranes. It can also affect other organs, including the kidneys, lungs, and blood vessels.

- Dry eye can be a symptom of chronic inflammation of the conjunctiva, the membrane lining the eyelid and covering the front part of the eye, or the lacrimal gland. Chronic conjunctivitis can be caused by certain eye diseases, infection, exposure to irritants such as chemical fumes and tobacco smoke, or drafts from air conditioning or heating.

- If the surface area of the eye is increased, as in thyroid disease when the eye protrudes forward or after cosmetic surgery if the eyelids are opened too widely, dry eye can result.

- Dry eye may occur from exposure keratitis, in which the eyelids do not close completely during sleep.

Treatment

How is dry eye treated?

Depending on the causes of dry eye, your doctor may use various approaches to relieve the symptoms.

Dry eye can be managed as an ongoing condition. The first priority is to determine if a disease is the underlying cause of the dry eye (such as Sjögren syndrome or lacrimal and meibomian gland dysfunction). If it is, then the underlying disease needs to be treated.

Cyclosporine, an anti-inflammatory medication, is the only prescription drug available to treat dry eye. It decreases corneal damage, increases basic tear production, and reduces symptoms of dry eye. It may take three to six months of twice-a-day dosages for the medication to work. In some cases of severe dry eye, short-term use of corticosteroid eye drops that decrease inflammation is required.

If dry eye results from taking a medication, your doctor may recommend switching to a medication that does not cause the dry eye side effect.

If contact lens wear is the problem, your eye care practitioner may recommend another type of lens or reducing the number of hours you wear your lenses. In the case of severe dry eye, your eye care professional may advise you not to wear contact lenses at all.

Another option is to plug the drainage holes, small circular openings at the inner corners of the eyelids where tears drain from the eye into the nose. Lacrimal plugs, also called punctal plugs, can be inserted painlessly by an eye care professional. The patient usually does not feel them. These plugs are made of silicone or collagen, are reversible, and are a temporary measure. In severe cases, permanent plugs may be considered.

In some cases, a simple surgery, called punctal cautery, is recommended to permanently close the drainage holes. The procedure helps keep the limited volume of tears on the eye for a longer period of time.

In some patients with dry eye, supplements or dietary sources (such as tuna fish) of omega-3 fatty acids (especially docosahexaenoic acid [DHA] and eicosapentaenoic acid [EPA]) may decrease symptoms of irritation. The use and dosage of nutritional supplements and vitamins should be discussed with your primary medical doctor.

What can I do to help myself?

- Use artificial tears, gels, gel inserts, and ointments—available over the counter—as the first line of therapy. They offer temporary relief and provide an important replacement of naturally produced tears in patients with aqueous tear deficiency. Avoid artificial tears with preservatives if you need to apply them more than four times a day, or preparations with chemicals that cause blood vessels to constrict.

- Wearing glasses or sunglasses that fit close to the face (wraparound shades) or that have side shields can help slow tear evaporation from the eye surfaces. Indoors, an air cleaner to filter dust and other particles helps prevent dry eyes. A humidifier also may help by adding moisture to the air.

- Avoid dry conditions and allow your eyes to rest when performing activities that require you to use your eyes for long periods of time. Instill lubricating eye drops while performing these tasks.

Section 22.3

Pinkeye (Infectious Conjunctivitis)

Excerpted from "Pinkeye (Conjunctivitis)," July 2009, reprinted with permission from www.kidshealth.org. Copyright © 2009 The Nemours Foundation. This information was provided by KidsHealth, one of the largest resources online for medically reviewed health information written for parents, kids, and teens. For more articles like this one, visit www.Kids Health.org, or www.TeensHealth.org.

What is it?

Conjunctivitis is an inflammation of the conjunctiva, the tissue covering the eye and inner surface of the eyelid. It can be infectious (mainly caused by bacteria or viruses) or noninfectious. The common types of noninfectious conjunctivitis are allergic conjunctivitis (caused by an allergic reaction) and irritant conjunctivitis (caused by anything that irritates the eyes, such as air pollution or chlorine in pools).

When people talk about pinkeye, they're usually referring to the infectious kind, which often is caused by the same bacteria and viruses responsible for colds and other infections, including ear infections, sinus infections, and sore throats.

It's also possible for the same types of bacteria that cause the sexually transmitted diseases (STDs) chlamydia and gonorrhea to cause conjunctivitis. If someone touches an infected person's genitals and then rubs his or her own eye or touches a contact lens, the infection can spread to the eye.

In most cases, infectious conjunctivitis causes only minor problems with no risk of damage to the eyes or vision. In very rare instances, though, it can cause permanent damage or even blindness, so be sure to see your doctor if you think you have pinkeye.

What are the signs and symptoms?

The incubation period for conjunctivitis (the length of time between when someone gets infected and when symptoms appear) depends on what's causing it, but usually ranges from a couple of days to a couple of weeks.

Conjunctivitis can affect one or both eyes. The most common symptom is discomfort in the eye, which may feel itchy or gritty. There often will be some discharge from the eyes and pain, swelling of the conjunctiva, and the very pink or red coloring that gives the infection its nickname.

It can be hard to tell whether the infection is caused by a virus or bacteria. In general, the discharge associated with viral conjunctivitis is watery, whereas it will be thicker and more pus-like when the infection is caused by bacteria. When you wake up in the morning, your eyelids may be stuck together (don't be alarmed, though—cleaning your eyes with a warm washcloth will loosen the dried crusts).

Itchiness and tearing are common with allergic conjunctivitis.

How long is conjunctivitis contagious?

Conjunctivitis that's caused by bacteria is contagious as soon as symptoms appear and remains so as long as there is a discharge from the eye—or until twenty-four hours after antibiotics are started. Conjunctivitis that's caused by a virus is generally contagious before symptoms appear and can remain so as long as the symptoms last.

Allergic and irritant conjunctivitis are not contagious.

Can I prevent it?

Because infectious conjunctivitis is highly contagious, wash your hands after interacting with anyone who has the infection. (It's a good idea to wash your hands regularly anyway!) Don't share potentially infected items like washcloths, towels, gauze, or cotton balls. This can be difficult among family members, so just do the best you can.

If you have pinkeye, it's important to wash your hands often, especially after touching your eyes. The infection can easily spread from one eye to the other on contaminated hands or tissues.

It's also wise not to share cosmetics, especially eye makeup. Conjunctivitis-causing bacteria can hang out on beauty products, so avoid using the testers at makeup counters directly on your eyes. And if you've already had a bout of pinkeye, throw away all your eye makeup and splurge on new stuff (but don't start using your new products until the infection is completely gone).

If you wear contact lenses and you've been diagnosed with conjunctivitis, your doctor or eye doctor may recommend that you not wear contact lenses while infected. After the infection is gone, clean your lenses carefully. Be sure to disinfect the lenses and case at least twice before wearing them again. If you wear disposable contact lenses, throw away your current pair and use a new pair.

If you know that you're prone to allergic conjunctivitis, limit allergy triggers in the home by keeping windows and doors closed on days when pollen is heavy and by not letting dust accumulate. Irritant conjunctivitis can only be prevented by avoiding the irritating causes.

Should I see a doctor?

Because it can be hard to tell which kind of conjunctivitis a person has, it's wise to visit a doctor if your eyes are red and irritated.

How is it treated?

Bacterial conjunctivitis is usually treated with prescription antibiotic drops or ointment. Drops—the form of treatment most commonly prescribed for teens—are used up to four times a day. They don't hurt, although they may cause a brief stinging sensation. Even though your eyes should feel and look better after a couple of days, it's important to use the drops for as long as the doctor has prescribed. The infection may come back if you stop too soon.

If a virus is causing conjunctivitis, antibiotic drops will not help. The eye infection will get better as the body fights off the virus.

If you have allergic conjunctivitis, your doctor may prescribe anti-allergy medication in pill or eye drop form.

What can I do to help myself feel better?

Placing cool or warm packs or washcloths over the infected eye (or eyes) can help. You can also take acetaminophen, if necessary. It may be helpful to clean the infected eye carefully with warm water and fresh, clean gauze or cotton balls.

Keep track of your symptoms, keep your hands clean, visit your doctor as needed, and follow your treatment instructions carefully. Within a week, your eyes should be feeling better.

Section 22.4

Pinguecula

"Pinguecula," © 2011 A.D.A.M., Inc. Reprinted with permission.

A pinguecula is a common, noncancerous growth of the clear, thin tissue (conjunctiva) that lays over the white part of the eye (sclera).

Causes

The cause is unknown, but long-term sunlight exposure and eye irritation may contribute to its development. Welding is a major job-related risk.

Symptoms

A pinguecula is a small, yellowish nodule on the conjunctiva near the cornea. It can appear on either side of the cornea, but tends to appear more on the nose (nasal) side. It may increase in size over many years.

Exams and Tests

An eye examination is often enough to diagnose this disorder.

Treatment

Usually no treatment is needed. Lubrication with artificial tears, and sometimes the temporary use of mild steroid eye drops, can be helpful. Rarely, the growth may need to be removed if you have discomfort or for cosmetic reasons.

Outlook (Prognosis)

This condition is noncancerous (benign) and the outlook is good.

Possible Complications

The pinguecula may grow over the cornea and impair vision.

When to Contact a Medical Professional

Call for an appointment with your healthcare provider if the size, shape, or color of a pinguecula changes.

Prevention

It is not known whether this condition can be prevented. It may help to wear good quality sunglasses and avoid eye irritants.

References

Farjo QA, Sugar A. Pterygium and conjunctival degenerations. In: Yanoff M, Duker JS, eds. *Ophthalmology. 3rd ed*. St. Louis, Mo: Mosby Elsevier; 2008:chap 4.9.

Section 22.5

Episcleritis

What Is Episcleritis?

An inflammation of the episclera, a membrane covering the sclera of the eye.

Causes, Incidence, and Risk Factors

The sclera is composed of collagenous fibers to form a white, hollow ball. It is the skeleton of the eyeball and is covered by the episclera, a thin layer of tissue containing many blood vessels that nourish the sclera. On the front of the eye, the episclera is covered by the conjunctiva. Inflammation of the episclera is usually mild and usually does not progress to scleritis. The cause is unknown, but certain diseases such as rheumatoid arthritis, Sjögren syndrome, syphilis, herpes zoster, and tuberculosis have been associated with episcleritis. It is a common condition.

Signs and Symptoms

Episcleritis presents as a relatively asymptomatic acute onset redness in one or both eyes. Typically, you'll observe a sectoral injection of the episcleral and overlying conjunctival vessels, although the redness may be diffuse throughout these tissues. Occasionally, there may be a translucent white nodule centrally within the inflamed area (nodular episcleritis). While some patients complain of mild pain or tenderness to the affected region, particularly upon manipulation, often there is no associated discomfort. The cornea remains clear in this condition, although long-standing or recurrent episcleritis may lead to dellen formation. There is no associated anterior chamber reaction. Other symptoms include:

- bloodshot eyes;
- a pink or purple coloration to the eyeball;
- eye pain;
- sensitivity to light;
- eye tenderness;
- tearing of the eye.

Pathophysiology

A benign inflammatory condition of the external eye, episcleritis is seen most commonly in young adults. Women appear to be affected slightly more often than men. The disorder is idiopathic in the majority of cases, however in certain instances there may be an association with some underlying systemic disease such as rheumatoid arthritis, polyarteritis nodosa, systemic lupus erythematosus, inflammatory bowel disease, sarcoidosis, Wegener granulomatosis, gout, herpes zoster virus, or syphilis.

Management

Most cases of episcleritis are self-limiting, meaning that they will resolve spontaneously within two to three weeks even if the patient does not undergo treatment. However, patients who are experiencing discomfort may benefit from a regimen of topical anti-inflammatory agents and lubricants.

Typically, prednisolone acetate 1 percent or fluorometholone acetate will speed resolution and decrease the tenderness. The patient may use cold compresses and artificial tears liberally if discomfort persists. More severe cases, particularly nodular episcleritis, may require oral nonsteroidal anti-inflammatory drugs (NSAIDs) to quell the inflammation.

Prevention

There is no known way to prevent this disorder.

Signs and Tests

Eye examination is usually sufficient to diagnose the disorder. No tests are usually necessary.

Treatment

The inflammation often runs its course without treatment in one to two weeks. Topical therapy with corticosteroid eye drops may hasten the resolution of inflammation in three or four days.

Expectations (Prognosis)

Episcleritis usually runs its course without treatment. It also responds well to treatment.

Complications

- Relapses may occur.
- Rarely, scleritis may develop.

Calling Your Healthcare Provider

Call your optometrist or doctor if symptoms of episcleritis persist, or if the eyes are very painful. Also, call if vision decreases.

Section 22.6

Scleritis

Overview

Scleritis is an inflammatory disease that affects the conjunctiva, sclera, and episclera (the connective tissue between the conjunctiva and sclera). It is associated with underlying systemic diseases in about half of the cases. The diagnosis of scleritis may lead to the detection of underlying systemic disease. Rarely, scleritis is associated with an infectious problem.

The affected area of the sclera may be confined to small nodules, or it may cause generalized inflammation. Necrotizing scleritis, a more rare, serious type, causes thinning of the sclera. Severe cases of scleritis may also involve inflammation of other ocular tissues.

Scleritis affects women more frequently then men. It most frequently occurs in those who are in their forties and fifties. The problem is usually confined to one eye, but may affect both.

Signs and Symptoms

- Severe, boring pain that can awaken the patient

- Local or general redness of the sclera and conjunctiva

- Extreme tenderness

- Light sensitivity and tearing (in some cases)

- Decreased vision (if other ocular tissues are involved)

Detection and Diagnosis

Along with visual acuity testing, measurement of intraocular pressure, slit lamp examination, and ophthalmoscopy, the doctor may order blood tests to rule out diseases affecting the body. If involvement of the back of the eye is suspected, the doctor may order imaging tests such as computed tomography (CT) scan, magnetic resonance imaging (MRI), or ultrasonography of the eye.

Treatment

Scleritis is treated with oral steroid and nonsteroidal anti-inflammatory medication to reduce inflammation. Eye drops alone do not provide adequate treatment. In very severe cases of necrotizing scleritis, surgery may be required to graft scleral or corneal tissue over the area of thinned sclera.

Section 22.7

Leukocoria

What is leukocoria?

Leukocoria literally means "white pupil." It occurs when the pupil (the round hole in the colored part of the eye) is white rather than the usual black.

How is leukocoria detected?

In more obvious cases the pupil may appear white on casual observation. In other situations the pupil may appear white only in certain circumstances such as when the pupil becomes larger in a darkened room. Sometimes leukocoria is detected from photographs when one pupil has an abnormal or "white reflex" compared to the other eye having a normal "red reflex."

What is a red reflex?

When light enters the eye through the pupil, the retina absorbs most of the light. A small amount of light, however, is reflected by the retina back out of the eye through the pupil. The light is reddish-orange, reflecting the color of normal retina. The red reflex is most easily seen when the observer's line of sight is very close to the direction of illumination into the eye. An example is a camera in which the flash is mounted very close to the lens, resulting in photographs with red pupillary reflexes.

The red reflex is either absent or white with leukocoria. This occurs as a result of abnormal reflection of light coming out of the eye.

How does an ophthalmologist detect leukocoria?

Ophthalmologists utilize a retinoscope to examine the red reflex from the eye and an ophthalmoscope to directly visualize the interior of the eye. Dilating eye drops are generally used to enlarge the pupil, which enables a more thorough examination.

What conditions cause leukocoria?

Many conditions cause leukocoria, including cataract, retinal detachment, retinopathy of prematurity, retinal malformation, intraocular infection (endophthalmitis), retinal vascular abnormality, and intraocular tumor (retinoblastoma).

Are any of these conditions serious?

All diseases which cause leukocoria represent a serious threat to vision and some pose a threat to life. Prompt evaluation of leukocoria by an ophthalmologist is always appropriate.

How is leukocoria treated?

Management of leukocoria involves treatment of the underlying condition (cataract, retinal detachment, infection, etc) responsible for the white-appearing pupil.

Part Four

Understanding and Treating Disorders of the Macula, Optic Nerve, Retina, Vitreous, and Uvea

Chapter 23

Age-Related Macular Degeneration

Chapter Contents

Section 23.1

Facts about Age-Related Macular Degeneration

Reprinted from the National Eye Institute,
National Institutes of Health, September 2009.

Age-Related Macular Degeneration (AMD) Defined

What is age-related macular degeneration?

Age-related macular degeneration (AMD) is a disease associated with aging that gradually destroys sharp, central vision. Central vision is needed for seeing objects clearly and for common daily tasks such as reading and driving.

AMD affects the macula, the part of the eye that allows you to see fine detail. AMD causes no pain.

In some cases, AMD advances so slowly that people notice little change in their vision. In others, the disease progresses faster and may lead to a loss of vision in both eyes. AMD is a leading cause of vision loss in Americans sixty years of age and older.

AMD occurs in two forms: wet and dry.

Where is the macula?

The macula is located in the center of the retina, the light-sensitive tissue at the back of the eye. The retina instantly converts light, or an image, into electrical impulses. The retina then sends these impulses, or nerve signals, to the brain.

What is wet AMD?

Wet AMD occurs when abnormal blood vessels behind the retina start to grow under the macula. These new blood vessels tend to be very fragile and often leak blood and fluid. The blood and fluid raise the macula from its normal place at the back of the eye. Damage to the macula occurs rapidly.

With wet AMD, loss of central vision can occur quickly. Wet AMD is also known as advanced AMD. It does not have stages like dry AMD.

An early symptom of wet AMD is that straight lines appear wavy. If you notice this condition or other changes to your vision, contact your eye care professional at once. You need a comprehensive dilated eye exam.

What is dry AMD?

Dry AMD occurs when the light-sensitive cells in the macula slowly break down, gradually blurring central vision in the affected eye. As dry AMD gets worse, you may see a blurred spot in the center of your vision. Over time, as less of the macula functions, central vision is gradually lost in the affected eye.

The most common symptom of dry AMD is slightly blurred vision. You may have difficulty recognizing faces. You may need more light for reading and other tasks. Dry AMD generally affects both eyes, but vision can be lost in one eye while the other eye seems unaffected.

One of the most common early signs of dry AMD is drusen.

What are drusen?

Drusen are yellow deposits under the retina. They often are found in people over age sixty. Your eye care professional can detect drusen during a comprehensive dilated eye exam.

Drusen alone do not usually cause vision loss. In fact, scientists are unclear about the connection between drusen and AMD. They do know that an increase in the size or number of drusen raises a person's risk of developing either advanced dry AMD or wet AMD. These changes can cause serious vision loss.

Dry AMD has three stages, all of which may occur in one or both eyes:

- **Early AMD:** People with early AMD have either several small drusen or a few medium-sized drusen. At this stage, there are no symptoms and no vision loss.

- **Intermediate AMD:** People with intermediate AMD have either many medium-sized drusen or one or more large drusen. Some people see a blurred spot in the center of their vision. More light may be needed for reading and other tasks.

- **Advanced dry AMD:** In addition to drusen, people with advanced dry AMD have a breakdown of light-sensitive cells and supporting tissue in the central retinal area. This breakdown can cause a blurred spot in the center of your vision. Over time, the blurred spot may get bigger and darker, taking more of your central vision. You may have difficulty reading or recognizing faces until they are very close to you.

If you have vision loss from dry AMD in one eye only, you may not notice any changes in your overall vision. With the other eye seeing clearly, you still can drive, read, and see fine details. You may notice changes in your vision only if AMD affects both eyes. If blurriness occurs in your vision, see an eye care professional for a comprehensive dilated eye exam.

Ninety percent of all people with AMD have this type. Scientists are still not sure what causes dry AMD.

Frequently Asked Questions about Wet and Dry AMD

Which is more common—the dry form or the wet form?

The dry form is much more common. More than 85 percent of all people with intermediate and advanced AMD combined have the dry form.

However, if only advanced AMD is considered, about two-thirds of patients have the wet form. Because almost all vision loss comes from advanced AMD, the wet form leads to significantly more vision loss than the dry form.

Can the dry form turn into the wet form?

Yes. All people who have the wet form had the dry form first.

The dry form can advance and cause vision loss without turning into the wet form. The dry form also can suddenly turn into the wet form, even during early-stage AMD. There is no way to tell if or when the dry form will turn into the wet form.

The dry form has early and intermediate stages. Does the wet form have similar stages?

No. The wet form is considered advanced AMD.

Can advanced AMD be either the dry form or the wet form?

Yes. Both the wet form and the advanced dry form are considered advanced AMD. Vision loss occurs with either form. In most cases, only advanced AMD can cause vision loss.

People who have advanced AMD in one eye are at especially high risk of developing advanced AMD in the other eye.

Causes and Risk Factors

Who is at risk for AMD?

The greatest risk factor is age. Although AMD may occur during middle age, studies show that people over age sixty are clearly at greater risk than other age groups. For instance, a large study found that people in middle age have about a 2 percent risk of getting AMD, but this risk increased to nearly 30 percent in those over age seventy-five.

Other risk factors include the following:

- **Smoking:** Smoking may increase the risk of AMD.

- **Obesity:** Research studies suggest a link between obesity and the progression of early- and intermediate-stage AMD to advanced AMD.

- **Race:** Whites are much more likely to lose vision from AMD than African Americans.

- **Family history:** Those with immediate family members who have AMD are at a higher risk of developing the disease.

- **Gender:** Women appear to be at greater risk than men.

Can my lifestyle make a difference?

Your lifestyle can play a role in reducing your risk of developing AMD:

- Eat a healthy diet high in green leafy vegetables and fish.
- Don't smoke.
- Maintain normal blood pressure.
- Watch your weight.
- Exercise.

Symptoms and Detection

What are the symptoms?

Both dry and wet AMD cause no pain.

For dry AMD, the most common early sign is blurred vision. As fewer cells in the macula are able to function, people will see details less clearly in front of them, such as faces or words in a book. Often this blurred vision will go away in brighter light. If the loss of these light-sensing cells becomes great, people may see a small—but growing—blind spot in the middle of their field of vision.

For wet AMD, the classic early symptom is that straight lines appear crooked. This results when fluid from the leaking blood vessels gathers and lifts the macula, distorting vision. A small blind spot may also appear in wet AMD, resulting in loss of one's central vision.

How is AMD detected?

Your eye care professional may suspect AMD if you are over age sixty and have had recent changes in your central vision. To look for signs of the disease, he or she will use eye drops to dilate, or enlarge, your pupils. Dilating the pupils allows your eye care professional to view the back of the eye better.

AMD is detected during a comprehensive eye exam that includes the following:

- **Visual acuity test:** This eye chart test measures how well you see at various distances.

- **Dilated eye exam:** Drops are placed in your eyes to widen, or dilate, the pupils. Your eye care professional uses a special magnifying lens to examine your retina and optic nerve for signs of AMD and other eye problems. After the exam, your close-up vision may remain blurred for several hours.

- **Tonometry:** An instrument measures the pressure inside the eye. Numbing drops may be applied to your eye for this test.

Your eye care professional also may do other tests to learn more about the structure and health of your eye.

During an eye exam, you may be asked to look at an Amsler grid. The pattern of the grid resembles a checkerboard. You will cover one eye and stare at a black dot in the center of the grid. While staring at the dot, you may notice that the straight lines in the pattern appear wavy. You may notice that some of the lines are missing. These may be signs of AMD.

If your eye care professional believes you need treatment for wet AMD, he or she may suggest a fluorescein angiogram. In this test, a special dye is injected into your arm. Pictures are taken as the dye passes through the blood vessels in your retina. The test allows your eye care professional to identify any leaking blood vessels and recommend treatment.

Treatment

How is wet AMD treated?

Wet AMD can be treated with laser surgery, photodynamic therapy, and injections into the eye. None of these treatments is a cure for wet AMD. The disease and loss of vision may progress despite treatment.

Laser surgery: This procedure uses a laser to destroy the fragile, leaky blood vessels. A high-energy beam of light is aimed directly onto the new blood vessels and destroys them, preventing further loss of vision. However, laser treatment may also destroy some surrounding healthy tissue and some vision. Only a small percentage of people with wet AMD can be treated with laser surgery. Laser surgery is more effective if the leaky blood vessels have developed away from the fovea, the central part of the macula. Laser surgery is performed in a doctor's office or eye clinic.

The risk of new blood vessels developing after laser treatment is high. Repeated treatments may be necessary. In some cases, vision loss may progress despite repeated treatments.

Photodynamic therapy: A drug called verteporfin is injected into your arm. It travels throughout the body, including the new blood vessels in your eye. The drug tends to "stick" to the surface of new blood vessels. Next, a light is shined into your eye for about ninety seconds. The light activates the drug. The activated drug destroys the new blood vessels and leads to a slower rate of vision decline. Unlike laser surgery, this drug does not destroy surrounding healthy tissue. Because the drug is activated by light, you must avoid exposing your skin or eyes to direct sunlight or bright indoor light for five days after treatment.

Photodynamic therapy is relatively painless. It takes about twenty minutes and can be performed in a doctor's office.

Photodynamic therapy slows the rate of vision loss. It does not stop vision loss or restore vision in eyes already damaged by advanced AMD. Treatment results often are temporary. You may need to be treated again.

Injections: Wet AMD can now be treated with new drugs that are injected into the eye (anti–vascular endothelial growth factor [anti-VEGF] therapy). Abnormally high levels of a specific growth factor occur in eyes with wet AMD and promote the growth of abnormal new blood vessels. This drug treatment blocks the effects of the growth factor.

You will need multiple injections that may be given as often as monthly. The eye is numbed before each injection. After the injection, you will remain in the doctor's office for a while and your eye will be monitored. This drug treatment can help slow down vision loss from AMD and in some cases improve sight.

How is dry AMD treated?

Once dry AMD reaches the advanced stage, no form of treatment can prevent vision loss. However, treatment can delay and possibly prevent intermediate AMD from progressing to the advanced stage, in which vision loss occurs.

The National Eye Institute's Age-Related Eye Disease Study (AREDS) found that taking a specific high-dose formulation of antioxidants and zinc significantly reduces the risk of advanced AMD and its associated vision loss. Slowing AMD's progression from the intermediate stage to the advanced stage will save the vision of many people.

Age-Related Eye Disease Study (AREDS)

What is the dosage of the AREDS formulation?

The specific daily amounts of antioxidants and zinc used by the study researchers were 500 milligrams of vitamin C, 400 international units of vitamin E, 15 milligrams of beta-carotene (often labeled as equivalent to 25,000 international units of vitamin A), 80 milligrams of zinc as zinc oxide, and two milligrams of copper as cupric oxide. Copper was added to the AREDS formulation containing zinc to prevent copper deficiency anemia, a condition associated with high levels of zinc intake.

Who should take the AREDS formulation?

People who are at high risk for developing advanced AMD should consider taking the formulation. You are at high risk for developing advanced AMD if you have either intermediate AMD in one or both eyes or advanced AMD (dry or wet) in one eye but not the other eye.

Your eye care professional can tell you if you have AMD, its stage, and your risk for developing the advanced form.

The AREDS formulation is not a cure for AMD. It will not restore vision already lost from the disease. However, it may delay the onset of advanced AMD. It may help people who are at high risk for developing advanced AMD keep their vision.

Can ceople with early-stage AMD take the AREDS formulation to help prevent the disease from progressing to the intermediate stage?

There is no apparent need for those diagnosed with early-stage AMD to take the AREDS formulation. The study did not find that the formulation provided a benefit to those with early-stage AMD. If you have early-stage AMD, a comprehensive dilated eye exam every year can help determine if the disease is progressing. If early-stage AMD progresses to the intermediate stage, discuss taking the formulation with your doctor.

Can diet alone provide the same high levels of antioxidants and zinc as the AREDS formulation?

No. The high levels of vitamins and minerals are difficult to achieve from diet alone. However, previous studies have suggested that people who have diets rich in green leafy vegetables have a lower risk of developing AMD.

Can a daily multivitamin alone provide the same high levels of antioxidants and zinc as the AREDS formulation?

No. The formulation's levels of antioxidants and zinc are considerably higher than the amounts in any daily multivitamin.

If you are already taking daily multivitamins and your doctor suggests you take the high-dose AREDS formulation, be sure to review all your vitamin supplements with your doctor before you begin. Because multivitamins contain many important vitamins not found in the AREDS formulation, you may want to take a multivitamin along with the AREDS formulation. For example, people with osteoporosis need to be particularly concerned about taking vitamin D, which is not in the AREDS formulation.

How can I take care of my vision now that I have AMD?

Dry AMD: If you have dry AMD, you should have a comprehensive dilated eye exam at least once a year. Your eye care professional can monitor your condition and check for other eye diseases. Also, if you have intermediate AMD in one or both eyes, or advanced AMD in one eye only, your doctor may suggest that you take the AREDS formulation containing the high levels of antioxidants and zinc.

Because dry AMD can turn into wet AMD at any time, you should get an Amsler grid from your eye care professional. Use the grid every day to evaluate your vision for signs of wet AMD. This quick test works best for people who still have good central vision. Check each eye separately. Cover one eye and look at the grid. Then cover your other eye and look at the grid. If you detect any changes in the appearance of this grid or in your everyday vision while reading the newspaper or watching television, get a comprehensive dilated eye exam.

Wet AMD: If you have wet AMD and your doctor advises treatment, do not wait. After laser surgery or photodynamic therapy, you will need frequent eye exams to detect any recurrence of leaking blood vessels. Studies show that people who smoke have a greater risk of recurrence than those who don't. In addition, check your vision at home with the Amsler grid. If you detect any changes, schedule an eye exam immediately.

What can I do if I have already lost some vision from AMD?

If you have lost some sight from AMD, don't be afraid to use your eyes for reading, watching TV, and other routine activities. Normal use of your eyes will not cause further damage to your vision.

If you have lost some sight from AMD, ask your eye care professional about low vision services and devices that may help you make the most of your remaining vision. Ask for a referral to a specialist in low vision. Many community organizations and agencies offer information about low vision counseling, training, and other special services for people with visual impairments. A nearby school of medicine or optometry may provide low vision services.

Current Research

What research is being done?

The National Eye Institute is conducting and supporting a number of studies to learn more about AMD. For example, scientists are doing the following:

- Studying the possibility of transplanting healthy cells into a diseased retina.

- Evaluating families with a history of AMD to understand genetic and hereditary factors that may cause the disease.

- Looking at certain anti-inflammatory treatments for the wet form of AMD.

This research should provide better ways to detect, treat, and prevent vision loss in people with AMD.

Section 23.2

Reducing the Risk of Macular Degeneration

Reducing the Risk of Wet AMD

Having a clear central visual field allows you to safely and easily accomplish tasks ranging from reading and driving to chopping an onion and playing fetch with your dog.

Screening for AMD

To detect AMD before symptoms appear, the following groups of people should be screened:

• People over sixty years of age

• People with hypertension or cardiovascular disease

• People who smoke

• People with a close family history (brother/sister or mother) of vision loss from AMD regardless of age

• People with aphakia or pre-1984 pseudophakia

• People with significant cumulative light exposure.

Signs of High Risk

During screening, your vision care provider will look for the following signs that you are at high risk of developing AMD-related low vision:

• **Number and size of drusen:** Drusen are yellow, fatlike deposits on the eye associated with macular degeneration. The presence of many drusen and at least one large drusen indicates an increased risk of developing advanced AMD.

- **Geographic atrophy in one or both eyes:** Geographic atrophy is a large central area of retinal atrophy that destroys the center of vision.

Risk Factors

Age

Wet AMD is the leading cause of low vision in Americans age sixty and older. Age is the single most important nonmodifiable risk factor.

Gender

Women are more likely than men to develop AMD. Because women have longer life expectancy, they are also more likely to develop AMD-related low vision.

Ethnicity

People of Caucasian descent, especially those age seventy-five and older, are much more likely than African Americans to develop low vision related to AMD. Of those with low vision, it is attributable to AMD in less than 5 percent of African Americans and less than 15 percent of Hispanics. By comparison, low vision is attributable to AMD in more than half of people who are Caucasian.

Hereditary Factors

Family history: Ten to twenty percent of people with AMD have one or more immediate family members (siblings, parents, or children) with AMD. Scientists have identified some of the specific genes believed to be responsible for causing macular degeneration. Researchers are working to develop genetic testing that might allow people to find out whether they are at high risk and should be closely monitored.

Eye color: People with light-colored eyes tend to have a higher risk of AMD than those with darker eyes.

Systemic Factors

Obesity: A body mass index of 30 or greater increases the likelihood that early- or intermediate-stage dry AMD will progress to advanced dry or wet AMD. Body mass index is a measure of body weight adjusted for height.

Nutrition: Low antioxidant levels may increase the risk of age-related conditions, including macular degeneration. One study conducted over a five-year interval showed that people with early or intermediate AMD who took a nutritional supplement of antioxidant vitamins and zinc had a 25 percent reduced risk that the disease would progress to an advanced stage. However, you should consult your primary care provider before taking a vitamin supplement, since high concentrations of zinc, vitamin K, and other vitamins and minerals can be harmful for some patients or can cause medication interactions.

It is also helpful, of course, to eat a diet high in antioxidants. People who eat five or more servings per week of dark leafy green vegetables, such as kale and spinach, have a reduced risk of developing AMD. In addition, researchers are investigating a possible link between AMD and diets high in saturated fats.

Ocular Factors

Severe hyperopia (farsightedness): People who are extremely hyperopic (farsighted) have up to two and a half times the risk of developing AMD.

Environmental Factors

Smoking: Smoking has a deleterious effect on virtually every body system, and your vision is no exception. The chemicals in tobacco are believed to keep your body from properly absorbing lutein, an antioxidant that helps shield the retina from age-related deterioration. In fact, smoking is the most important preventable risk factor for AMD, increasing the risk to two to three times that of a person who has never smoked.

Evidence shows, however, that quitting reduces your risk of developing AMD, a benefit that continues to build each year that you do not smoke, especially in the first several years after quitting. Speak with your doctor about your options for smoking cessation.

Modifying Your Risk Factors

You're stuck with your age and genetics, but you can reduce your other risk factors. Here's how:

- Stop smoking.

- Eat a diet high in antioxidant vitamins, especially fish, nuts, and dark leafy green vegetables such as spinach and kale.

- Get moving! Aerobic physical activity doesn't have to involve leg warmers and Spandex. It just means you need to get your heart rate up to your target range at least three times a week. You can do this with brisk walking, swimming, bicycling, Rollerblading, or any other activity that's powered by you.

- Stay out of the sun. You already knew that getting a tan causes wrinkles and age spots, not to mention skin cancer. Now you know that sunlight can contribute to the development of cataracts, AMD, and other eye diseases. If you can't avoid the sun, use a high–sun protection factor (SPF) sunscreen, a wide-brimmed hat, and ultraviolet (UV)–filtering sunglasses.

- Control high blood pressure and reduce your blood cholesterol.

When to Seek Care

If you have wet AMD, don't put off having the treatment recommended by your vision care provider. Vision loss occurs rapidly with wet AMD but can improve with prompt treatment unless the macula has been permanently damaged by delay in treatment.

If you have dry AMD, you need to monitor your vision so that you can seek treatment if it progresses to wet AMD. If you have no blank spots in your central vision, ask your provider for an Amsler grid. Look at the grid every day, covering each eye separately, and see your provider right away if the grid lines begin to look wavy, blurry, or gray. If your ability to read declines or if your vision deteriorates in any other way, an immediate visit to your vision care provider is in order.

Section 23.3

Nutrition and Age-Related Macular Degeneration

You've been hearing a lot about vitamins to "reverse" macular degeneration or a diet that can prevent it.

The truth is that although we know a great deal about what seems to be helpful, no one has the whole answer. Beware of companies that claim to have a "cure" or a supplement to reverse macular degeneration. There is no research to support this type of "miracle."

The good news is that valid scientific research *does* show that your diet can affect your eyes. And, if you have macular degeneration, there is a proven supplement that may slow down the progression and the vision loss.

Facts:

- People who eat a diet high in vegetables and fruit have a lower incidence of age-related macular degeneration. Dark green, leafy vegetables are particularly helpful.

- People who eat fish three times a week have a lower incidence of macular degeneration.

- People who eat a lot of saturated fats have a higher risk of AMD.

Eat Lots of Vegetables and Fruits

Antioxidants protect against oxidation, which is a part of the process of AMD. Dark green leafy vegetables like spinach, kale, mustard greens, and collard greens contain high levels of lutein, a critical antioxidant. Antioxidants are also present in fruits and vegetables with bright color, including red grapes, peppers, corn, oranges, cantaloupe, and mango. Look for fresh produce in a variety of colors to get a wide range of vitamins in your diet. We don't have all the answers, so eating a varied diet is wise.

Eat five to nine servings a day. While this may sound like a lot, a serving is really only half a cup of most foods or one cup of leafy greens.

Eat Fish

People who eat fish two to three times a week have a lower risk for AMD. Fish contain omega-3, which seems to be a critical nutrient for the heart and eyes. The best fish are either wild salmon or small fish like sardines. If you cannot tolerate fish or obtain it easily, an omega-3 supplement is another option. Fish oil capsules are widely available.

Limit Your Fat Intake

In reviewing studies on fat, researchers found that while the amount of fat consumed makes a difference, the real issue for AMD is the amount of saturated fats in the diet.

The biggest source of saturated fat is animal products—beef, lamb, pork, lard, butter, cream, whole milk, and high-fat cheese. Plant oils also have saturated fat, including coconut oil, cocoa butter, palm oil, and palm kernel oil.

Read the labels on processed foods and baked goods, as they often have high amounts of saturated fats.

Ask Your Doctor about Supplements

If you have intermediate AMD already, your doctor may recommend taking a supplement that has been proven to slow the progression and vision loss from AMD. The Age-Related Eye Disease Study (AREDS) was a ten-year study of 3,500 people with AMD. The supplement contains:

- 500 mg Vitamin C
- 400 IU Vitamin E
- 15 mg beta-carotene
- 80 mg zinc
- 2 mg copper

The AREDS formula did not prevent AMD and was not effective in people with early AMD. But for those with intermediate AMD, it slowed the progression by 25 percent and slowed the vision loss by 19 percent. This is a high-dose vitamin, so you should only take it if your doctor recommends it. You should also inform all your doctors of every supplement or herbal remedy you use.

Additional research findings have led scientists to consider changing the AREDS formula. The level of zinc has been thought to be too high and we now know more about lutein, zeaxanthin, and omega-3.

There is currently an AREDS II project underway, which reduces the zinc, eliminates the beta-carotene, and adds lutein, zeaxanthin, and omega-3. It will be several years before we have the results of this study. In the meantime, your doctor may suggest that you take some of these nutrients.

We don't have any evidence that a particular vitamin prevents macular degeneration. However, there is good research on lutein, zeaxanthin, and omega-3. If your diet is very low in these substances, you might ask your doctor about taking supplements. They have been proven to have an effect on other body systems, like the heart, circulation, and skin.

Section 23.4

Treatment and Care of Age-Related Macular Degeneration

Americans like to fix things. When our knees, hips, or shoulders give out, we replace them. Presto! Hank's old golf swing is back and Lillian is rolling strikes again. When our jowls sag or our frown lines deepen, a facelift or a little Botox does the trick. So when the eye doctor tells us we have age-related macular degeneration (AMD)—and that neither a spare part nor a nip and tuck will make it go away—we may be left feeling frustrated and vulnerable.

It's important to acknowledge these feelings and talk about them with your vision care provider and loved ones. But rather than move to the sidelines, learn what you can do to prevent vision loss or to adjust successfully to having low vision. Educating yourself is always a good place to start, so let's take a look at the available treatment options.

Treatment

Age-related macular degeneration destroys the macula, a cluster of light-sensitive cells in the central part of the retina. The retina is responsible for converting images into electrical signals and transmitting them to the brain via the optic nerve. The macula gives you crisp central vision and allows you to perceive fine detail.

Dry AMD is a condition in which central vision gradually deteriorates as the light-sensitive cells and supportive tissues of the macula break down over time. In advanced dry AMD, a blank spot of geographic atrophy may develop in the center of the visual field. Dry AMD may progress to become wet AMD, which is always considered to be advanced because it poses a serious threat to vision. Wet AMD is caused by the abnormal growth of blood vessels under and into the retina, a process called neovascularization, and sometimes by the detachment of a layer of cells that lies between the choroid and the retina.

Whether treatment is useful depends on the size, location, and specific type of blood vessel migration or geographic atrophy of the retina. Progress or further decline is measured in terms of how many letters you can read on a standard eye chart after a period of weeks, months, or years. For example, a person might lose the ability to read fifteen letters (three lines) in an eighteen-month period.

Anti–Vascular Endothelial Growth Factor (Anti-VEGF) Medication

The word *vascular* simply refers to vessels, which need a special substance called endothelial growth factor (EGF) to thrive. Think of EGF as fertilizer for blood vessels. Depriving the vascular network of EGF chokes off new growth, which turns out to be a fairly effective therapy for wet AMD. In fact, Lucentis is the only treatment that can marginally improve vision in those with AMD. The drug is injected directly into the eye every four weeks or so.

Lucentis

Lucentis (ranibizumab), a drug recently approved by the U.S. Food and Drug Administration (FDA), has been shown to improve vision over one to two years in at least one-third of those treated. This is the most important drug in the treatment of macular degeneration, and is used by the vast majority of retinal specialists. It has revolutionized the treatment of the disease.

Investigational Treatments

There are two new drugs under investigation for dry AMD that have some possibility of success.

New Drugs

Retaane (anecortave), an injectable drug for wet AMD currently in late-stage clinical trials, may stabilize or improve vision in nearly three-quarters of people treated. Zybrestat (fosbretabulin), a drug also undergoing clinical trials, works by collapsing the newly formed vessels in the retina. It has shown some promise in people who have AMD related to myopia (nearsightedness). A topical formulation of Zybrestat is being developed.

When to Seek Care

If you have wet AMD, don't put off having the treatment recommended by your vision care provider. With this form of AMD, vision loss occurs rapidly and will be permanent if the macula has been damaged.

If you have dry AMD, you must monitor your vision so that you can seek immediate treatment if it progresses to wet AMD. If you have geographic atrophy, you should receive a comprehensive eye examination every six months if you have no new symptoms. You should visit a vision care specialist within twenty-four hours of the onset of any new symptoms.

If you have no geographic atrophy and no evidence of neovascularization, you may need to see your vision care specialist only once a year. Ask your provider for an Amsler grid. Look at the grid every day, covering each eye separately, and see your provider right away if the grid lines begin to look wavy, blurry, or gray. If you have trouble reading or watching television, or if your vision deteriorates in any other way, an immediate examination is in order.

Of course, no treatment option for AMD will give us back the vision we once had. We can't pick up a spare retina on our lunch hour or fill a prescription that will give us sharp eyesight. But there are things you can do to maximize your remaining vision.

Living with Low Vision

Wet AMD, if left untreated, leads to low vision—and for those who have it, that's the only symptom that matters. People with advanced

AMD lose vision in the central visual field but keep their peripheral vision. Learning to accommodate low vision takes patience, support, and determination, but it can be done with the help of low-vision devices and a few simple adjustments.

Visual Adjustments

Using your eyes after they have been damaged by AMD will not cause further deterioration, so you should continue to engage in any activities you can perform comfortably and safely. If you have a blur or blank spot in your central visual field, try adjusting your gaze. Instead of looking at things head-on, try looking at them obliquely—to one side, above, or below the mark. This allows you to see your real target using your peripheral vision.

Low-Vision Devices

Many low-vision devices are available to help people go about their activities as normally as possible. Below are just a few examples:

- **Magnification:** Magnifying lenses mounted as spectacles, hand held or stand-based magnifiers, telescopic lenses, or electronics can be used to produce magnified images.

- **Large numbers:** Telephones and television remote controls are made with jumbo keypads, or you can purchase overlays for existing devices. You can also purchase clocks, watches, and timers with extra-large dials or digital readouts.

- **Large print:** Large-print and audio editions of books, newspapers, and magazines are available.

Low-Vision Services

Teaching hospitals at local universities may offer ophthalmic or optometric services. These schools, as well as community centers, senior centers, community organizations, and government agencies, may also offer low-vision counseling to help you learn to live safely, comfortably, and productively at home. Vision rehabilitation therapists can show you, for example, how to organize your pantry so that you don't open the peaches when you want carrots. They can help you arrange your clothes so that you can easily find a matching shirt and slacks, and they can identify any hazards posed by flooring, rugs, furniture, and appliances.

Section 23.5

Stem Cell Therapy for Age-Related Macular Degeneration

The notion of transplanting adult stem cells to treat or even cure age-related macular degeneration has taken a significant step toward becoming a reality. In a study published on March 24, 2011, in *Stem Cells*, Georgetown University Medical Center (GUMC) researchers have demonstrated, for the first time, the ability to create retinal cells derived from human-induced pluripotent stem cells that mimic the eye cells that die and cause loss of sight.

Age-related macular degeneration (AMD) is a leading cause of visual impairment and blindness in older Americans and worldwide. AMD gradually destroys sharp, central vision needed for seeing objects clearly and for common daily tasks such as reading and driving. AMD progresses with death of retinal pigment epithelium (RPE), a dark-colored layer of cells which nourishes the visual cells in the retina.

While some treatments can help slow its progression, there is no cure. The discovery of human-induced pluripotent stem (hiPS) cells has opened a new avenue for the treatment of degenerative diseases, like AMD, by using a patient's own stem cells to generate tissues and cells for transplantation.

For transplantation to be viable in age-related macular degeneration, researchers have to first figure out how to program the naïve hiPS cells to function and possess the characteristics of the native retinal pigment epithelium, RPE, the cells that die off and lead to AMD.

The research conducted by the Georgetown scientists shows that this critical step in regenerative medicine for AMD has greatly progressed.

"This is the first time that hiPS-RPE cells have been produced with the characteristics and functioning of the RPE cells in the eye. That makes these cells promising candidates for retinal regeneration therapies in age-related macular degeneration," says the study's lead author

Nady Golestaneh, Ph.D., assistant professor in GUMC's Department of Biochemistry and Molecular and Cellular Biology.

Using an established laboratory stem cell line, Golestaneh and her colleagues show that RPE generated from hiPS cells under defined conditions exhibit ion transport, membrane potential, polarized vascular endothelial growth factor (VEGF) secretion and gene expression profile similar to those of a normal eye's RPE.

"This isn't ready for prime time though. We also identified some issues that need to be worked out before these cells are ready for transplantation but overall, this is a tremendous step forward in regenerative medicine," Golestaneh adds.

She explains that the hiPS-derived RPE cells show rapid telomere shortening, deoxyribonucleic acid (DNA) chromosomal damage, and increased p21 expression that cause cell growth arrest. This might be due to the random integration of viruses in the genome of skin fibroblasts during the reprogramming of iPS cells. Therefore, generation of viral-free iPS cells and their differentiation into RPE will be a necessary step towards implementation of these cells in clinical application, Golestaneh says.

"The next step in this research is to focus on a generation of 'safe' as well as viable hiPS-derived somatic cells," Golestaneh concludes.

Chapter 24

Other Macular Disorders

Chapter Contents

Section 24.1

Macular Hole

"Facts about Macular Hole," National Eye Institute,
National Institutes of Health, August 2009.

Macular Hole Defined

What is a macular hole?

A macular hole is a small break in the macula, located in the center of the eye's light-sensitive tissue called the retina. The macula provides the sharp, central vision we need for reading, driving, and seeing fine detail.

A macular hole can cause blurred and distorted central vision. Macular holes are related to aging and usually occur in people over age sixty.

Are there different types of a macular hole?

Yes. There are three stages to a macular hole:

- **Foveal detachments (stage I):** Without treatment, about half of stage I macular holes will progress.

- **Partial-thickness holes (stage II):** Without treatment, about 70 percent of stage II macular holes will progress.

- **Full-thickness holes (stage III).**

The size of the hole and its location on the retina determine how much it will affect a person's vision. When a stage III macular hole develops, most central and detailed vision can be lost. If left untreated, a macular hole can lead to a detached retina, a sight-threatening condition that should receive immediate medical attention.

Frequently Asked Question about Macular Hole

Is a macular hole the same as age-related macular degeneration?

No. Macular holes and age-related macular degeneration are two separate and distinct conditions, although the symptoms for each are similar. Both conditions are common in people sixty and over. An eye care professional will know the difference.

Causes and Risk Factors

What causes a macular hole?

Most of the eye's interior is filled with vitreous, a gel-like substance that fills about 80 percent of the eye and helps it maintain a round shape. The vitreous contains millions of fine fibers that are attached to the surface of the retina. As we age, the vitreous slowly shrinks and pulls away from the retinal surface. Natural fluids fill the area where the vitreous has contracted. This is normal. In most cases, there are no adverse effects. Some patients may experience a small increase in floaters, which are little "cobwebs" or specks that seem to float about in your field of vision.

However, if the vitreous is firmly attached to the retina when it pulls away, it can tear the retina and create a macular hole. Also, once the vitreous has pulled away from the surface of the retina, some of the fibers can remain on the retinal surface and can contract. This increases tension on the retina and can lead to a macular hole. In either case, the fluid that has replaced the shrunken vitreous can then seep through the hole onto the macula, blurring and distorting central vision.

Macular holes can also occur from eye disorders, such as high myopia (nearsightedness), macular pucker, and retinal detachment; eye disease, such as diabetic retinopathy and Best disease; and injury to the eye.

Is my other eye at risk?

If a macular hole exists in one eye, there is a 10 to15 percent chance that a macular hole will develop in your other eye over your lifetime. Your doctor can discuss this with you.

Symptoms

What are the symptoms of a macular hole?

Macular holes often begin gradually. In the early stage of a macular hole, people may notice a slight distortion or blurriness in their straight-ahead vision. Straight lines or objects can begin to look bent or wavy. Reading and performing other routine tasks with the affected eye becomes difficult.

Treatment

How is a macular hole treated?

Although some macular holes can seal themselves and require no treatment, surgery is necessary in many cases to help improve vision. In this surgical procedure—called a vitrectomy—the vitreous gel is removed to prevent it from pulling on the retina and replaced with a bubble containing a mixture of air and gas. The bubble acts as an internal, temporary bandage that holds the edge of the macular hole in place as it heals. Surgery is performed under local anesthesia and often on an outpatient basis.

Following surgery, patients must remain in a face-down position, normally for a day or two but sometimes for as long as two to three weeks. This position allows the bubble to press against the macula and be gradually reabsorbed by the eye, sealing the hole. As the bubble is reabsorbed, the vitreous cavity refills with natural eye fluids.

Maintaining a face-down position is crucial to the success of the surgery. Because this position can be difficult for many people, it is important to discuss this with your doctor before surgery.

What are the risks of surgery?

The most common risk following macular hole surgery is an increase in the rate of cataract development. In most patients, a cataract can progress rapidly, and often becomes severe enough to require removal. Other less common complications include infection and retinal detachment either during surgery or afterward, both of which can be immediately treated.

For a few months after surgery, patients are not permitted to travel by air. Changes in air pressure may cause the bubble in the eye to expand, increasing pressure inside the eye.

How successful is this surgery?

Vision improvement varies from patient to patient. People that have had a macular hole for less than six months have a better chance of recovering vision than those who have had one for a longer period. Discuss vision recovery with your doctor before your surgery. Vision recovery can continue for as long as three months after surgery.

What if I cannot remain in a face-down position after the surgery?

If you cannot remain in a face-down position for the required period after surgery, vision recovery may not be successful. People who are unable to remain in a face-down position for this length of time may not be good candidates for a vitrectomy. However, there are a number of devices that can make the "face-down" recovery period easier on you. There are also some approaches that can decrease the amount of "face-down" time. Discuss these with your doctor.

Section 24.2

Macular Pucker

"Facts about Macular Pucker," National Eye Institute,
National Institutes of Health, August 2009.

Macular Pucker Defined

What is a macular pucker?

A macular pucker is scar tissue that has formed on the eye's macula, located in the center of the eye's light-sensitive tissue called the retina. The macula provides the sharp, central vision we need for reading, driving, and seeing fine detail. A macular pucker can cause blurred and distorted central vision.

Macular pucker is also known as epiretinal membrane, preretinal membrane, cellophane maculopathy, retina wrinkle, surface wrinkling retinopathy, premacular fibrosis, and internal limiting membrane disease.

Frequently Asked Questions about Macular Pucker

Is a macular pucker the same as age-related macular degeneration?

No. A macular pucker and age-related macular degeneration are two separate and distinct conditions, although the symptoms for each are similar. An eye care professional will know the difference.

Can macular pucker get worse?

For most people, vision remains stable and does not get progressively worse. Usually macular pucker affects one eye, although it may affect the other eye later.

Is a macular pucker similar to a macular hole?

A macular pucker and a macular hole are different conditions, although they both result from the same reason: The pulling on the retina from a shrinking vitreous. When the "pulling" causes microscopic damage, the retina can heal itself; scar tissue, or a macular pucker, can be the result. If the shrinking vitreous pulls too hard, it can tear the retina, creating a macular hole, which is more serious. Both conditions have similar symptoms—distorted and blurred vision. Also, a macular pucker will not "develop" into a macular hole. An eye care professional will know the difference.

Cause

What causes a macular pucker?

Most of the eye's interior is filled with vitreous, a gel-like substance that fills about 80 percent of the eye and helps it maintain a round shape. The vitreous contains millions of fine fibers that are attached to the surface of the retina. As we age, the vitreous slowly shrinks and pulls away from the retinal surface. This is called a vitreous detachment, and is normal. In most cases, there are no adverse effects, except for a small increase in floaters, which are little "cobwebs" or specks that seem to float about in your field of vision.

However, sometimes when the vitreous pulls away from the retina, there is microscopic damage to the retina's surface (Note: This is not a macular hole). When this happens, the retina begins a healing process to the damaged area and forms scar tissue, or an epiretinal membrane, on the surface of the retina. This scar tissue is firmly attached to the retina surface. When the scar tissue contracts, it causes the retina to wrinkle, or pucker, usually without any effect on central vision. However, if the scar tissue has formed over the macula, our sharp, central vision becomes blurred and distorted.

Symptoms

What are the symptoms of a macular pucker?

Vision loss from a macular pucker can vary from no loss to severe loss, although severe vision loss is uncommon. People with a macular pucker may notice that their vision is blurry or mildly distorted, and straight lines can appear wavy. They may have difficulty in seeing fine detail and reading small print. There may be a gray area in the center of your vision, or perhaps even a blind spot.

Treatment

How is a macular pucker treated?

A macular pucker usually requires no treatment. In many cases, the symptoms of vision distortion and blurriness are mild, and no treatment is necessary. People usually adjust to the mild visual distortion, since it does not affect activities of daily life, such as reading and driving. Neither eye drops, medications, nor nutritional supplements will improve vision distorted from macular pucker. Sometimes the scar tissue—which causes a macular pucker—separates from the retina, and the macular pucker clears up.

Rarely, vision deteriorates to the point where it affects daily routine activities. However, when this happens, surgery may be recommended. This procedure is called a vitrectomy, in which the vitreous gel is removed to prevent it from pulling on the retina and replaced with a salt solution (Because the vitreous is mostly water, you will notice no change between the salt solution and the normal vitreous). Also, the scar tissue which causes the wrinkling is removed. A vitrectomy is usually performed under local anesthesia.

After the operation, you will need to wear an eye patch for a few days or weeks to protect the eye. You will also need to use medicated eye drops to protect against infection.

How successful is this surgery?

Surgery to repair a macular pucker is very delicate, and while vision improves in most cases, it does not usually return to normal. On average, about half of the vision lost from a macular pucker is restored; some people have significantly more vision restored, some less. In most cases, vision distortion is significantly reduced. Recovery of vision can take up to three months. Patients should talk with their eye care professional about whether treatment is appropriate.

What are the risks of surgery?

The most common complication of a vitrectomy is an increase in the rate of cataract development. Cataract surgery may be needed within a few years after the vitrectomy. Other, less common complications are retinal detachment either during or after surgery, and infection after surgery. Also, the macular pucker may grow back, but this is rare.

Current Research

What research is being done?

Research studies are being conducted to determine other treatments for macular pucker. Please note that both of the procedures described below need additional clinical testing. We suggest you share this information with your eye care professional.

Some physicians are researching the use of a surgical procedure in which scar tissue is peeled off without performing the vitrectomy.

Other doctors are researching a new surgical technique to remove the internal limiting membrane (a layer of the retina) for patients with both macular pucker and macular hole. This surgical technique is called fluidic internal limiting membrane separation (FILMS). After a vitrectomy, fluid is injected between the membrane and the retina that causes the membrane, along with the scar tissue, to lift away. It is then removed with forceps.

Chapter 25

Glaucoma

Chapter Contents

Section 25.1

Facts about Glaucoma

Reprinted from the National Eye Institute,
National Institutes of Health, September 2009.

Glaucoma Defined

What is glaucoma?

Glaucoma is a group of diseases that can damage the eye's optic nerve and result in vision loss and blindness. Glaucoma occurs when the normal fluid pressure inside the eyes slowly rises. However, with early treatment, you can often protect your eyes against serious vision loss.

What is the optic nerve?

The optic nerve is a bundle of more than one million nerve fibers. It connects the retina to the brain. The retina is the light-sensitive tissue at the back of the eye. A healthy optic nerve is necessary for good vision.

What are some other forms of glaucoma?

Open-angle glaucoma is the most common form. Some people have other types of the disease.

Low-tension or normal-tension glaucoma: Optic nerve damage and narrowed side vision occur in people with normal eye pressure. Lowering eye pressure at least 30 percent through medicines slows the disease in some people. Glaucoma may worsen in others despite low pressures.

A comprehensive medical history is important in identifying other potential risk factors, such as low blood pressure, that contribute to low-tension glaucoma. If no risk factors are identified, the treatment options for low-tension glaucoma are the same as for open-angle glaucoma.

Angle-closure glaucoma: The fluid at the front of the eye cannot reach the angle and leave the eye. The angle gets blocked by part of the iris. People with this type of glaucoma have a sudden increase in eye pressure. Symptoms include severe pain and nausea, as well as redness of the eye and blurred vision. If you have these symptoms, you need to seek treatment immediately.

This is a medical emergency. If your doctor is unavailable, go to the nearest hospital or clinic. Without treatment to improve the flow of fluid, the eye can become blind in as few as one or two days. Usually, prompt laser surgery and medicines can clear the blockage and protect sight.

Congenital glaucoma: Children are born with a defect in the angle of the eye that slows the normal drainage of fluid. These children usually have obvious symptoms, such as cloudy eyes, sensitivity to light, and excessive tearing. Conventional surgery typically is the suggested treatment, because medicines may have unknown effects in infants and be difficult to administer. Surgery is safe and effective. If surgery is done promptly, these children usually have an excellent chance of having good vision.

Secondary glaucomas: These can develop as complications of other medical conditions. These types of glaucomas are sometimes associated with eye surgery or advanced cataracts, eye injuries, certain eye tumors, or uveitis (eye inflammation). Pigmentary glaucoma occurs when pigment from the iris flakes off and blocks the meshwork, slowing fluid drainage. A severe form, called neovascular glaucoma, is linked to diabetes. Corticosteroid drugs used to treat eye inflammations and other diseases can trigger glaucoma in some people. Treatment includes medicines, laser surgery, or conventional surgery.

Causes and Risk Factors

How does open-angle glaucoma damage the optic nerve?

In the front of the eye is a space called the anterior chamber. A clear fluid flows continuously in and out of the chamber and nourishes nearby tissues. The fluid leaves the chamber at the open angle where the cornea and iris meet. When the fluid reaches the angle, it flows through a spongy meshwork, like a drain, and leaves the eye.

Sometimes, when the fluid reaches the angle, it passes too slowly through the meshwork drain. As the fluid builds up, the pressure inside the eye rises to a level that may damage the optic nerve. When the optic nerve is damaged from increased pressure, open-angle glaucoma—and vision loss—may result. That's why controlling pressure inside the eye is important.

Does increased eye pressure mean that I have glaucoma?

Not necessarily. Increased eye pressure means you are at risk for glaucoma, but does not mean you have the disease. A person has glaucoma only if the optic nerve is damaged. If you have increased eye pressure but no damage to the optic nerve, you do not have glaucoma. However, you are at risk. Follow the advice of your eye care professional.

Can I develop glaucoma if I have increased eye pressure?

Not necessarily. Not every person with increased eye pressure will develop glaucoma. Some people can tolerate higher eye pressure better than others. Also, a certain level of eye pressure may be high for one person but normal for another.

Whether you develop glaucoma depends on the level of pressure your optic nerve can tolerate without being damaged. This level is different for each person. That's why a comprehensive dilated eye exam is very important. It can help your eye care professional determine what level of eye pressure is normal for you.

Can I develop glaucoma without an increase in my eye pressure?

Yes. Glaucoma can develop without increased eye pressure. This form of glaucoma is called low-tension or normal-tension glaucoma. It is not as common as open-angle glaucoma.

Who is at risk for glaucoma?

Anyone can develop glaucoma. Some people are at higher risk than others. They include the following:

- African Americans over age forty
- Everyone over age sixty, especially Mexican Americans
- People with a family history of glaucoma

Among African Americans, studies show that glaucoma is:

- five times more likely to occur than in Caucasians;
- about four times more likely to cause blindness than in Caucasians;

- fifteen times more likely to cause blindness between the ages of forty-five and sixty-four than in Caucasians of the same age group.

A comprehensive dilated eye exam can reveal more risk factors, such as high eye pressure, thinness of the cornea, and abnormal optic nerve anatomy. In some people with certain combinations of these high-risk factors, medicines in the form of eye drops reduce the risk of developing glaucoma by about half.

Medicare covers an annual comprehensive dilated eye exam for some people at high risk for glaucoma.

What can I do to protect my vision?

Studies have shown that the early detection and treatment of glaucoma, before it causes major vision loss, is the best way to control the disease. So, if you fall into one of the high-risk groups for the disease, make sure to have your eyes examined through dilated pupils every two years by an eye care professional.

If you are being treated for glaucoma, be sure to take your glaucoma medicine every day. See your eye care professional regularly.

You also can help protect the vision of family members and friends who may be at high risk for glaucoma—African Americans over age forty; everyone over age sixty, especially Mexican Americans; and people with a family history of the disease. Encourage them to have a comprehensive dilated eye exam at least once every two years. Remember: Lowering eye pressure in glaucoma's early stages slows progression of the disease and helps save vision.

Symptoms and Detection

What are the symptoms of glaucoma?

At first, there are no symptoms. Vision stays normal, and there is no pain.

However, as the disease progresses, a person with glaucoma may notice his or her side vision gradually failing. That is, objects in front may still be seen clearly, but objects to the side may be missed.

As glaucoma remains untreated, people may miss objects to the side and out of the corner of their eye. Without treatment, people with glaucoma will slowly lose their peripheral (side) vision. They seem to be looking through a tunnel. Over time, straight-ahead vision may decrease until no vision remains.

Glaucoma can develop in one or both eyes.

How is glaucoma detected?

Glaucoma is detected through a comprehensive eye exam that includes the following:

- **Visual acuity test:** This eye chart test measures how well you see at various distances. A tonometer measures pressure inside the eye to detect glaucoma.

- **Visual field test:** This test measures your side (peripheral) vision. It helps your eye care professional tell if you have lost side vision, a sign of glaucoma.

- **Dilated eye exam:** Drops are placed in your eyes to widen, or dilate, the pupils. Your eye care professional uses a special magnifying lens to examine your retina and optic nerve for signs of damage and other eye problems. After the exam, your close-up vision may remain blurred for several hours.

- **Tonometry:** An instrument measures the pressure inside the eye. Numbing drops may be applied to your eye for this test.

- **Pachymetry:** A numbing drop is applied to your eye. Your eye care professional uses an ultrasonic wave instrument to measure the thickness of your cornea.

Treatment

Can glaucoma be treated?

Yes. Immediate treatment for early-stage, open-angle glaucoma can delay progression of the disease. That's why early diagnosis is very important.

Glaucoma treatments include medicines, laser trabeculoplasty, conventional surgery, or a combination of any of these. While these treatments may save remaining vision, they do not improve sight already lost from glaucoma.

Medicines: Medicines, in the form of eye drops or pills, are the most common early treatment for glaucoma. Some medicines cause the eye to make less fluid. Others lower pressure by helping fluid drain from the eye.

Before you begin glaucoma treatment, tell your eye care professional about other medicines you may be taking. Sometimes the drops can interfere with the way other medicines work.

Glaucoma medicines may be taken several times a day. Most people have no problems. However, some medicines can cause headaches or other side effects. For example, drops may cause stinging, burning, and redness in the eyes. Many drugs are available to treat glaucoma. If you have problems with one medicine, tell your eye care professional. Treatment with a different dose or a new drug may be possible.

Because glaucoma often has no symptoms, people may be tempted to stop taking, or may forget to take, their medicine. You need to use the drops or pills as long as they help control your eye pressure. Regular use is very important. Make sure your eye care professional shows you how to put the drops into your eye.

Laser trabeculoplasty: Laser trabeculoplasty helps fluid drain out of the eye. Your doctor may suggest this step at any time. In many cases, you need to keep taking glaucoma drugs after this procedure.

Laser trabeculoplasty is performed in your doctor's office or eye clinic. Before the surgery, numbing drops will be applied to your eye. As you sit facing the laser machine, your doctor will hold a special lens to your eye. A high-intensity beam of light is aimed at the lens and reflected onto the meshwork inside your eye. You may see flashes of bright green or red light. The laser makes several evenly spaced burns that stretch the drainage holes in the meshwork. This allows the fluid to drain better.

Like any surgery, laser surgery can cause side effects, such as inflammation. Your doctor may give you some drops to take home for any soreness or inflammation inside the eye. You need to make several follow-up visits to have your eye pressure monitored.

If you have glaucoma in both eyes, only one eye will be treated at a time. Laser treatments for each eye will be scheduled several days to several weeks apart.

Studies show that laser surgery is very good at reducing the pressure in some patients. However, its effects can wear off over time. Your doctor may suggest further treatment.

Conventional surgery: Conventional surgery makes a new opening for the fluid to leave the eye. Your doctor may suggest this treatment at any time. Conventional surgery often is done after medicines and laser surgery have failed to control pressure.

Conventional surgery is performed in an eye clinic or hospital. Before the surgery, you will be given medicine to help you relax. Your doctor will make small injections around the eye to numb it. A small piece of tissue is removed to create a new channel for the fluid to drain from the eye.

For several weeks after the surgery, you must put drops in the eye to fight infection and inflammation. These drops will be different from those you may have been using before surgery.

As with laser surgery, conventional surgery is performed on one eye at a time. Usually the operations are four to six weeks apart. Conventional surgery is about 60 to 80 percent effective at lowering eye pressure. If the new drainage opening narrows, a second operation may be needed. Conventional surgery works best if you have not had previous eye surgery, such as a cataract operation.

In some instances, your vision may not be as good as it was before conventional surgery. Conventional surgery can cause side effects, including cataract, problems with the cornea, and inflammation or infection inside the eye. The buildup of fluid in the back of the eye may cause some patients to see shadows in their vision. If you have any of these problems, tell your doctor so a treatment plan can be developed.

Conventional surgery makes a new opening for the fluid to leave the eye.

How should I use my glaucoma eye drops?

If eye drops have been prescribed for treating your glaucoma, you need to use them properly and as instructed by your eye care professional. Proper use of your glaucoma medication can improve the medicine's effectiveness and reduce your risk of side effects. To properly apply your eye drops, follow these steps:

- First, wash your hands.

- Hold the bottle upside down.

- Tilt your head back.

- Hold the bottle in one hand and place it as close as possible to the eye.

- With the other hand, pull down your lower eyelid. This forms a pocket.

- Place the prescribed number of drops into the lower eyelid pocket. If you are using more than one eye drop, be sure to wait at least five minutes before applying the second eye drop.

- Close your eye *or* press the lower lid lightly with your finger for at least one minute. Either of these steps keeps the drops in the eye and helps prevent the drops from draining into the tear duct, which can increase your risk of side effects.

What can I do if I already have lost some vision from glaucoma?

If you have lost some sight from glaucoma, ask your eye care professional about low vision services and devices that may help you make the most of your remaining vision. Ask for a referral to a specialist in low vision.

Many community organizations and agencies offer information about low vision counseling, training, and other special services for people with visual impairments. A nearby school of medicine or optometry may provide low vision services.

Current Research

What research is being done?

A large amount of research is being done in the United States to learn what causes glaucoma and to improve its diagnosis and treatment. For instance, the National Eye Institute (NEI) is funding a number of studies to find out what causes fluid pressure to increase in the eye. By learning more about this process, doctors may be able to find the exact cause of the disease and learn better how to prevent and treat it. The NEI also supports clinical trials of new drugs and surgical techniques that show promise against glaucoma.

Section 25.2

Reducing the Risk of Glaucoma

When it comes to glaucoma, risk reduction is a simple matter of damage control. Aside from following healthy-lifestyle recommendations, we have little control over whether we develop glaucoma.

If your vision care provider discovers you have elevated eye pressure, he or she may label you a "glaucoma suspect" and will be monitoring you closely to check your eye pressure and test for damage to your optic nerve.

Risk Factors

Researchers have identified a number of factors that indicate you are at increased risk of developing glaucoma.

Nonmodifiable Risk Factors

- **Advancing age:** Adults over age sixty are at increased risk of developing glaucoma. Elderly adults over age eighty have three to ten times the risk of developing glaucoma as those in their forties.

- **Ethnicity:** People of certain ethnic backgrounds have a greater risk of developing glaucoma and of having vision loss associated with the disease:

  - Black Americans, in particular, have a magnified risk. They're five times more likely than whites to be diagnosed with glaucoma and four times more likely to lose their sight to the disease.

  - Hispanic Americans also have an enhanced risk for open-angle glaucoma.

  - Asian Americans have a heightened risk of angle-closure glaucoma.

- **Family history:** Having an immediate family member with glaucoma—that is, a parent, child, brother, or sister who has the disease, boosts your risk of developing it as well.

- **Poor eyesight:** Nearsighted (myopic) people have a two- to threefold risk of glaucoma compared with non-nearsighted people. Farsighted people have recently been shown to have a steeper risk as well. People with either of these conditions, which vision care providers call refractive errors, should be monitored carefully.

- **Thin corneas:** The human cornea is so thin, it's measured in microns. One study showed that people with thin corneas—555 microns or less—have three times the risk of developing glaucoma, compared with people whose corneas measure 588 microns or more. Researchers are working to confirm this intriguing finding, but it's likely that having thin corneas will prove to be an independent risk factor for glaucoma.

Modifiable Risk Factors

- **Elevated eye pressure:** Calling elevated eye pressure a risk factor for glaucoma is like saying that having elevated blood sugar is a risk factor for diabetes. In other words, this risk factor is so closely associated with the disease itself that it's difficult to distinguish one from the other. On the other hand, the human body is idiosyncratic. An eye pressure that would destroy the optic nerve in one person might do no damage at all in another. Some folks can just tolerate a higher pressure with no ill effects. If your eye pressure is high, but you have no evidence of the disease, you should receive careful follow-up exams.

- **Having diabetes:** Researchers believe that if you have diabetes, you're twice as likely to develop glaucoma, although some studies are beginning to question that conclusion. Likewise, people who have glaucoma are more likely to develop diabetes. Systemic high blood pressure (as opposed to high eye pressure) is thought to coexist frequently with glaucoma. Scientists are still investigating the reason for this. Similarly, an unexplained association has been demonstrated between glaucoma and the endocrine disorder hypothyroidism.

- **Use of corticosteroid medications:** Certain corticosteroid medications, such as those found in some asthma inhalers, can block the ducts through which the aqueous fluid exits the eye. The optic nerve can be damaged if the drug is not discontinued promptly.

- **Eye injuries:** A type of glaucoma called traumatic glaucoma is associated with eye injuries. Such injuries can be caused by blunt trauma, such as being punched in a fight or being struck with a hockey puck, tennis racket, rock, or even a snowball or baton. In everyday terms, it's the kind of injury that gives you a black eye. Penetrating trauma occurs when a sharp object penetrates the eye. Objects that cause penetrating trauma include knives, metal fragments, BB gun pellets, glass, plastic, and even animal bites or scratches.

Risk Reduction

Doing damage control requires knowing whether you have glaucoma and, if so, keeping your eye pressure within the normal range to keep your optic nerve cells intact. Be sure to have your eyes examined at the recommended intervals. If your eye pressure is elevated, your provider may use a special tool to determine your risk that the condition will progress to glaucoma. If it does, following your prescribed treatment regimen, including using your eye drops as instructed, will help preserve your vision.

Glaucoma Screening

If you have diabetes or a family history of glaucoma, or if you are a black American age fifty or older or a Hispanic American age sixty-five and older, Medicare will cover a comprehensive dilated eye exam every year to check for diseases such as glaucoma, diabetic retinopathy, macular degeneration, and cataracts.

Follow the Recommended Treatment Regimen

Patients and doctors often wish there were a magic bullet that could make a disease go away. In glaucoma treatment, medicated eye drops aren't quite a magic bullet, but they're close. One convincing study reports that eye drops reduce eye pressure by more than 20 percent. In some patients with elevated pressure, daily use of eye drops cuts in half the risk of developing glaucoma.

Remember, vision loss from glaucoma can occur so slowly that you don't notice it, so continue to use your eye drops as prescribed even if you think your vision is tip-top.

Follow Healthy Lifestyle Recommendations to Prevent Diabetes and Obesity

Your risk of developing type 2 diabetes doubles for every 20 percent increase over your healthy body weight. Controlling your weight, then, reduces your risk of both diabetes and glaucoma, as well as many other obesity-related diseases. You should engage in moderate-intensity aerobic activity for at least 2.5 hours per week if you're able to do so. Not many of us can do headstands after age ten or so, but in case you're tempted, be aware that such activities can raise your eye pressure temporarily.

Stock your kitchen with fresh fruits and veggies, or with canned, frozen, or dried ones if you can't get out to the grocery store often. Aim for a low-fat, high-fiber diet consistent with the U.S. Department of Agriculture's most recent Dietary Guidelines for Americans.

Wear Recommended Eye Protection

It's not practical, of course, to wear safety goggles while playing with a cat or twirling a baton in the marching band. But those who are engaged in any activity that poses a serious threat of eye injury, such as drilling, sawing, riveting, and even lawn mowing, should wear safety glasses.

At work, pipe fitters, carpenters, and others who require protective eyewear should follow the guidelines issued by the Occupational Safety and Health Administration (OSHA). Glaucoma may develop soon after the injury or years later, so it's important for those who have suffered such injuries to receive regular screenings.

Living with Glaucoma

Being diagnosed with glaucoma or being told you are at risk for the disease means taking responsibility for your remaining vision, in concert with your vision care professional. The usual order of things, however, is reversed. Instead of patient relying on practitioner, your vision care provider is counting on you.

Section 25.3

Alternative Treatments for Glaucoma

Homeopathic Remedies: Herbs

Proponents of homeopathic medicine believe that symptoms represent the body's attack against disease, and that substances which induce the symptoms of a particular disease or diseases can help the body ward off illness.

Holistic Treatments

Holistic medicine is a system of health care designed to assist individuals in harmonizing mind, body, and spirit. Some of the more popular therapies include good nutrition, physical exercise, and self-regulation techniques including meditation, biofeedback, and relaxation training. While holistic treatments can be part of a good physical regimen, there is no proof of their usefulness in glaucoma therapy.

Eating and Drinking

No conclusive studies prove a connection between specific foods and glaucoma, but it is reasonable to assume that what you eat and drink and your general health have an effect on the disease.

Some studies have shown that significant caffeine intake over a short time can slightly elevate intraocular eye pressure (IOP) for one to three hours. However, other studies indicate that caffeine has no meaningful impact on IOP. To be safe, people with glaucoma are advised to limit their caffeine intake to moderate levels.

Studies have also shown that as many as 80 percent of people with glaucoma who consume an entire quart of water over the course of twenty minutes experience elevated IOP, as compared to only 20 percent of people who don't have glaucoma. Since many commercial diet programs stress the importance of drinking at least eight glasses of water each day, to be safe, people with glaucoma are encouraged to consume water in small amounts throughout the day.

Good Nutrition

The ideal way to ensure a proper supply of essential vitamins and minerals is by eating a balanced diet. If you are concerned about your own diet, you may want to consult with your doctor about taking a multivitamin or multimineral nutritional supplement.

Some of the vitamins and minerals important to the eye include zinc and copper, antioxidant vitamins C, E, and A (as beta-carotene), and selenium, an antioxidant mineral.

Bilberry

An extract of the European blueberry, bilberry is available through the mail and in some health food stores. It is most often advertised as an antioxidant eye health supplement that advocates claim can protect and strengthen the capillary walls of the eyes, and thus is especially effective in protecting against glaucoma, cataracts, and macular degeneration. There is some data indicating that bilberry may improve night vision and recovery time from glare, but there is no evidence that it is effective in the treatment or prevention of glaucoma.

Remember that the Food and Drug Administration (FDA) has not tested homeopathic remedies for safety or effectiveness. There is no guarantee that they contain consistent ingredients, or that dosage recommendations are accurate. It would be a serious mistake to use homeopathic remedies and dismiss valid therapies, delaying proven treatment for serious conditions.

Physical Exercise

There is some evidence suggesting that regular exercise can reduce eye pressure on its own, and can also have a positive impact on other glaucoma risk factors including diabetes and high blood pressure.

In a recent study, people with glaucoma who exercised regularly for three months reduced their IOPs an average of 20 percent. These people rode stationary bikes four times per week for forty minutes. Measurable improvements in eye pressure and physical conditioning were seen at the end of three months. These beneficial effects were maintained by continuing to exercise at least three times per week; lowered IOP was lost if exercise was stopped for more than two weeks.

In an ongoing study, glaucoma patients who walked briskly four times per week for forty minutes were able to lower their IOP enough to eliminate the need for beta blockers. Final results are not available, but there is hope that glaucoma patients with extremely high IOP who maintain an exercise schedule and continue beta-blocker therapy could significantly reduce their IOP.

Regular exercise may be a useful addition to the prevention of visual loss from glaucoma, but only your eye doctor can assess the effects of exercise on your eye pressure. Some forms of glaucoma (such as closed-angle) are not responsive to the effects of exercise, and other forms of glaucoma (for example, pigmentary glaucoma) may actually develop a temporary increase in IOP after vigorous exercise. And remember—exercise cannot replace medications or doctor visits!

Yoga and Recreational Body Inversion

The long-term effects of repeatedly assuming a head-down or inverted position on the optic nerve head (the nerve that carries visual images to the brain) have not been adequately demonstrated, but due to the potential for increased IOP, people with glaucoma should be careful about these kinds of exercises.

Glaucoma patients should let their doctors know if yoga shoulder and headstands or any other recreational body inversion exercises that result in head-down or inverted postures over extended periods of time are part of their exercise routines.

Self-Regulation Techniques

The results of studies regarding changes in IOP following relaxation and biofeedback sessions have generated some optimism in controlling selected cases of open-angle glaucoma, but further research is needed.

However, findings that reduced blood pressure and heart rate can be achieved with relaxation and biofeedback techniques show promise that nonmedicinal and nonsurgical techniques may be effective methods of treating and controlling open-angle glaucoma.

Section 25.4

Medical Marijuana to Treat Glaucoma

Glaucoma is a disease of the optic nerve, the cable that carries visual information from the eye to the brain. Damage to the optic nerve from glaucoma can result in vision loss and blindness.

Treatments that lower the pressure in the eye lower both the risk of developing the optic nerve damage that defines glaucoma, and the risk of preexisting damage getting worse.

Despite the treatments available for lowering eye pressure, such as eye drop medication, laser treatment, and operating room surgery, there are some individuals for whom these treatments either do not sufficiently lower the eye pressure, or cause unacceptable side effects. In these situations, both glaucoma patient and physician look for alternative therapies.

Treatment Alternative?

One of the commonly discussed alternatives for the treatment of glaucoma is the smoking of marijuana, because smoking marijuana does lower the eye pressure. Less often appreciated is the fact that marijuana's effect on eye pressure lasts only three to four hours, meaning that to lower the eye pressure around the clock it would have to be smoked six to eight times a day.

Furthermore, marijuana's mood-altering effects prevent the patient who is using it from driving, operating heavy machinery, and functioning at maximum mental capacity. Marijuana cigarettes also contain hundreds of compounds that damage the lungs, and the chronic, frequent use of marijuana can damage the brain.

Other means of administering the active ingredient of marijuana, tetrahydrocannabinol (THC), include by mouth and under the tongue. These methods avoid the harmful effect of marijuana smoke on the lungs, but are limited by the other systemic side effects, such as drowsiness and loss of judgment. In one study in which doctors offered some of their patients with worsening glaucoma the option of pills containing tetrahydrocannabinol and/or smoking marijuana, nine of nine patients discontinued use by either or both methods within nine months due to side effects. The use of eye drops containing THC or related compounds has been investigated, but it has not yet been possible to formulate an eye drop that is able to introduce the drug into the eye in sufficient concentration to be effective.

Lower Pressure

Although marijuana does lower the eye pressure, it also lowers blood pressure. Lower blood pressure could result in reduced blood supply to the optic nerve, which in turn might harm the optic nerve. Therefore it is possible that even though marijuana does lower the eye pressure, its use could conceivably make the vision loss from glaucoma worse! For this reason, marijuana cannot be recommended without a long-term clinical trial that evaluates the health of the optic nerve as well as the eye pressure.

The take-home message is that although marijuana can lower the eye pressure, recommending this drug in any form for the treatment of glaucoma at the present time does not make sense, given its side effects and short duration of action, coupled with a lack of evidence that its use alters the course of glaucoma.

Chapter 26

Other Disorders of the Optic Nerve

Chapter Contents

Section 26.1

Optic Nerve Atrophy

Optic nerve atrophy is damage to the optic nerve. The optic nerve carries images of what we see from the eye to the brain.

Causes

There are many unrelated causes of optic atrophy. The most common cause is poor blood flow, called ischemic optic neuropathy, which most often affects elderly people. The optic nerve can also be damaged by shock, various toxic substances, radiation, and trauma.

Various eye diseases, most commonly glaucoma, can also cause a form of optic nerve atrophy. In addition, the condition can be caused by diseases of the brain and central nervous system, such as:

- brain tumor;

- cranial arteritis (sometimes called temporal arteritis);

- multiple sclerosis;

- stroke.

There are also several rare forms of hereditary optic nerve atrophy that affect children and young adults.

Symptoms

Optic nerve atrophy causes vision to dim and reduces the field of vision. The ability to see fine detail will also be lost. Colors will seem faded. The pupil reaction to light will diminish and may eventually be lost.

Exams and Tests

Optic nerve atrophy can be seen during a complete examination of the eyes. The examination will include tests of:

- color loss;
- tonometry;
- pupil light reflex;
- visual acuity.

You may need a complete physical examination and specific tests.

Treatment

Damage from optic nerve atrophy cannot be reversed. The underlying disease must be found and treated, if possible, to prevent further loss.

Rarely, conditions that lead to optic atrophy may be treatable.

Outlook (Prognosis)

Vision lost to optic nerve atrophy cannot be recovered. If the cause can be found and controlled, further vision loss and blindness may be prevented. It is very important to protect the other eye.

Possible Complications

Complications are related to the disease that causes the atrophy.

When to Contact a Medical Professional

Patients with optic nerve atrophy will be closely monitored by an ophthalmologist who has experience in neuro-ophthalmology. Tell your doctor right away about any change in vision.

Prevention

Many causes of optic nerve atrophy cannot be prevented.
Ways to protect yourself include:

- Older adults should have their healthcare provider carefully manage their blood pressure.

- Prevent injuries to the face by using standard safety precautions. Most injuries to the face are related to motor vehicle accidents and can be prevented by using seat belts.

- Schedule a routine annual eye exam to check for glaucoma.

Methanol, which is found in home-brewed alcohol, can cause optic nerve atrophy in both eyes. Never drink home-brewed alcohol and forms of alcohol that are not intended for drinking.

Alternative Names

Optic atrophy; optic neuropathy

References

Balcer LJ, Brasad S. Abnormalities of the optic nerve and retina. In: Bradley WG, Daroff RB, Fenichel GM, Jankovic J, eds. *Neurology in Clinical Practice. 5th ed*. Philadelphia, Pa: Butterworth-Heinemann;2008:chap 15.

Arnold AC. Ischemic optic neuropathies. In: Yanoff M, Duker JS, eds. *Ophthalmology. 3rd ed*. St. Louis, Mo: Mosby Elsevier;2008:chap 9.7.

Wax M, Clark A, Civan MM. Mechanisms of glaucoma. In: Yanoff M, Duker JS, eds. *Ophthalmology. 3rd ed*. St. Louis, Mo: Mosby Elsevier;2008:chap 10.3.

Section 26.2

Optic Nerve Drusen

Your doctor has diagnosed you with optic disc drusen. Optic disc drusen are abnormal deposits of protein-like material in the optic disc—the front part of the optic nerve. We do not know the exact cause of optic disc drusen but they are thought to come from abnormal flow of material in optic nerve cells.

Optic disc drusen occur in about 1 percent of the population and are found more frequently in Caucasians. In three-quarters of cases they appear in both eyes. Optic disc drusen may be inherited or may occur without any family history. Familial drusen are inherited as an autosomal dominant trait, which means your mother or father or child is likely to have the condition.

Optic disc drusen are usually not visible at birth and are rarely found in infants and children. The drusen tend to develop slowly over time as the abnormal material collects in the optic nerve head and calcifies. The average age when optic disc drusen first appear is about twelve. Often, the optic disc has an unusual appearance, with multiple branches of the major blood vessels as they emerge on the optic disc.

As time passes, optic disc drusen can calcify and become more prominent. Optic disc drusen are rarely associated with any systemic disease or eye disease.

Symptoms

Optic disc drusen often come to medical attention during a routine eye examination. Patients usually have no symptoms and do not notice any problem with their vision. Occasionally, patients may have flickering or graying out of vision that lasts a few seconds or they may notice subtle visual field loss. The elevation of the optic disc with drusen may be mistaken for papilledema, which is swelling of the optic nerve from high pressure in the brain. This prompts referral to a neurologist, neurosurgeon, or even the emergency room.

Diagnosis

Optic disc drusen either can be buried within the substance of the optic nerve head or located superficially on the surface of the optic nerve head. When the drusen are superficial, they appear as glistening yellow bodies just below the surface of the optic nerve head and can be seen by ophthalmoscopic examination. When the optic disc drusen are buried deep in the disc, the drusen are hidden from direct view by the ophthalmoscope but can be identified by ultrasound.

If the drusen have become calcified, they also can be detected with computer tomography (CT) scanning. Visual field testing is important to detect defects in peripheral vision.

Prognosis

Most patients with optic disc drusen retain normal central vision. However, over time 70 percent of patients lose some peripheral vision. The amount of peripheral visual field loss varies from none to severe constriction of the peripheral visual field. The visual field should be followed periodically with formal visual field testing. Patients with optic disc drusen may also be at an increased risk for developing nonarteritic anterior ischemic optic neuropathy (NAION), branch retinal vein occlusion (BRVO), and central retinal vein occlusion (CRVO).

Although these conditions are uncommon, they may cause permanent visual loss.

Management and Treatment

There is no proven or standard treatment for optic disc drusen. Nevertheless, careful monitoring of the visual field is important to detect progression of visual field loss. Rarely, a small area of new blood vessels called a choroidal neovascular membrane [CNV] can develop adjacent to the optic disc. A CNV has a tendency to bleed and cause sudden visual loss. Early detection of the presence of CNV is extremely important because prompt treatment can often prevent serious complications from bleeding.

Frequently Asked Questions

Why did I develop optic disc drusen?

Optic disc drusen are caused by an abnormal deposition of a protein-like material in the optic nerve. The cause of this material is unknown. In some individuals, the deposition of this material can be inherited, while in others it occurs without a family history.

How does my doctor diagnose this condition?

Your doctor can diagnosis this condition either by an ophthalmoscopic examination or with the aid of ultrasound or computer tomography (CT) scanning.

Will the drusen get worse?

The number and size of the optic disc drusen tend to increase over time.

Can this condition affect any of my family members?

Yes, optic disc drusen can occur as an inherited family trait and may affect first-degree relatives. Patients diagnosed with optic disc drusen should consider discussing their diagnosis with their family members so that they undergo screening evaluation. Optic disc drusen usually do not show up in infants and children younger than four years.

Should I let other physicians who may be caring for me or other family members know about my condition?

Yes, it would be helpful for other physicians who are involved with your care or the care of a family member to know that you have diagnosed with optic disc drusen. You should inform them that you do not have papilledema.

Is there anything I can do to prevent the drusen from getting worse?

No, there is no proven or standard way, no medicine nor diet, to prevent the optic disc drusen from increasing in size.

Is there any treatment for this condition?

No, there is no proven treatment for optic disc drusen at this time.

If there is no treatment for optic disc drusen, why should I have regular ophthalmic examinations?

Some patients with optic disc drusen may rarely develop a growth of new abnormal blood vessels (choroidal neovascularization) adjacent to the optic nerve, which may be prone to bleeding. If new blood vessels develop, they may need laser treatment to prevent bleeding. Periodic examination is recommended to detect this potentially serious complication. Additionally, regular visual field testing is necessary to track any progression of peripheral visual field loss.

Section 26.3

Optic Nerve Hypoplasia

Introduction

A person with optic nerve hypoplasia (ONH) has small eye nerves
(optic nerves) from the eye to the brain. Some people with optic nerve
hypoplasia also have an abnormal brain and a poorly functioning pituitary gland. This section explains the problems that can occur in
children with optic nerve hypoplasia. Your child may have none, any,
or all of these problems in a mild or more serious form. Depending
on the person's problem, sometimes the disease is called optic nerve
hypoplasia (ONH), septo-optic dysplasia, or de Morsier syndrome.

How the Eye Works

The eyes receive light from the outside world and send these pictures to the brain along the optic nerves.

The Vision of People with Optic Nerve Hypoplasia

A person with optic nerve hypoplasia has optic nerves which are
small and poorly developed. Instead of having over one million connections (nerve fiber) from each eye to the brain, people with optic nerve
hypoplasia have far fewer connections. The more connections between
the eye and brain, the better vision. Some people with ONH have near
normal vision in one eye, others have decreased vision in both eyes,
and others are severely affected and nearly blind.

The Eye Examination

An eye doctor (ophthalmologist) can diagnose optic nerve hypoplasia
by looking inside the eye with an ophthalmoscope. The front of the optic

nerve (optic disc) appears smaller than normal. Your child will undergo a number of eye examinations to determine his or her vision. The younger the child the more difficult it is to tell the amount of vision present. Depending on your child's ability to cooperate with the examination, an experienced ophthalmologist can usually tell your child's ability to see. However, this usually cannot be done with children under the age of three to four years. It takes a number of years to be able to tell what a child's vision will be like. The vision does not usually worsen over time from optic nerve hypoplasia. It may, however, improve over time. Most children with optic nerve hypoplasia have unusual eye movements (nystagmus). They may have eyes that seem to move around with no real pattern or purpose. This occurs because the eyes are not able to focus well enough to hold still; this pattern is often seen with children who have poor vision.

The Brain: Formation and Function

Many people with optic nerve hypoplasia have abnormalities of the brain. These abnormalities may include how the brain is formed (brain structure) and how the brain works (brain function). While both usually occur, sometimes a child has a problem only with the structure of the brain and at other times, a child has a problem only with the function of the brain. All the problems with the brain can range from minor to very serious. The normal brain is made up of two equal parts (hemispheres), which are connected by nerve fibers (corpus callosum) and are separated by fluid-filled spaces (ventricles). The ventricles have dividers between them (septum pellucidum). Some people with optic nerve hypoplasia have a problem with the formation of the septum pellucidum; this is called septo-optic dysplasia or DeMorsier syndrome. Others have an abnormal corpus callosum. Some people also have other parts of the brain which are abnormally formed. These can be seen with the CT (computerized tomography) or MRI (magnetic resonance imaging). Problems with the formation of the brain can be quite varied, often involving the hemispheres and the ventricles. These can lead to small brains, excessively large ventricles, and fluid filled sacs (cysts) in the ventricles. In some people with optic nerve hypoplasia, these brain problems are minor and do not cause abnormal brain function. In others, brain function is affected, ranging from mild to severe. The major areas which can be involved are the use of large muscle (gross motor) and small muscle (fine motor), intelligence and learning, speech, and interacting with people. Many of these problems can be helped with therapy. Some children with optic nerve hypoplasia also have seizures (fits, convulsions) and may need to take medicines to control the seizures.

Brain Evaluation and Tests

When your child is diagnosed, and at regular times during your child's life, he or she will undergo a number of evaluations and brain function tests (neurologic tests). These are usually done by a brain specialist (neurologist). To show the structure of the brain, radiologic tests such as CT or MRI can be done by an imaging specialist (radiologist). Testing to determine how your child is developing and to screen for learning problems can be done by specialists in child development (pediatricians, psychologists, occupational/physical therapists, and or teachers). Testing can be done in several settings, including schools, hospitals, or other clinical settings. At the time your child is diagnosed with optic nerve hypoplasia your doctors should be able to tell you if there are major problems with your child's brain structure. Doctors cannot always predict if a child will or will not have problems with brain function. When a child is less than three to four years of age, it is often difficult to predict future brain functions such as speech, intelligence, and learning. All of these brain problems may worsen if your child has poor vision (is visually impaired). It is sometimes difficult to assess the brain function and overall development of a child with poor vision. Visually impaired children must be taught and tested in different ways. Be sure that your child is tested and treated by professionals who have experience working with children with poor vision.

The Pituitary Gland

The pituitary gland is found at the base of the brain and serves as the body's "master control gland" because it makes important chemicals (hormones) and directs the making of hormones in glands located in other parts of the body. These hormones are required for growth, energy control (metabolism), and sexual development. Many children with ONH have problems with their pituitary gland ranging from very minor problems with almost no effect on the child, to problems making one or more very important hormones. When a person has problems making hormones in the pituitary gland, it is called hypopituitarism. Your child will be tested to see if there are any problems making hormones. This is done by a doctor who specializes in gland problems (endocrinologist). Tests are done at the time of diagnosis and regularly as your child grows up. A child who initially does not have hormone problems may develop them at a later time. Therefore, it is very important for your child to be tested regularly as he or she grows up.

Services

Children with optic nerve hypoplasia (ONH) may need many special evaluations, tests, and services. As the parent of child with optic nerve hypoplasia, it is important to have a healthcare team that is knowledgeable about your child's condition. The medical team should include a primary care provider, an ophthamologist, an endocrinologist, a psychologist, a neurologist, and perhaps a social worker.

During preschool years, your child will need a developmental assessment. This must be done by someone who is skilled in working with children with poor vision. When your child is about to start school, testing for the most appropriate school placement should be performed. All children are entitled to receive education which meets their needs. To start the process for school placement, contact your local elementary school or local center for children with developmental problems (for example, regional center) both in person and in writing. You will need to request an individualized education plan (IEP) for your child. This process includes an assessment of your child by either the school district or a center for children with developmental problems with a specific educational program for your child. You will need to let the professionals know that your child has ONH and any other problems. Keep track of all letters and phone calls made to the district or developmental center. If your child is too young to start an in-school program (for example, if he or she is an infant), services may be provided on a weekly or monthly basis in your home via the local developmental disabilities center or visually impaired program. To make your child's educational experience the best it can be, repeat assessments must be done to insure that your child is learning and developing as expected.

Many children require placement in programs for children with poor sight (visually handicapped). As your child gets older, he or she may benefit from visual aids such as an enlarger (to increase the size of print) and/or a special computer for the visually impaired (e.g., a scanner which would take written words and turn them into spoken words).

If your child is not progressing well, additional services might be helpful. Other services may include language therapy (provided by a speech/ language pathologist) and vision therapy. If you have concerns about your child's development in any of these areas, contact the school or developmental disabilities center and request an assessment in these specific areas.

You should become aware of state and local programs that can help your child, such as early intervention programs (funded by state and federal funds), supplemental insurance programs, and special resources.

Section 26.4

Optic Neuritis

Your doctor thinks that you have had an episode of optic neuritis. This is the most common cause of sudden visual loss in a young patient. It is often associated with discomfort in or around the eye, particularly with eye movement.

Anatomy

We do not see with our eyes. Our eyes send a message via the optic nerves to the back part of the brain (occipital lobes), where the information is interpreted as an image. The optic nerve fibers are coated with myelin to help them conduct the electrical signals back to your brain.

Physiology

In the most common form of optic neuritis, the optic nerve has been attacked by the body's overactive immune system. The immune system is very important to our well-being. It is responsible for fighting off bacteria and viruses that can cause infection. In optic neuritis and other autoimmune diseases, the body's immune system has decided that otherwise normal tissues are foreign and therefore has attacked it. In the case of optic neuritis, the myelin coating the optic nerve has been targeted as foreign material. A viral infection that may have occurred years, or even decades, earlier may have set the stage for an acute episode of optic neuritis. What triggers the sudden loss of vision and optic nerve dysfunction at this time is unknown but probably occurs in individuals with a certain type of immune system. The inflammation associated with optic neuritis can result in discomfort (particularly with movement of the eye). In some cases of optic neuritis there may be more extensive involvement, including the other optic nerve, the chiasm (where the two optic nerves come together), or other tissues in the brain.

Symptoms

The most common symptom of optic neuritis is sudden decrease in vision. Patients may describe this as blurred vision, dark vision, dim vision, or simply loss of vision in the center or part or all of the visual field. In mild cases, it may look like "the contrast is turned down" or that colors appear "washed out." This may vary and, not infrequently, will progress from the time it is first noticed. The second most common symptom associated with optic neuritis is discomfort in or around the eye, often made worse by movement of the eye.

Signs

Optic neuritis may be difficult to diagnose, as your eye looks perfectly normal. Often the inside of your eye also looks normal. A few patients with optic neuritis have swelling of the optic disc (the beginning of the optic nerve) at the back of the eye. This is referred to as papillitis. One sign usually detected by your eye doctor is the presence of an afferent pupillary defect. This indicates that there is less light being sensed by the affected eye than the opposite eye. This is found by swinging a bright light back and forth between your two eyes while observing how your pupil reacts.

Prognosis

The pain will go away, usually in a few days. The vision problems will improve in the majority (92 percent) of patients. There are rare patients who have continued progressive loss of vision. Even in the 92 percent that improve, often they do not return completely to normal. Patients may be left with blurred, dark, dim, or distorted vision. Frequently colors look different or "washed out." Visual recovery usually takes place over a period of weeks to months, although both earlier and later improvement is possible.

Late variations in vision are common, often associated with exercise or taking a hot shower or bath. This is known as Uhthoff phenomena and is probably related to damage to the myelin coating. Patients who notice this problem are not more likely to get worse.

Optic neuritis can recur involving the same eye, the other eye, or other parts of the central nervous system (brain and spinal cord). This may result in recurrent episodes of decreased or loss of vision or problems with weakness, numbness, or other signs of brain involvement. A magnetic resonance imaging (MRI) scan can give us a rough guess as to the likelihood of recurrence.

It will not completely exclude the possibility of future episodes or guarantee that they will happen.

Other testing techniques are sometimes used to confirm the suspicion of optic neuritis. These may include visual evoked potentials (a test where you are shown a checkerboard of light and signals are recorded from electrodes on your scalp) that can show a delay in conduction due to the damage to the myelin.

Treatment

A study (the Optic Neuritis Treatment Trial [ONTT]) suggested that the likelihood of recovery at six months was equal whether they were treated with steroids or sugar pills. Patients treated with oral (pills) steroids seemed to have a higher chance of recurrent episodes. Therefore, steroid pills are not recommended as treatment. Patients who were treated with intravenous (IV; given by needle) steroids did have a slightly more rapid recovery of their vision, although the final visual outcome was not better than in those who were not treated. Thus, IV steroids can be recommended for patients with severe involvement or involvement of both eyes. The ONTT also suggested that IV steroids in those patients at high risk (as determined by their MRI scan) could have a reduction in the chances of a second episode over the next three years. Recent studies have suggested that the chance of developing a recurrent episode may be reduced by starting other medications after IV steroids in those patients at high risk. MRI is important in suggesting the chance of recurrence or progression. Your doctor can address questions about possible treatment with you.

Frequently Asked Questions

What caused this to happen?

We don't have a complete understanding of optic neuritis at this time. It is likely that it represents a combination of a particular form of immune system combined with a previous stimulation, possibly a virus.

What's going to happen to my vision?

In the vast majority of patients, your vision will improve. It may not improve to normal, but it is likely that there will be a substantial improvement whether or not you are treated.

Can treatment with steroids make this better?

Treatment with IV steroids has been demonstrated to accelerate recovery but it will not change the ultimate level of recovery on average. We have no way to guarantee that vision will recover and in some patients it will not.

Do I have multiple sclerosis?

Multiple sclerosis (MS) is a disease process where the body's immune system attacks multiple areas in multiple episodes. An episode of optic neuritis may be the first indication of multiple sclerosis. With a single episode, without other evidence of involvement, we usually cannot make the diagnosis at that time. An MRI scan may be helpful in dividing those patients into high and low risks. Finding evidence of other areas of inflammation on MRI scanning suggests you may be at higher risk for recurrent episodes and thus MS. Your doctor may suggest consultation with a neurologist to discuss treatments that might reduce the risk of recurrent disease. Even a normal scan does not guarantee that episodes may not recur over years. Whether or not this turns out to be MS in the future, the prognosis in terms of visual recovery is still good for this particular episode.

Can I prevent MS?

The ONTT demonstrated that the use of high-dose intravenous steroids in patients at high risk (two or more spots on MRI scan) may delay the onset of MS. Recent data suggests that some of the newer medications may also decrease the chance of having another neurologic event. Thus it may be important to recognize those patients at higher risk to start earlier treatment. This is best determined by MRI. There is no treatment that will absolutely prevent the development of multiple sclerosis.

Chapter 27

Disorders of the Retina

Chapter Contents

Section 27.1

Retinal Detachment

"Facts about Retinal Detachment," National Eye Institute,
National Institutes of Health, October 2009.

Retinal Detachment Defined

What is retinal detachment?

The retina is the light-sensitive layer of tissue that lines the inside of the eye and sends visual messages through the optic nerve to the brain. When the retina detaches, it is lifted or pulled from its normal position. If not promptly treated, retinal detachment can cause permanent vision loss.

In some cases there may be small areas of the retina that are torn. These areas, called retinal tears or retinal breaks, can lead to retinal detachment.

Frequently Asked Questions about Retinal Detachment

What are the different types of retinal detachment?

There are three different types of retinal detachment:

- **Rhegmatogenous [reg-ma-TAH-jenous]:** A tear or break in the retina allows fluid to get under the retina and separate it from the retinal pigment epithelium (RPE), the pigmented cell layer that nourishes the retina. These types of retinal detachments are the most common.

- **Tractional:** In this type of detachment, scar tissue on the retina's surface contracts and causes the retina to separate from the RPE. This type of detachment is less common.

- **Exudative:** Frequently caused by retinal diseases, including inflammatory disorders and injury/trauma to the eye. In this type, fluid leaks into the area underneath the retina, but there are no tears or breaks in the retina.

Causes and Risk Factors

Who is at risk for retinal detachment?

A retinal detachment can occur at any age, but it is more common in people over age forty. It affects men more than women, and whites more than African Americans.

A retinal detachment is also more likely to occur in people who have the following characteristics:

- Are extremely nearsighted

- Have had a retinal detachment in the other eye

- Have a family history of retinal detachment

- Have had cataract surgery

- Have other eye diseases or disorders, such as retinoschisis, uveitis, degenerative myopia, or lattice degeneration

- Have had an eye injury

Symptoms and Detection

What are the symptoms of retinal detachment?

Symptoms include a sudden or gradual increase in either the number of floaters, which are little "cobwebs" or specks that float about in your field of vision, and/or light flashes in the eye. Another symptom is the appearance of a curtain over the field of vision. A retinal detachment is a medical emergency. Anyone experiencing the symptoms of a retinal detachment should see an eye care professional immediately.

Treatment

How is retinal detachment treated?

Small holes and tears are treated with laser surgery or a freeze treatment called cryopexy. These procedures are usually performed in the doctor's office. During laser surgery tiny burns are made around the hole to "weld" the retina back into place. Cryopexy freezes the area around the hole and helps reattach the retina.

Retinal detachments are treated with surgery that may require the patient to stay in the hospital. In some cases a scleral buckle, a tiny synthetic band, is attached to the outside of the eyeball to gently push the wall of the eye against the detached retina. If necessary, a vitrectomy may also be performed. During a vitrectomy, the doctor makes a tiny incision in the sclera (white of the eye). Next, a small instrument is placed into the eye to remove the vitreous, a gel-like substance that fills the center of the eye and helps the eye maintain a round shape. Gas is often injected into the eye to replace the vitreous and reattach the retina; the gas pushes the retina back against the wall of the eye. During the healing process, the eye makes fluid that gradually replaces the gas and fills the eye. With all of these procedures, either laser or cryopexy is used to "weld" the retina back in place.

With modern therapy, over 90 percent of those with a retinal detachment can be successfully treated, although sometimes a second treatment is needed. However, the visual outcome is not always predictable. The final visual result may not be known for up to several months following surgery. Even under the best of circumstances, and even after multiple attempts at repair, treatment sometimes fails and vision may eventually be lost. Visual results are best if the retinal detachment is repaired before the macula (the center region of the retina responsible for fine, detailed vision) detaches. That is why it is important to contact an eye care professional immediately if you see a sudden or gradual increase in the number of floaters and/or light flashes, or a dark curtain over the field of vision.

Current Research

What research is being done?

The National Eye Institute (NEI) supported the Silicone Study, a nationwide clinical trial that compared the use of silicone oil with long-acting intraocular gas for repairing a retinal detachment caused by proliferative vitreoretinopathy (PVR). With PVR, cells grow on the surface of the retina, causing it to detach. This is a serious complication that sometimes follows retinal detachment surgery and is difficult to treat. The results indicate that both treatments are effective and give the surgeons more options for treating these difficult cases.

Section 27.2

Retinal Vein Occlusions

What Is Retinal Vein Occlusion?

Retinal vein occlusion (RVO) results from the blockage of a branch of retinal veins or the central retinal vein by a blood clot. The occlusion of the retinal veins leads to backup of the blood into the retina. The blood that has backed up becomes stagnant and leads to lack of oxygen getting to the retina.

Symptoms

RVO can cause sudden or gradual (days to weeks) painless vision loss, sensitivity to light, or it can be present without any symptoms at all.

RVO does not have a racial predilection. It is slightly more common in males than females. A majority of cases of RVO occur in people over the age of fifty, but it can occur in all age groups.

The common signs of RVO include: bleeding throughout the retina, engorged blood vessels, retinal swelling, and growth of new blood vessels in the retina or iris. In branch retinal vein occlusions, the signs only affect one quadrant of the retina, whereas in central retinal vein occlusions, the signs affect the entire retina.

Risk Factors

How RVO develop is not exactly known, but various risk factors contribute to the occlusion of the retinal veins.

Risk factors include:

- age;
- high blood pressure;
- diabetes;

349

- increased blood viscosity;

- use of oral contraceptives;

- glaucoma;

- cardiovascular disorders;

- bleeding disorders;

- clotting disorders;

- autoimmune disorders;

- inflammation of blood vessels

- closed head trauma.

The fellow eye may develop RVO in about 7 percent of cases within two years. There is a 2.5 percent risk of developing another RVO in the same eye and about 12 percent risk in the fellow eye within four years.

Treatment

Proper evaluation and management by an eye doctor is essential to correctly diagnose retinal vein occlusions. The diagnosis of RVO is made by a dilated eye exam.

Although there are no known effective treatments for RVO itself, there are treatments available to manage the complications associated with RVO, such as laser surgery to stop new blood vessel growth or injections to resolve swelling in the macula. It is also important to see a primary medical doctor to treat the underlying systemic medical conditions to reduce further complications.

Currently in clinical trials, the National Eye Institute is funding research throughout the country to evaluate the effects of an injection steroid treatment versus traditional treatment for treating macular swelling (observation for central retinal vein occlusion [CRVO]; laser surgery for branch retinal vein occlusion [BRVO]). The patients will be followed for three years to determine the long-term safety and efficacy of the treatment.

Section 27.3

Retinitis Pigmentosa

Retinitis pigmentosa (RP) is the name given to a group of hereditary retinal diseases characterized by progressive loss of visual field, night blindness, and reduced or absent electroretinogram (ERG test) recording, which indicates that a large portion of the retina is damaged.

RP causes the degeneration of photoreceptor cells in the retina. Photoreceptor cells capture and process light, helping us to see. As these cells degenerate and die, patients experience progressive vision loss.

There are two types of photoreceptor cells: rod cells and cone cells. Rod cells are concentrated along the outer perimeter of the retina. Rod cells help us to see images that come into our peripheral or side vision. They also help us to see in dark and dimly lit environments. Cone cells are concentrated in the macula, the center of the retina, and allow us to see fine visual detail in the center of our vision. Cone cells also allow us to perceive color. Together, rods and cones are the cells responsible for converting light into electrical impulses that are transmitted to the brain, where "seeing" actually occurs.

What Are the Different Types of Retinitis Pigmentosa?

Genetics of RP

Within the nucleus of every human cell reside a host of genes. Genes are the fundamental building blocks of life. Inherited from our parents, genes carry family traits like eye and hair color, the shape of our face, and even diseases like RP.

Genes are like computer programs containing sets of coded instructions. Each gene instructs the cell to create a specialized protein that performs a specific task for the cell. In retinal cells, some genes encode proteins that allow the cell to process light. Other genes encode proteins that uptake nutrients and eliminate waste. Still other genes encode proteins that form the cell walls and other structures within the cell.

Sometimes, the coded instructions within a gene become altered. These alterations, known as mutations, can confer a benefit, allowing the organism to better adapt to its environment. However, mutations can also interfere with the proper encoding of a protein. The resulting protein cannot perform its job within the cell, thereby hampering the cell's well-being and leading to disease.

Retinal cells are among the most specialized cells in the human body and depend on a number of unique genes to create vision. A disease-causing mutation in any one of these genes can lead to vision loss. To date, researchers have discovered over one hundred genes that can contain mutations leading to RP.

RP can be passed to succeeding generations by one of three genetic inheritance patterns—autosomal dominant, autosomal recessive, or X-linked inheritance.

Each type of inheritance causes a different pattern of affected and unaffected family members. For example, in families with autosomal recessive RP, unaffected parents can have both affected and unaffected children. In recessive RP, there is often no prior family history. In families with the autosomal dominant RP, an affected parent can have both affected and unaffected children. In families with the X-linked type, only males are affected, while females carry the genetic trait but do not experience serious vision loss.

It is very important to remember that because RP is an inherited disorder, it can potentially affect another member of the family. If one member of a family is diagnosed with a hereditary retinal degeneration, it is strongly advised that all members of that family contact an ophthalmologist.

Related Diseases

Other inherited diseases share some of the clinical symptoms of RP. Some of these conditions are complicated by other symptoms besides loss of vision. The most common of these is Usher syndrome, which causes both hearing and vision loss. Other rare syndromes include Bardet-Biedl (Laurence-Moon) syndrome, rod-cone dystrophy, choroideremia, gyrate-atrophy, Leber congenital amaurosis, and Stargardt disease.

RP and related diseases are rare and difficult to accurately diagnose. Only a specialist can properly distinguish between the subtle clinical features of these diseases. Therefore, it is important that patients who are symptomatic see an ophthalmologist who specializes in retinal degenerative diseases.

Symptoms

- Normal visual acuity in early stages, possibly—but not usually—progressing to no light perception
- Doughnut-shaped visual field loss progressing to severe constriction (loss of peripheral vision)
- Night blindness
- Decreased response to magnification
- Need for more light

The most common feature of all forms of RP is a gradual degeneration of the rods and cones. Most forms of RP first cause the degeneration of rod cells. These forms of RP, sometimes called rod-cone dystrophy, usually begin with night blindness. Night blindness is somewhat like the experience normally sighted individuals encounter when entering a dark movie theatre on a bright, sunny day. However, patients with RP cannot adjust well to dark and dimly lit environments.

As the disease progresses and more rod cells degenerate, patients lose their peripheral vision. Patients with RP often experience a ring of vision loss in their mid-periphery with small islands of vision in their very far periphery. Others report the sensation of tunnel vision, as though they see the world through the opening of a straw. Many patients with RP retain a small degree of central vision throughout their life.

Other forms of RP, sometimes called cone-rod dystrophy, first affect central vision. Patients first experience a loss of central vision that cannot be corrected with glasses or contact lenses. With the loss of cone cells also comes disturbance in color perception. As the disease progresses, rod cells also degenerate, causing night blindness and loss of peripheral vision.

Symptoms of RP are most often recognized in children, adolescents, and young adults, with progression of the disease continuing throughout the individual's life. The pattern and degree of visual loss are variable.

Diagnosis

These special tests can be used to help diagnose RP:

- **Acuity tests:** These tests measure the accuracy of your central vision at specific distances in specific lighting situations.

- **Color testing:** This can help determine the status of your cone cells, the retinal cells that interpret color.

- **Visual field test:** This test uses a machine to measure how much peripheral vision you have.

- **Dark adaptation test:** This test will measure how well your eyes adjust to changes in lighting and can help the doctor better understand the current function of your rod cells, which are the retinal cells responsible for night vision.

- **Electroretinogram (ERG) test:** The ERG test records the electrical currents produced by the retina due to a light stimulus. The intensity and speed of the electrical signal becomes reduced as the photoreceptor cells degenerate.

Risk Factors

Recent research findings suggest that in some forms of RP, prolonged, unprotected exposure to sunlight may accelerate vision loss.

Some women feel that their vision loss progressed more rapidly during pregnancy. However, the effect of pregnancy on RP has not been clinically studied.

RP is an inherited, genetic disease. It is caused by mutations in genes that are active in retinal cells. Gene mutations are programmed into your cells at the time of conception. RP is not caused by injury, infection, or exposure to any toxic substance.

What You Can Do to Reduce Risk

Reducing your exposure to sunlight is important for keeping the eye protected. However, since RP is an inherited disorder and it runs in families, the disease is not preventable. If someone in your family is diagnosed with a retinal degeneration, it is strongly advised that all members of the family contact an eye care professional.

Treatment

As yet, there is no known cure for RP. However, intensive research is currently under way to discover the cause, prevention, and treatment of RP.

Researchers have identified some of the genes that cause RP. It is now possible, in some families with X-linked RP or autosomal dominant RP, to perform a test on genetic material from blood and other cells to determine if members of an affected family have one of several RP genes.

Section 27.4

Retinoblastoma

Excerpted from PDQ® Cancer Information Summary. National Cancer Institute; Bethesda, MD. "Retinoblastoma Treatment (PDQ)—Patient Version." Updated November 2010. Available at: http://cancer.gov. Accessed March 27, 2011.

General Information about Retinoblastoma

What Is Retinoblastoma?

Retinoblastoma is a disease in which malignant (cancer) cells form in the tissues of the retina.

The retina is the nerve tissue that lines the inside of the back of the eye. The retina senses light and sends images to the brain by way of the optic nerve.

Although retinoblastoma may occur at any age, it usually occurs in children younger than five years, most often younger than two years. The tumor may be in one eye or in both eyes. Retinoblastoma rarely spreads from the eye to nearby tissue or other parts of the body.

Causes

Retinoblastoma is sometimes caused by a gene mutation passed from the parent to the child. Retinoblastoma that is caused by an inherited gene mutation is called hereditary retinoblastoma. It usually occurs at a younger age than retinoblastoma that is not inherited. Retinoblastoma that occurs in only one eye is usually not inherited. Retinoblastoma that occurs in both eyes is thought to be inherited.

When hereditary retinoblastoma first occurs in only one eye, there is a chance it will develop later in the other eye. After diagnosis of retinoblastoma in one eye, regular follow-up exams of the healthy eye should be done every two to four months for at least twenty-eight months. After treatment for retinoblastoma is finished, it is important that follow-up exams continue until the child is five years old.

Treatment for both types of retinoblastoma should include genetic counseling (a discussion with a trained professional about inherited diseases). The parents of a child with retinoblastoma should have an eye exam by an ophthalmologist (a doctor with special training in diseases of the eye) and genetic counseling about whether they should be tested for the gene that causes retinoblastoma and the risk of the child's brothers or sisters developing retinoblastoma. The child's brothers and sisters also should have regular eye exams by an ophthalmologist until age five years.

Additional Risks

A child who has hereditary retinoblastoma is at risk for developing pineal tumors in the brain. This is called trilateral retinoblastoma and usually occurs more than twenty months after retinoblastoma is diagnosed. Regular screening using MRI (magnetic resonance imaging) every six months for five years may be recommended for a child with hereditary retinoblastoma or with retinoblastoma in one eye and a family history of the disease. CT scans (computerized tomography) should not be used for routine screening to avoid exposing the child to ionizing radiation. Hereditary retinoblastoma also increases the child's risk of developing other types of cancer such as bone or soft tissue sarcoma or melanoma in later years. Regular follow-up exams are important.

Signs and Symptoms

Possible signs of retinoblastoma include "white pupil" and eye pain or redness.

These and other symptoms may be caused by retinoblastoma. Other conditions may cause the same symptoms. A doctor should be consulted if any of the following problems occur:

- Pupil of the eye appears white instead of red when light shines into it. This may be seen in flash photographs of the child.

- Eyes appear to be looking in different directions.

- Pain or redness in the eye.

Diagnosis

Tests that examine the retina are used to detect (find) and diagnose retinoblastoma.

The following tests and procedures may be used:

- **Physical exam and history:** An exam of the body to check general signs of health, including checking for signs of disease, such as lumps or anything else that seems unusual. A history of the patient's health habits and past illnesses and treatments will also be taken. The doctor will ask if there is a family history of retinoblastoma.

- **Eye exam with dilated pupil:** An exam of the eye in which the pupil is dilated (opened wider) with medicated eye drops to allow the doctor to look through the lens and pupil to the retina. The inside of the eye, including the retina and the optic nerve, is examined with a light. Depending on the age of the child, this exam may be done under anesthesia.

- **Ultrasound exam:** A procedure in which high-energy sound waves (ultrasound) are bounced off internal tissues or organs and make echoes. The echoes form a picture of body tissues called a sonogram.

- **Computed tomography (CT scan or CAT scan):** A procedure that makes a series of detailed pictures of areas inside the body, such as the eye, taken from different angles. The pictures are made by a computer linked to an x-ray machine. A dye may be injected into a vein or swallowed to help the organs or tissues show up more clearly. This procedure is called computed tomography, computerized tomography, or computerized axial tomography.

- **Magnetic resonance imaging (MRI):** A procedure that uses a magnet, radio waves, and a computer to make a series of detailed pictures of areas inside the body, such as the eye. This procedure is also called nuclear magnetic resonance imaging (NMRI).

Retinoblastoma is usually diagnosed without a biopsy (removal of cells or tissues so they can be viewed under a microscope to check for signs of cancer).

Prognosis

Certain factors affect prognosis (chance of recovery) and treatment options.

The prognosis (chance of recovery) and treatment options depend on the following:

- The stage of the cancer

- The age of the patient

- How likely it is that vision can be saved in one or both eyes

- The size and number of tumors
- Whether the patient has glaucoma
- Whether trilateral retinoblastoma occurs

Stages of Retinoblastoma

Testing for Spread of the Disease

After retinoblastoma has been diagnosed, tests are done to find out if cancer cells have spread within the eye or to other parts of the body.

The process used to find out if cancer has spread within the eye or to other parts of the body is called staging. The information gathered from the staging process determines the stage of the disease. It is important to know the stage in order to plan treatment. The following tests and procedures may be used in the staging process:

- Eye exam with dilated pupil
- Ultrasound exam
- CT scan (CAT scan)
- Magnetic resonance imaging (MRI)
- Lumbar puncture (spinal tap)
- Bone marrow aspiration and biopsy

There are several staging systems for retinoblastoma. For treatment, retinoblastoma is classified as intraocular (within the eye) or extraocular (outside the eye).

Stages

The following stages are used for retinoblastoma:

- **Intraocular retinoblastoma:** In intraocular retinoblastoma, cancer is found in the eye and may be only in the retina or may also be in other parts of the eye, such as the choroid, ciliary body, or part of the optic nerve. Cancer has not spread to tissues around the outside of the eye or to other parts of the body.

- **Extraocular retinoblastoma:** In extraocular (metastatic) retinoblastoma, cancer has spread beyond the eye. It may be found in tissues around the eye or it may have spread to the central nervous system (brain and spinal cord) or to other parts of the body such as the bone marrow or lymph nodes.

There are three ways that cancer spreads in the body. They are:

- **Through tissue:** Cancer invades the surrounding normal tissue.

- **Through the lymph system:** Cancer invades the lymph system and travels through the lymph vessels to other places in the body.

- **Through the blood:** Cancer invades the veins and capillaries and travels through the blood to other places in the body.

When cancer cells break away from the primary (original) tumor and travel through the lymph or blood to other places in the body, another (secondary) tumor may form. This process is called metastasis. The secondary (metastatic) tumor is the same type of cancer as the primary tumor. For example, if breast cancer spreads to the bones, the cancer cells in the bones are actually breast cancer cells. The disease is metastatic breast cancer, not bone cancer.

Recurrent Retinoblastoma

Recurrent retinoblastoma is cancer that has recurred (come back) after it has been treated. The cancer may recur in the eye, in tissues around the eye, or in other places in the body.

Treatment Option Overview

Types of Treatment

Different types of treatment are available for patients with retinoblastoma. Some treatments are standard (the currently used treatment), and some are being tested in clinical trials. A treatment clinical trial is a research study meant to help improve current treatments or obtain information on new treatments for patients with cancer. When clinical trials show that a new treatment is better than the standard treatment, the new treatment may become the standard treatment.

Because cancer in children is rare, taking part in a clinical trial should be considered. Some clinical trials are open only to patients who have not started treatment.

Side Effects

Some cancer treatments cause side effects months or years after treatment has ended. Side effects from cancer treatment that begin during or after treatment and continue for months or years are called late effects. Late effects of cancer treatment may include the following:

- Physical problems such as problems with seeing clearly

- Changes in mood, feelings, thinking, learning, or memory

- Second cancers (new types of cancer)

Some late effects may be treated or controlled. It is important to talk with your child's doctors about the effects cancer treatment can have on your child.

Children with the inherited form of retinoblastoma have an increased risk of developing second cancers. Children, especially those younger than twelve years, who have been treated for retinoblastoma with radiation therapy have a risk of developing second cancers. Regular follow-up by health professionals who are expert in finding and treating late effects is important.

Standard Treatments

Six types of standard treatment are used.

Enucleation: Enucleation is surgery to remove the eye and part of the optic nerve. The eye will be checked with a microscope to see if there are any signs that the cancer is likely to spread to other parts of the body. This is done if the tumor is large and there is little or no chance that vision can be saved. The patient will be fitted for an artificial eye after this surgery. Close follow-up is needed for two years or more to check the other eye and to check for signs of recurrence in the area around the eye.

Radiation therapy: Radiation therapy is a cancer treatment that uses high-energy x-rays or other types of radiation to kill cancer cells or keep them from growing. There are two types of radiation therapy. External radiation therapy uses a machine outside the body to send radiation toward the cancer. Internal radiation therapy uses a radioactive substance sealed in needles, seeds, wires, plaques, or catheters that are placed directly into or near the cancer. The way the radiation therapy is given depends on the type and stage of the cancer being treated. Methods of radiation therapy used to treat retinoblastoma include the following:

- **Intensity-modulated radiation therapy (IMRT):** A type of three-dimensional (3-D) radiation therapy that uses a computer to make pictures of the size and shape of the tumor. Thin beams of radiation of different intensities (strengths) are aimed at the tumor from many angles. This type of radiation therapy causes less damage to healthy tissue near the tumor.

- **Stereotactic radiation therapy:** Radiation therapy that uses a rigid head frame attached to the skull to aim high-dose radiation beams directly at the tumors, causing less damage to nearby healthy tissue. It is also called stereotactic external-beam radiation and stereotaxic radiation therapy.

- **Proton beam radiation therapy:** Radiation therapy that uses protons made by a special machine. A proton is a type of high-energy radiation that is different from an x-ray.

- **Plaque radiotherapy:** Radioactive seeds are attached to one side of a disk, called a plaque, and placed directly on the outside wall of the eye near the tumor. The side of the plaque with the seeds on it faces the eyeball, aiming radiation at the tumor. The plaque helps protect other nearby tissue from the radiation.

- **Cryotherapy:** Cryotherapy is a treatment that uses an instrument to freeze and destroy abnormal tissue, such as carcinoma in situ. This type of treatment is also called cryosurgery.

- **Thermotherapy:** Thermotherapy is the use of heat to destroy cancer cells. Thermotherapy may be given using a laser beam aimed through the dilated pupil or onto the outside of the eyeball, or using ultrasound, microwaves, or infrared radiation (light that cannot be seen but can be felt as heat). Thermotherapy may be used alone for small tumors or combined with chemotherapy for larger tumors.

- **Chemotherapy:** Chemotherapy is a cancer treatment that uses drugs to stop the growth of cancer cells, either by killing the cells or by stopping them from dividing. When chemotherapy is taken by mouth or injected into a vein or muscle, the drugs enter the bloodstream and can reach cancer cells throughout the body (systemic chemotherapy). When chemotherapy is placed directly into the cerebrospinal fluid, an organ (such as the eye), or a body cavity such as the abdomen, the drugs mainly affect cancer cells in those areas (regional chemotherapy). The way the chemotherapy is given depends on the type and stage of the cancer being treated. A form of chemotherapy called chemoreduction is used to treat retinoblastoma. Chemoreduction reduces the size of the tumor so it may be treated with local treatment (such as radiation therapy, cryotherapy, or thermotherapy).

Experimental Treatments

New types of treatment are being tested in clinical trials.

This summary section describes treatments that are being studied in clinical trials. It may not mention every new treatment being studied. Information about clinical trials is available from the National Cancer Institute website.

Subtenon chemotherapy: Subtenon chemotherapy is the use of drugs injected through the membrane covering the muscles and nerves at the back of the eyeball. This is a type of regional chemotherapy. It is usually combined with systemic chemotherapy and local treatment (such as radiation therapy, cryotherapy, or thermotherapy).

Ophthalmic arterial infusion therapy: Ophthalmic arterial infusion therapy is a type of regional chemotherapy used to deliver anticancer drugs directly to the eye. A catheter is put into an artery that leads to the eye and the anticancer drug is given through the catheter. During this treatment, a small balloon may be inserted into the artery to block it and keep most of the anticancer drug trapped near the tumor.

High-dose chemotherapy with stem cell rescue: High-dose chemotherapy with stem cell rescue is a way of giving high doses of chemotherapy and replacing blood-forming cells destroyed by the cancer treatment. Stem cells (immature blood cells) are removed from the blood or bone marrow of the patient or a donor and are frozen and stored. After the chemotherapy is completed, the stored stem cells are thawed and given back to the patient through an infusion. These reinfused stem cells grow into (and restore) the body's blood cells.

Biologic therapy: Biologic therapy is a treatment that uses the patient's immune system to fight cancer. Substances made by the body or made in a laboratory are used to boost, direct, or restore the body's natural defenses against cancer. This type of cancer treatment is also called biotherapy or immunotherapy. Clinical trials for retinoblastoma are studying a biologic therapy called gene therapy. This is a treatment that changes a gene to improve the body's ability to fight the disease.

Clinical Trials

For some patients, taking part in a clinical trial may be the best treatment choice. Clinical trials are part of the cancer research process. Clinical trials are done to find out if new cancer treatments are safe and effective or better than the standard treatment.

Many of today's standard treatments for cancer are based on earlier clinical trials. Patients who take part in a clinical trial may receive the standard treatment or be among the first to receive a new treatment.

Patients who take part in clinical trials also help improve the way cancer will be treated in the future. Even when clinical trials do not lead to effective new treatments, they often answer important questions and help move research forward.

Patients can enter clinical trials before, during, or after starting their cancer treatment.

Some clinical trials only include patients who have not yet received treatment. Other trials test treatments for patients whose cancer has not gotten better. There are also clinical trials that test new ways to stop cancer from recurring (coming back) or reduce the side effects of cancer treatment.

Follow-Up Tests

Some of the tests that were done to diagnose the cancer or to find out the stage of the cancer may be repeated. Some tests will be repeated in order to see how well the treatment is working. Decisions about whether to continue, change, or stop treatment may be based on the results of these tests. This is sometimes called re-staging.

Some of the tests will continue to be done from time to time after treatment has ended. The results of these tests can show if your condition has changed or if the cancer has recurred (come back). These tests are sometimes called follow-up tests or check-ups.

Treatment Options for Retinoblastoma

Intraocular Retinoblastoma

If the cancer is in one eye and the tumor is large, treatment is usually enucleation. Chemotherapy may be given to shrink the tumor before surgery or after surgery to lower the risk that the cancer will spread to other parts of the body.

If the cancer is in one eye and it is expected that vision can be saved, treatment may include one or more of the following:

- External-beam radiation therapy or plaque radiotherapy

- Cryotherapy

- Thermotherapy

- Chemotherapy (chemoreduction)

- A clinical trial of chemotherapy using more than one anticancer drug

- A clinical trial of intensity-modulated radiation therapy, stereotactic radiotherapy, or proton beam radiation therapy.

If the cancer is in both eyes, treatment may include one or more of the following:

- Chemotherapy (chemoreduction) followed by local treatment such as cryotherapy, thermotherapy, or plaque radiotherapy. This may be done if there is a chance to save vision in both eyes.

- Enucleation of one or both eyes, when vision cannot be saved.

- A clinical trial of subtenon chemotherapy combined with systemic chemotherapy and local treatment.

- A clinical trial of new combinations of chemotherapy and other treatments to the eye.

- A clinical trial of higher doses of systemic chemotherapy combined with regional chemotherapy, local treatment, and lower doses of radiation therapy to the eye.

- A clinical trial of gene therapy.

- A clinical trial of ophthalmic arterial infusion therapy.

Extraocular Retinoblastoma

There is no standard treatment for extraocular retinoblastoma. In the past, radiation therapy and intrathecal chemotherapy have been used. If treatment is enucleation, chemotherapy to shrink the tumor may be given before surgery. Treatment may be a clinical trial of chemotherapy followed by high-dose chemotherapy and stem cell rescue with radiation therapy.

Recurrent Retinoblastoma

If the cancer is small and in the eye only, treatment is usually local therapy (enucleation, plaque radiotherapy, cryotherapy, or thermotherapy). If the cancer is large and in the eye only, treatment is usually chemotherapy followed by radiation therapy.

If the cancer comes back outside of the eye, treatment will depend on many things and may be within a clinical trial of chemotherapy combined with high-dose chemotherapy and stem cell rescue with radiation therapy.

Section 27.5

Retinopathy of Prematurity

"Facts about Retinopathy of Prematurity," National Eye
Institute, National Institutes of Health, October 2009.

Retinopathy of Prematurity Defined

What is retinopathy of prematurity?

Retinopathy of prematurity (ROP) is a potentially blinding eye
disorder that primarily affects premature infants weighing about 2.75
pounds (1250 grams) or less that are born before thirty-one weeks of
gestation (A full-term pregnancy has a gestation of thirty-eight to
forty-two weeks). The smaller a baby is at birth, the more likely that
baby is to develop ROP. This disorder—which usually develops in both
eyes—is one of the most common causes of visual loss in childhood and
can lead to lifelong vision impairment and blindness. ROP was first
diagnosed in 1942.

Frequently Asked Questions about Retinopathy of Prematurity

How many infants have retinopathy of prematurity?

Today, with advances in neonatal care, smaller and more premature
infants are being saved. These infants are at a much higher risk for
ROP. Not all babies who are premature develop ROP. There are approximately 3.9 million infants born in the United States each year; of
those, about 28,000 weigh 2.75 pounds or less. About 14,000 to 16,000
of these infants are affected by some degree of ROP. The disease improves and leaves no permanent damage in milder cases of ROP. About
90 percent of all infants with ROP are in the milder category and do
not need treatment. However, infants with more severe disease can
develop impaired vision or even blindness. About 1,100 to 1,500 infants
annually develop ROP that is severe enough to require medical treatment. About 400 to 600 infants each year in the United States become
legally blind from ROP.

Are there different stages of ROP?

Yes. ROP is classified in five stages, ranging from mild (stage I) to severe (stage V):

- **Stage I:** Mildly abnormal blood vessel growth. Many children who develop stage I improve with no treatment and eventually develop normal vision. The disease resolves on its own without further progression.

- **Stage II:** Moderately abnormal blood vessel growth. Many children who develop stage II improve with no treatment and eventually develop normal vision. The disease resolves on its own without further progression.

- **Stage III:** Severely abnormal blood vessel growth. The abnormal blood vessels grow toward the center of the eye instead of following their normal growth pattern along the surface of the retina. Some infants who develop stage III improve with no treatment and eventually develop normal vision. However, when infants have a certain degree of Stage III and "plus disease" develops, treatment is considered. "Plus disease" means that the blood vessels of the retina have become enlarged and twisted, indicating a worsening of the disease. Treatment at this point has a good chance of preventing retinal detachment.

- **Stage IV:** Partially detached retina. Traction from the scar produced by bleeding, abnormal vessels pull the retina away from the wall of the eye.

- **Stage V:** Completely detached retina and the end stage of the disease. If the eye is left alone at this stage, the baby can have severe visual impairment and even blindness.

Most babies who develop ROP have stages I or II. However, in a small number of babies, ROP worsens, sometimes very rapidly. Untreated ROP threatens to destroy vision.

Can ROP cause other complications?

Yes. Infants with ROP are considered to be at higher risk for developing certain eye problems later in life, such as retinal detachment, myopia (nearsightedness), strabismus (crossed eyes), amblyopia (lazy eye), and glaucoma. In many cases, these eye problems can be treated or controlled.

Causes and Risk Factors

What causes ROP?

ROP occurs when abnormal blood vessels grow and spread throughout the retina, the tissue that lines the back of the eye. These abnormal blood vessels are fragile and can leak, scarring the retina and pulling it out of position. This causes a retinal detachment. Retinal detachment is the main cause of visual impairment and blindness in ROP.

Several complex factors may be responsible for the development of ROP. The eye starts to develop at about sixteen weeks of pregnancy, when the blood vessels of the retina begin to form at the optic nerve in the back of the eye. The blood vessels grow gradually toward the edges of the developing retina, supplying oxygen and nutrients. During the last twelve weeks of a pregnancy, the eye develops rapidly. When a baby is born full-term, the retinal blood vessel growth is mostly complete (The retina usually finishes growing a few weeks to a month after birth). But if a baby is born prematurely, before these blood vessels have reached the edges of the retina, normal vessel growth may stop. The edges of the retina—the periphery—may not get enough oxygen and nutrients.

Scientists believe that the periphery of the retina then sends out signals to other areas of the retina for nourishment. As a result, new abnormal vessels begin to grow. These new blood vessels are fragile and weak and can bleed, leading to retinal scarring. When these scars shrink, they pull on the retina, causing it to detach from the back of the eye.

Are there other risk factors for ROP?

In addition to birth weight and how early a baby is born, other factors contributing to the risk of ROP include anemia, blood transfusions, respiratory distress, breathing difficulties, and the overall health of the infant.

An ROP epidemic occurred in the 1940s and early 1950s when hospital nurseries began using excessively high levels of oxygen in incubators to save the lives of premature infants. During this time, ROP was the leading cause of blindness in children in the United States. In 1954, scientists funded by the National Institutes of Health determined that the relatively high levels of oxygen routinely given to premature infants at that time were an important risk factor, and that reducing the level of oxygen given to premature babies reduced the incidence of ROP. With newer technology and methods to monitor the oxygen levels of infants, oxygen use as a risk factor has diminished in importance.

Although it had been suggested as a factor in the development of ROP, researchers supported by the National Eye Institute (NEI) determined that lighting levels in hospital nurseries have no effect on the development of ROP.

Treatment

How is ROP treated?

The most effective proven treatments for ROP are laser therapy or cryotherapy. Laser therapy "burns away" the periphery of the retina, which has no normal blood vessels. With cryotherapy, physicians use an instrument that generates freezing temperatures to briefly touch spots on the surface of the eye that overlie the periphery of the retina. Both laser treatment and cryotherapy destroy the peripheral areas of the retina, slowing or reversing the abnormal growth of blood vessels. Unfortunately, the treatments also destroy some side vision. This is done to save the most important part of our sight—the sharp, central vision we need for "straight ahead" activities such as reading, sewing, and driving.

Both laser treatments and cryotherapy are performed only on infants with advanced ROP, particularly stage III with "plus disease." Both treatments are considered invasive surgeries on the eye, and doctors don't know the long-term side effects of each.

In the later stages of ROP, other treatment options include:

- **Scleral buckle:** This involves placing a silicone band around the eye and tightening it. This keeps the vitreous gel from pulling on the scar tissue and allows the retina to flatten back down onto the wall of the eye. Infants who have had a scleral buckle need to have the band removed months or years later, since the eye continues to grow; otherwise they will become nearsighted. Scleral buckles are usually performed on infants with stage IV or V.

- **Vitrectomy:** Vitrectomy involves removing the vitreous and replacing it with a saline solution. After the vitreous has been removed, the scar tissue on the retina can be peeled back or cut away, allowing the retina to relax and lay back down against the eye wall. Vitrectomy is performed only at stage V.

What happens if treatment does not work?

While ROP treatment decreases the chances for vision loss, it does not always prevent it. Not all babies respond to ROP treatment, and the disease may get worse. If treatment for ROP does not work, a retinal detachment may develop. Often, only part of the retina detaches (stage IV). When this happens, no further treatments may be needed, since a partial detachment may remain the same or go away without treatment. However, in some instances, physicians may recommend treatment to try to prevent further advancement of the retinal detachment (stage V). If the center of the retina or the entire retina detaches, central vision is threatened, and surgery may be recommended to reattach the retina.

Current Research

What research is being done?

The NEI-supported clinical studies on ROP include:

- The Cryotherapy for Retinopathy of Prematurity (CRYO-ROP)– Outcome Study of Cryotherapy for Retinopathy of Prematurity Study examined the safety and effectiveness of cryotherapy (freezing treatment) of the peripheral retina in reducing the risk of blindness in certain low birth weight infants with ROP. Follow-up results confirm that applying a freezing treatment to the eyes of premature babies with ROP helps save their sight. The follow-up results also give researchers more information about how well the babies can see in the years after cryotherapy.

- The Effects of Light Reduction on Retinopathy of Prematurity (Light-ROP) Study evaluated the effect of ambient light reduction on the incidence of ROP. The study determined that light reduction has no effect on the development of a potentially blinding eye disorder in low birth weight infants. The study determined that light reduction in hospital nurseries has no effect on the development of ROP.

- The Supplemental Therapeutic Oxygen for Prethreshold Retinopathy of Prematurity (the STOP-ROP) Multicenter Trial tested the efficacy, safety, and costs of providing supplemental oxygen in moderately severe retinopathy of prematurity (prethreshold ROP). Results showed that modest supplemental oxygen given to premature infants with moderate cases of ROP may not significantly improve ROP, but definitely does not make it worse.

- The Early Treatment for Retinopathy of Prematurity Study (ETROP) is designed to determine whether earlier treatment in carefully selected cases of ROP will result in an overall better visual outcome than treatment at the conventional disease threshold point used in the CRYO-ROP study.

369

Section 27.6

Retinoschisis

What is juvenile retinoschisis?

Juvenile retinoschisis is an inherited disease diagnosed in childhood that causes progressive loss of central and peripheral (side) vision due to degeneration of the retina.

What are the symptoms?

Juvenile retinoschisis, also known as X-linked retinoschisis, occurs almost exclusively in males. Although the condition begins at birth, symptoms do not typically become apparent until after the age of ten. About half of all patients diagnosed with juvenile retinoschisis first notice a decline in vision. Other early symptoms of the disease include an inability of both eyes to focus on an object (strabismus) and roving, involuntary eye movements (nystagmus).

Vision loss associated with juvenile retinoschisis is caused by the splitting of the retina into two layers. This retinal splitting most notably affects the macula, the central portion of the retina responsible for fine visual detail and color perception. On examination, the fovea (the center of the macula) has spoke-like streaks. The spaces created by the separated layers are often filled with blisters and ruptured blood vessels that can leak blood into the vitreous body (the transparent, colorless mass of jelly-like material filling the center of the eye). The presence of blood in the vitreous body causes further visual impairment. The vitreous body degenerates and may eventually separate from the retina. The entire retina may also separate from underlying tissue layers, causing retinal detachments.

The extent and rate of vision loss vary greatly among patients with juvenile retinoschisis. Central vision is almost always affected. Peripheral (side) vision loss occurs in about half of all cases. Some patients retain useful vision well into adulthood, while others experience a rapid decline during childhood.

Is it an inherited disease?

Juvenile retinoschisis is genetically passed through families by the X-linked pattern of inheritance. In this type of inheritance, the gene for the disease is located on the X chromosome. Females have two X chromosomes and can carry the disease gene on one of their X chromosomes. Because they have a healthy version of the gene on their other X chromosome, carrier females typically are not affected by X-linked diseases such as juvenile retinoschisis. Sometimes, however, when carrier females are examined, the retina shows minor signs of the disease.

Males have only one X chromosome (paired with one Y chromosome) and are therefore genetically susceptible to X-linked diseases. Males cannot be carriers of X-linked diseases. Males affected with an X-linked disease always pass the gene on the X chromosome to their daughters, who then become carriers. Affected males never pass an X-linked disease gene to their sons because fathers pass the Y chromosome to their sons.

Female carriers have a 50 percent chance (or one chance in two) of passing the X-linked disease gene to their daughters, who become carriers, and a 50 percent chance of passing the gene to their sons, who are then affected by the disease.

What treatment is available?

In 1997, researchers identified mutations in a gene on the X chromosome that cause juvenile retinoschisis. Scientists are now studying the gene to determine its function in the retina. This information will greatly enhance efforts to develop treatments for juvenile retinoschisis.

A recent study showed that a drug called dorzolamide may improve retinal health and restore some vision in people with retinoschisis.

Individuals with juvenile retinoschisis may also benefit from the use of low-vision aids, including electronic, computer-based, and optical aids. Orientation and mobility training, adaptive training skills, job placement, and income assistance are available through community resources.

Are there any other related diseases?

Juvenile retinoschisis can resemble other retinal degenerative diseases such as retinitis pigmentosa (RP), Goldmann-Favre vitreoretinal dystrophy, Wagner vitreoretinal dystrophy, and Sticklers syndrome. A thorough ophthalmologic examination, including diagnostic tests measuring retinal function and visual field, combined with an accurate documentation of family history, can distinguish between these diseases.

Chapter 28

Disorders of the Vitreous

Chapter Contents

Section 28.1

Floaters

Excerpted from "Facts about Floaters," National Eye Institute,
National Institutes of Health, October 2009.

Floaters Defined

What are floaters?

Floaters are little "cobwebs" or specks that float about in your field of vision. They are small, dark, shadowy shapes that can look like spots, threadlike strands, or squiggly lines. They move as your eyes move and seem to dart away when you try to look at them directly. They do not follow your eye movements precisely, and usually drift when your eyes stop moving.

Frequently Asked Questions about Floaters

What are the differences between floaters and retinal detachment and sight-threatening concerns?

Sometimes a section of the vitreous pulls the fine fibers away from the retina all at once, rather than gradually, causing many new floaters to appear suddenly. This is called a vitreous detachment, which in most cases is not sight-threatening and requires no treatment.

However, a sudden increase in floaters, possibly accompanied by light flashes or peripheral (side) vision loss, could indicate a retinal detachment. A retinal detachment occurs when any part of the retina, the eye's light-sensitive tissue, is lifted or pulled from its normal position at the back wall of the eye.

A retinal detachment is a serious condition and should always be considered an emergency. If left untreated, it can lead to permanent visual impairment within two or three days or even blindness in the eye.

Those who experience a sudden increase in floaters, flashes of light in peripheral vision, or a loss of peripheral vision should have an eye care professional examine their eyes as soon as possible.

Causes and Risk Factors

What causes floaters?

Floaters occur when the vitreous, a gel-like substance that fills about 80 percent of the eye and helps it maintain a round shape, slowly shrinks.

As the vitreous shrinks, it becomes somewhat stringy, and the strands can cast tiny shadows on the retina. These are floaters.

In most cases, floaters are part of the natural aging process and simply an annoyance. They can be distracting at first, but eventually tend to "settle" at the bottom of the eye, becoming less bothersome. They usually settle below the line of sight and do not go away completely.

However, there are other, more serious causes of floaters, including infection, inflammation (uveitis), hemorrhaging, retinal tears, and injury to the eye.

Who is at risk for floaters?

Floaters are more likely to develop as we age and are more common in people who are very nearsighted, have diabetes, or who have had a cataract operation.

Symptoms and Detection

Floaters are little "cobwebs" or specks that float about in your field of vision. They are small, dark, shadowy shapes that can look like spots, threadlike strands, or squiggly lines. They move as your eyes move and seem to dart away when you try to look at them directly. They do not follow your eye movements precisely, and usually drift when your eyes stop moving.

Treatment

How are floaters treated?

For people who have floaters that are simply annoying, no treatment is recommended.

On rare occasions, floaters can be so dense and numerous that they significantly affect vision. In these cases, a vitrectomy, a surgical procedure that removes floaters from the vitreous, may be needed.

A vitrectomy removes the vitreous gel, along with its floating debris, from the eye. The vitreous is replaced with a salt solution. Because the vitreous is mostly water, you will not notice any change between the salt solution and the original vitreous.

This operation carries significant risks to sight because of possible complications, which include retinal detachment, retinal tears, and cataract. Most eye surgeons are reluctant to recommend this surgery unless the floaters seriously interfere with vision.

Section 28.2

Vitreous Detachment

"Facts about Vitreous Detachment," National Eye Institute, National Institutes of Health, August 2009.

Vitreous Detachment Defined

What is vitreous detachment?

Most of the eye's interior is filled with vitreous, a gel-like substance that helps the eye maintain a round shape. There are millions of fine fibers intertwined within the vitreous that are attached to the surface of the retina, the eye's light-sensitive tissue. As we age, the vitreous slowly shrinks, and these fine fibers pull on the retinal surface. Usually the fibers break, allowing the vitreous to separate and shrink from the retina. This is a vitreous detachment.

In most cases, a vitreous detachment, also known as a posterior vitreous detachment, is not sight-threatening and requires no treatment.

Risk Factors

Who is at risk for vitreous detachment?

A vitreous detachment is a common condition that usually affects people over age fifty, and is very common after age eighty. People who are nearsighted are also at increased risk. Those who have a vitreous detachment in one eye are likely to have one in the other, although it may not happen until years later.

Symptoms and Detection

What are the symptoms of vitreous detachment?

As the vitreous shrinks, it becomes somewhat stringy, and the strands can cast tiny shadows on the retina that you may notice as floaters, which appear as little "cobwebs" or specks that seem to float about in your field of vision. If you try to look at these shadows they appear to quickly dart out of the way.

One symptom of a vitreous detachment is a small but sudden increase in the number of new floaters. This increase in floaters may be accompanied by flashes of light (lightning streaks) in your peripheral, or side, vision. In most cases, either you will not notice a vitreous detachment, or you will find it merely annoying because of the increase in floaters.

How is vitreous detachment detected?

The only way to diagnose the cause of the problem is by a comprehensive dilated eye examination. If the vitreous detachment has led to a macular hole or detached retina, early treatment can help prevent loss of vision.

Treatment

How does vitreous detachment affect vision?

Although a vitreous detachment does not threaten sight, once in a while some of the vitreous fibers pull so hard on the retina that they create a macular hole or lead to a retinal detachment. Both of these conditions are sight-threatening and should be treated immediately.

If left untreated, a macular hole or detached retina can lead to permanent vision loss in the affected eye. Those who experience a sudden increase in floaters or an increase in flashes of light in peripheral vision should have an eye care professional examine their eyes as soon as possible.

Chapter 29

Disorders of the Uvea

Chapter Contents

Section 29.1

Uveal Coloboma

Excerpted from "Facts about Uveal Coloboma," National Eye
Institute, National Institutes of Health, September 2009.

Coloboma Defined

What is a coloboma?

Coloboma comes from a Greek word which means "curtailed." It is
used to describe conditions where normal tissue in or around the eye
is missing from birth.

What is a uveal coloboma?

This coloboma can present as an iris coloboma (the iris is the colored
part of the eye), with the traditional "keyhole" or "cat-eye" appearance
to the iris, and/or as a chorioretinal coloboma, where the retina in the
lower inside corner of the eye is missing.

How common is uveal coloboma?

Uveal coloboma is a rare condition that is not always well documented. Depending on the study and where the study was conducted,
estimates range from 0.5 to 2.2 cases per 10,000 births. Some cases
may go unnoticed because uveal coloboma does not always affect vision
or the outside appearance of the eye.

Uveal coloboma is a significant cause of blindness.

Frequently Asked Questions about Coloboma

What are the different kinds of coloboma?

There are different kinds of coloboma, depending on which part of the
eye is missing. Coloboma can affect the following parts of the eye:

- Eyelid
- Lens

- Macula

- Optic nerve

- Uvea

Eyelid coloboma: In eyelid coloboma a piece of either the upper or lower eyelid is absent. Eyelid coloboma may be part of a genetic syndrome, or happen as a result of a disruption of eyelid development in a baby. A syndrome is a specific grouping of birth defects or symptoms present in one person.

Lens coloboma: In this type of coloboma, a piece of the lens is absent. The lens, which helps focus light on the retina, will typically appear with a notch.

Macular coloboma: This happens when the center of the retina, called the macula, does not develop normally. The macula is responsible for daylight, fine, and color vision. Macular coloboma may be caused when normal eye development is interrupted or following an inflammation of the retina during development of the baby.

Optic nerve coloboma: Optic nerve coloboma refers to one of two distinct things. They are as follows:

- An abnormal optic nerve that is deeply "excavated" or hollowed out. In some cases it can also be referred to as an optic nerve pit. The optic nerve is the bundle of nerve fibers that relays the light signals from the eye to the brain.

- A uveal coloboma that is large enough to involve the optic nerve, either the inferior portion or the entire optic disc.

Are there other diseases or conditions associated with coloboma?

In the eye: Coloboma is sometimes found in association with other eye features. These may include the following:

- Difference in eye color between the two eyes (heterochromia)

- Small eye (microphthalmia)

- Increased thickness of the cornea. The cornea is the clear front part of the eye.

- Clouding of the lens (cataract)

- Elevated pressure in the eye (glaucoma)

- Retinal malformation (retinal dysplasia)

- Nearsightedness (myopia)

- Involuntary eye movements (nystagmus)

- Protrusion of the back of the eyeball (posterior staphyloma)

In other parts of the body: Coloboma may be an isolated feature, or may be found with other features. Sometimes these other features may be few and minor, such as skin tags near the ear. Sometimes they may be more numerous and severe, such as a heart or a kidney defect. A few of these associations may be genetic syndromes. These include (but are not limited to) the following:

- CHARGE syndrome

- Cat-eye syndrome

- Kabuki syndrome

- 13q deletion syndrome

- Wolf-Hirschhorn syndrome

Causes

What causes uveal coloboma?

It is believed that uveal coloboma is primarily genetic in origin. "Genetic" means that the coloboma was caused by a gene that was not working properly when the eye was forming. Sometimes coloboma is part of a specific genetic syndrome, for which the genetics are known. For instance, coloboma is one feature of CHARGE syndrome, which is associated with a change in, or a complete deletion of a gene called CHD7.

Researchers have found genes associated with coloboma in a few cases. To date, however, we still do not know which genes explain most cases of coloboma.

Some researchers have proposed that certain environmental factors may contribute to developing coloboma, either in humans or in animals. These findings have been published over time in the research literature, but there has been no systematic analysis of possible links. For instance, it is known that babies exposed to alcohol during pregnancy can develop coloboma—but they also have other anomalies. There are no known strong links between environmental exposures and isolated coloboma.

It is always possible that coloboma happens strictly by chance. In summary, there is little data to presently say why coloboma happened to a person in a family where no one else is affected.

How does uveal coloboma happen?

To understand how uveal coloboma happens, we first have to understand how the eye forms in the developing baby. The eyes start as stalks coming out of the brain. The tip of each stalk will become the eye itself, while the rest of the stalk will become the optic nerve linking the eye to the brain. There is a seam at the bottom of each stalk, where blood vessels originally run. This seam is known as the optic fissure, or the choroidal fissure, or the embryonic fissure. Starting at the fifth week of gestation (pregnancy), this seam must close. The closure starts roughly in the middle of the developing eye, and runs in both directions. This process is finished by the seventh week of gestation. If, for some reason, the closure does not happen, a uveal coloboma is formed.

Depending on where the closure did not happen, the baby can have an iris coloboma (front of the fissure), a chorioretinal coloboma (back of the fissure), or any combination of these. Uveal coloboma can affect one eye (unilateral) or both eyes (bilateral). The condition can be the same in both eyes (symmetric) or different in both eyes (asymmetric). A uveal coloboma may go from front to back (continuous) or have "skip lesions." The fact that the seam runs at the bottom of the stalk is the reason why uveal coloboma is always located in the lower inside corner of the eye.

How can uveal coloboma be inherited?

Isolated coloboma can follow all possible patterns of single gene inheritance, namely autosomal dominant, autosomal recessive, and X-linked. In one family, however, coloboma will follow only one pattern. For instance, in case of an autosomal dominant pattern, a person with coloboma would have a fifty-fifty chance of passing on the coloboma to each of his or her offspring. In families with a single case of coloboma, it is not possible to say what pattern of inheritance is involved; therefore it is not possible to give an exact recurrence risk number. The recurrence risk of coloboma computed from averaging data across many families (empiric risk) is about 10 percent. This is an imperfect number, as it mixes information from families where this risk may be close to 0 percent with information from families where the actual risk may be 25 percent or even 50 percent.

The topic of inheritance of coloboma is complicated by several factors:

- Sometimes a person who is at risk for developing coloboma may not develop the condition, or it may be so minor that it goes unnoticed. This may appear in the family history as an inconsistent, noninterpretable pattern of inheritance.

- Knowing the pattern of inheritance of coloboma in a family does not give information on how severely an at-risk person will be affected (e.g., how good their visual acuity will be).

- There may be more than one gene involved in being at risk for coloboma, which makes predicting inheritance even more difficult.

For coloboma due to a known syndrome, such as CHARGE syndrome, inheritance is based on what is known about that particular syndrome. However, it is rarely, if ever, possible to say whether coloboma will be a feature of the syndrome in a person inheriting the genetic background responsible for this syndrome.

Symptoms

What are the symptoms of uveal coloboma?

There may or may not be any symptoms related to coloboma; it all depends on the amount and location of the missing tissue. People with a coloboma affecting the macula and the optic nerve will likely have reduced vision. In general, it is difficult to exactly predict what level of vision a baby will have only by looking at how much of the retina is missing.

People with a coloboma affecting any part of the retina will have what is called a "field defect." A field defect means that a person is missing vision in a specific location. Because coloboma is located in the lower part of the retina, vision in the upper part of the field of vision will be missing. This may or may not be noticeable to the affected person.

A person with a coloboma affecting the front of the eye only will not have any decreased vision from it. Some people, however, have reported being more sensitive to light.

Treatment

Can uveal coloboma be treated?

Patients with uveal coloboma should have yearly follow-up exams by an eye care professional. However, there is currently no medication or surgery that can cure or reverse coloboma and make the eye whole again. Treatment consists of helping patients adjust to vision problems and make the most of the vision they have by doing the following:

- Correcting any refractive error with glasses or contact lenses.

- Maximizing the vision of the most affected eye in asymmetric cases. This may involve patching or using drops to temporarily blur vision in the stronger eye for a limited period of time.

- Ensuring that amblyopia (lazy eye) does not develop in childhood in case of asymmetry. Sometimes amblyopia treatment (patching, glasses, and/or drops) can improve vision in eyes even with severe colobomas.

- Treating any other eye condition that may be present with coloboma, such as cataracts.

- Treating any complications that might arise from a retinal coloboma later in life, such as the growth of new blood vessels at the back of the eye (neovascularization) and/or retinal detachment.

- Using low vision devices, as needed.

- Making use of rehabilitation services, such as early intervention programs.

- Offering genetic counseling to the patient and family members.

If the eye with the coloboma is very small (microphthalmia), other follow-ups may be needed. Conformers and expanders may be used to help support the face and encourage the eye socket to grow. Children may also be fitted for a prosthetic (artificial) eye to improve appearance. As the face develops, new conformers will need to be made.

For people who wish to alter the appearance of a coloboma affecting the front of the eye, two options are currently available:

- Colored contact lenses that make the black part of the eye (pupil) round.

- Surgery to make the pupil rounder. This procedure pulls and sutures together the lower edges of the iris.

Is genetic testing available for uveal coloboma?

Testing may be available in cases where the coloboma is part of a specific genetic syndrome. This testing would look for the gene(s) causing whole syndrome and not just the coloboma. Genetic testing is done on a blood sample and may involve looking at the patient's chromosomes, or looking at a specific gene on one of the chromosomes.

There is no specific recommended testing for isolated coloboma. Testing for some of the genes that were reported in the medical literature might be performed as part of research projects. However, results from such testing will likely be negative, since these genes explain very few cases of uveal coloboma.

Section 29.2

Uveal Melanoma

PDQ® Cancer Information Summary. National Cancer Institute; Bethesda, MD. "Intraocular (Eye) Melanoma Treatment (PDQ)— Health Professional Version." Updated December 2007. Available at: http://cancer.gov. Accessed March 27, 2011. Reviewed by David A. Cooke, MD, FACP, December 2011.

Melanoma of the uveal tract (iris, ciliary body, and choroid), though rare, is the most common primary intraocular malignancy in adults. The mean age-adjusted incidence of uveal melanoma in the United States is approximately 4.3 new cases per million population.[1] The age-adjusted incidence of this cancer has remained stable for the past fifty years.

Uveal melanoma is diagnosed mostly at older ages, with a progressively rising age-specific incidence rate that peaks near the age of seventy.[1] Host susceptibility factors associated with the development of this cancer include Caucasian race, light eye color, fair skin color, and the ability to tan.[1,2] In view of these susceptibility factors, numerous observational studies have attempted to explore the relationship between sunlight exposure and risk of uveal melanoma. To date, these studies have found only weak associations or yielded contradictory results.[1] Similarly, there is no consistent evidence that occupational exposure to ultraviolet (UV) light or other agents is a risk factor for uveal melanoma.[1]

Uveal melanomas can arise in the anterior (iris) or the posterior (ciliary body or choroid) uveal tract. Iris melanomas have the best prognosis, whereas melanomas of the ciliary body have the worst. Most uveal tract melanomas originate in the choroid. The ciliary body is less commonly a site of origin, and the iris is the least common. The comparatively low incidence of iris melanomas has been attributed to the characteristic features of these tumors (i.e., they tend to be small, slow growing, and relatively dormant in comparison with their posterior counterparts). Iris melanomas rarely metastasize.[3] Melanomas of the posterior uveal tract are cytologically more malignant, detected later, and metastasize more frequently than iris melanomas. The typical choroidal melanoma is a brown, elevated, dome-shaped subretinal mass. The degree of pigmentation ranges from dark brown to totally amelanotic.

Most uveal melanomas are initially completely asymptomatic. As the tumor enlarges, it may cause distortion of the pupil (iris melanoma), blurred vision (ciliary body melanoma), or markedly decreased visual acuity caused by secondary retinal detachment (choroidal melanoma). Serous detachment of the retina frequently complicates tumor growth. If extensive retinal detachment occurs, secondary angle-closure glaucoma occasionally develops. Clinically, several lesions simulate uveal melanoma, including metastatic carcinoma, posterior scleritis, and benign tumors, such as nevi and hemangiomas.[4]

Careful examination by an experienced clinician remains the most important test to establish the presence of intraocular melanoma. Ancillary diagnostic testing, including fluorescein angiography and ultrasonography, can be extremely valuable in establishing and/or confirming the diagnosis.[5]

A number of factors influence prognosis. The most important are cell type, tumor size, location of the anterior margin of the tumor, the degree of ciliary body involvement, and extraocular extension. Cell type, however, remains the most often used predictor of outcome.[6] The selection of treatment depends on the site of origin (choroid, ciliary body, or iris), the size and location of the lesion, the age of the patient, and whether extraocular invasion, recurrence, or metastasis has occurred. Extraocular extension, recurrence, and metastasis are associated with an extremely poor prognosis, and long-term survival cannot be expected.[7] The five-year mortality rate caused by metastasis from ciliary body or choroidal melanoma is approximately 30 percent, compared with a rate of 2 percent to 3 percent for iris melanomas.[8] In a group of patients with large tumors of the choroid or choroid and ciliary body, the concurrent presence of abnormalities in chromosomes 3 and 8 was also associated with a poor outcome.[9]

In the past, enucleation (eye removal) was the accepted standard treatment for primary choroidal melanoma, and it remains the most commonly used treatment for large tumors. Because of the effect of enucleation on the appearance of the patient, the diagnostic uncertainty encountered by the ophthalmologist (particularly in the case of smaller tumors), and the potential for tumor spread, alternative treatments, such as radiation therapy (i.e., brachytherapy or external-beam, charged-particle radiation therapy), transpupillary thermotherapy, photocoagulation, and cryotherapy have been developed in an attempt to spare the affected eye and possibly retain useful vision.[10,11] One of the clinical trials of the randomized Collaborative Ocular Melanoma Study compared iodine 125 (125I) episcleral-plaque brachytherapy to enucleation in treating patients with medium-sized choroidal tumors.[12] Eighty-five percent of the patients treated with 125I brachytherapy retained their eye for five years or more, and 37 percent had visual acuity better than 20/200 in the irradiated eye five years after treatment.[12] No significant differences in mortality were observed between the two study arms after twelve years of follow-up, whether considering death from all causes or death with histopathologically confirmed melanoma metastasis.[13]

References

1. Singh AD, Bergman L, Seregard S, Uveal melanoma: epidemiologic aspects. *Ophthalmol Clin North Am* 18 (1): 75–84, viii, 2005.

2. Weis E, Shah CP, Lajous M, et al., The association between host susceptibility factors and uveal melanoma: a meta-analysis. *Arch Ophthalmol* 124 (1): 54–60, 2006.

3. Yap-Veloso MI, Simmons RB, Simmons RJ: Iris melanomas: diagnosis and management. *Int Ophthalmol Clin* 37 (4): 87–100, 1997 Fall.

4. Eye and ocular adnexa. In: Rosai J, *Ackerman's Surgical Pathology*. 8th ed. St. Louis, Mo: Mosby, 1996, 2449–2508.

5. Avery RB, Mehta MP, Auchter RM, et al., Intraocular melanoma. In: DeVita VT Jr, Hellman S, Rosenberg SA, eds., *Cancer: Principles and Practice of Oncology*. 7th ed. Philadelphia, Pa: Lippincott Williams & Wilkins, 2005, 1800–24.

6. McLean IW, Prognostic features of uveal melanoma. *Ophthalmol Clin North Am* 8 (1): 143–53, 1995.

7. Gragoudas ES, Egan KM, Seddon JM, et al., Survival of patients with metastases from uveal melanoma. *Ophthalmology* 98 (3): 383–89; discussion 390, 1991.

8. Introduction to melanocytic tumors of the uvea. In: Shields JA, Shields CL, *Intraocular Tumors: A Text and Atlas*. Philadelphia, Pa: Saunders, 1992, 45–59.

9. White VA, Chambers JD, Courtright PD, et al., Correlation of cytogenetic abnormalities with the outcome of patients with uveal melanoma. *Cancer* 83 (2): 354–59, 1998.

10. Zimmerman LE, McLean IW, Foster WD, Statistical analysis of follow-up data concerning uveal melanomas, and the influence of enucleation. *Ophthalmology* 87 (6): 557–64, 1980.

11. De Potter P, Shields CL, Shields JA, New treatment modalities for uveal melanoma. *Curr Opin Ophthalmol* 7 (3): 27–32, 1996.

12. Diener-West M, Earle JD, Fine SL, et al., The COMS randomized trial of iodine 125 brachytherapy for choroidal melanoma, III: initial mortality findings. COMS Report No. 18. *Arch Ophthalmol* 119 (7): 969–82, 2001.

13. Collaborative Ocular Melanoma Study Group.: The COMS randomized trial of iodine 125 brachytherapy for choroidal melanoma: V. Twelve-year mortality rates and prognostic factors: COMS report No. 28. *Arch Ophthalmol* 124 (12): 1684–93, 2006.

Section 29.3

Uveitis

What Is Uveitis?

The term uveitis covers a range of conditions which affect the inside of the eye. Uveitis is inflammation of the uvea. The uvea is the part of the eye consisting collectively of the iris, the choroid, and the ciliary body. The iris is the circular, colored center of the front of the eye that surrounds the pupil. The choroid is a thin layer of the eye that is situated between the sclera (the white of the eye) and the retina (the nerve layer that lines the back of the eye, senses light, and creates impulses that travel through the optic nerve to the brain). The ciliary body is the tissue that connects the iris with the choroid and includes a group of muscles which help to change the shape of the lens, in order to see different distances. The word "uvea" comes from the Latin word "uva" for grape. If you remove the stem from a grape, the hole left looks like the pupil and the grape looks like the eyeball. "Itis" means inflammation. Therefore, uveitis means inflammation of any part of the uvea (iris, choroid, or ciliary body).

Uveitis can be controlled with early treatment, but if left untreated may cause serious problems and sight loss.

Types of Uveitis

There are different types of uveitis and there can be many different causes. It is very important to know which type you have.

Uveitis can be divided into 4 main groups:

- **Anterior uveitis:** Affects the front of the eye, including the iris and ciliary body. (Sometimes called iritis.)

- **Intermediate uveitis:** Affects the middle of the eye, mainly the vitreous or vitreous humor. (Sometimes called iridocyclitis, cyclitis, vitreitis, or pars planitis.)

- **Posterior uveitis:** Affects the choroid layer at the back of the eye and often involves the retina. (Sometimes called choroiditis, retinitis, or vasculitis.)

- **Panuveitis:** When inflammation affects both the front and back of the eye. (Sometimes called diffuse uveitis.)

Uveitis can be acute or chronic:

- **Acute:** the inflammation comes in short episodes of up to about six weeks, but it may recur from time to time.

- **Chronic:** the inflammation may persist for months or years, possibly flaring up at times. It may have to be controlled by taking medication for long periods.

Why Is It Important to Know What Type of Uveitis I Have?

The symptoms, causes, and treatment may be completely different depending on what type you have.

Causes of Uveitis

There are many possible causes of uveitis. Uveitis may also be associated with other medical conditions. The types of causes may be divided into the following categories.

Autoimmune

The immune system's job in our body is to detect and attack foreign bodies such as bacteria or viruses. To do this it needs to be able to tell "self" and "foreign" apart. In autoimmune disease this process goes wrong and a part of our body (self) is mistaken as foreign. That part of the body is attacked by its own immune system. The result is inflammation.

Infection

A variety of infections may cause uveitis. This is not a very common cause of uveitis. It is very important to establish whether the uveitis is infectious or not, as the treatment will be very different. If you receive the wrong treatment it may not improve your condition. In fact, it may make your condition worse.

Trauma

This includes some form of eye injury and/or eye surgery.

Idiopathic

This means no specific cause or association with other medical conditions can be found, Up to 50 percent of uveitis cases are in this group but are still likely to be autoimmune in nature.

Associated Medical Condition

Some patients will have a medical condition which is known to be linked with uveitis (e.g., sarcoidosis, Crohn disease, ulcerative colitis, juvenile forms of rheumatoid arthritis, and ankylosing spondylitis).

Symptoms of Uveitis

Symptoms of uveitis will depend on the type of uveitis. The main symptoms are as follows.

Anterior Uveitis

- Pain
- Redness
- Sensitivity to light
- Blurring of vision

Intermediate and Posterior Uveitis

- Painless
- Floaters (black dots or wispy lines)
- Impairment of vision

With anterior uveitis, some people will only ever get a single episode of anterior uveitis. For many, the uveitis will recur in the future or be chronic and require treatment over a longer period of time.

With intermediate or posterior uveitis, it is more likely that the condition will last for a longer time or will be chronic.

The eye contains delicate structures and is easily damaged. Inflammation must *not* be allowed to remain for any length of time because it may damage your vision.

If you experience or suspect a recurrence of any of the symptoms above, you should report straight away to the eye clinic.

Ensure that you receive a follow-up appointment and ensure you keep seeing your specialist until you and your specialist are absolutely sure there is no more inflammation. For some people, even when there is no inflammation present, they will need to continue seeing specialists, particularly if the uveitis is deemed to be autoimmune.

Tests and Diagnosis

To diagnose the exact type of uveitis and to find its possible cause, different methods should be used.

Medical History

Some questions about any past medical problems can suggest possible causes or associations with other medical conditions at an early stage.

Thorough Eye Examination

First, your vision should be measured with any glasses you wear. The eye chart that we know from the optometrist is used. This measures visual acuity. Your near, or reading, vision should also be checked. It is a good idea to get the nurse who measures these to write the results down for you. Anyone you contact about your eye problem (e.g., patient group, employer) will then know how your vision has been affected.

You should then have drops placed in your eyes to dilate the pupil. This is important so that the back of the eye can be examined for signs of inflammation or complications. The eyes will be examined with a "slit lamp," a type of microscope found in eye clinics and at optometrists. Depending on the type of uveitis found or if certain complications are suspected, other more specialized tests such as a fluorescein angiogram or an optical coherence tomography (OCT), which is a useful and non-invasive investigation), may be used.

Medical Tests

As a result of the questions asked and the eye examination, a variety of medical tests may be carried out to follow up any "leads." This may include blood tests and x-rays.

Some of the medical conditions associated with uveitis include: sarcoidosis, Crohn disease, ulcerative colitis, ankylosing spondylitis, and juvenile forms of arthritis.

It is not unusual to worry about what caused your uveitis. You should remember the following things:

- You couldn't have done anything to avoid getting uveitis.

- It is not contagious.

- It is very rare to pass it on to your children.

Treatment of Uveitis

Treatment of uveitis will depend on the following factors:

- **Type:** Anterior and posterior uveitis have completely different treatments (see below)

- **Severity:** Is the uveitis thought to be sight threatening or non–sight threatening?

- **Chronic/Acute:** Treatment may need to carry on for a long time if chronic.

- **Cause:** Treatment will be different depending on what caused the uveitis (e.g., infection).

- **Complications:** Treatment may be necessary for complications such as raised pressure or macula edema.

It is a good idea to ask which of these applies to you. The treatment of the different types are summarized below.

Anterior Uveitis

- This is usually treated with eye drops only. These must be given as soon as the uveitis starts and should include the following:

  - Dilating drop: This will dilate the pupil, and is given to relieve pain and also prevent the iris sticking to the lens.

  - Steroid eye drops to control the inflammation: These must usually be given very frequently at first and for long enough to completely control the inflammation.

- If the uveitis is more severe, injections around the eye or steroid tablets may be necessary.

- Hot compresses may be very useful to relieve symptoms and to treat synechiae (iris sticking to lens).

- You must take all the drops and continue to take them for the whole course (usually at least six weeks) and not stop them if the eyes feel better. *Never* stop taking any form of steroids suddenly unless told by your doctors. This can be dangerous.

- Make sure you are followed up to check things are all clear after an attack.

- Make sure you are given information about the treatment you are prescribed, including name of drug, exactly how it should be taken, how often it should be taken, and how it should be stored.

Intermediate Uveitis

This type may vary a lot between cases which can be either:

- mild, requiring more monitoring than treatment if there are no complications; or

- more severe, and/or develop complications, especially macula edema.

Treatment may include injections around or even inside the eye, sometime tablets and sometimes eye drops if the front of the eye is involved.

Posterior Uveitis

Treatment depends on the different forms of posterior uveitis and severity.

Eye drops cannot reach the back of the eye, so tablets and sometimes injections must be used. The main drug used is a steroid, (a corticosteroid, not related to those misused by athletes), called prednisolone. Taking tablets is called a systemic treatment.

Steroid treatment starts with high doses (e.g., 80 mg prednisolone), which are tapered down when the uveitis is under control.

If the steroids alone cannot control the uveitis or if the steroid dose cannot be reduced down to below about 7.5mg within a reasonable time without the inflammation "flaring up," then a "second line" immunosuppressant drug may be introduced.

These "second line" drugs are used to reduce (or "spare") the amount of steroids used and/or to control the uveitis if this cannot be achieved by short-term steroid use. There are a number of "immunosuppressant" drugs which can be used and these should be discussed with your eye specialist to understand what is involved. They can be very useful to control difficult cases and to decrease a patient's dependence on high doses of steroids.

Side Effects of Treatment

All treatments may have some side effects.

Make sure you are given information about this by your doctors and make sure you ask your doctors about any concerns you have about the treatments.

Always report all side effects.

Complications of Uveitis

Some other eye problems may arise in patients with uveitis. These may be caused by the effects of the inflammation inside the eye, but also can result from steroid treatment to control the inflammation. It must be remembered that using sufficient steroids to control the uveitis will generally give a better outcome than using too little steroid and not controlling the inflammation:

- **Cataract:** Caused by uveitis but also by steroid treatment.

- **Secondary glaucoma:** Caused by a rise in the pressure inside the eye. Can be caused by uveitis and steroid use.

- **Macula edema:** Fluid which builds up in the back of the eye and can be sight threatening.

- **Posterior synechiae (anterior uveitis):** The iris "sticks" to the lens—this can be avoided or sometimes removed by use of dilating drops and hot towels/compresses.

It is very important that these complications are picked up very early on, as they can be more sight threatening than the underlying uveitis. Complications can only be picked up by thorough examination, which should always include the back of the eye.

Section 29.4

Iritis

Overview

Iritis is an inflammatory problem of the iris, the colored part of the
eye. It often occurs for unknown reasons, but it may be linked to certain
diseases affecting the body, infections, previous eye surgery, or injury.

Iritis may affect one or both eyes. It is sometimes a chronic, recurring condition.

Signs and Symptoms

- Red eye
- Light sensitivity
- Pain that may range from aching or soreness to intense discomfort
- Small pupil
- Tearing

Detection and Diagnosis

The doctor can detect iritis during an examination of the eye with
a slit lamp microscope. Among other things, the doctor will look for
microscopic white cells floating inside the eye which are a sign of inflammation. The doctor will also carefully examine inside the eye to
determine if other parts of the eye are involved.

Treatment

Steroids and anti-inflammatory drops are prescribed to reduce
inflammation in the eye. Dilating drops also make the eye more
comfortable by relaxing the muscle that constricts the pupil.

Iritis must be treated to avoid permanent problems such as scarring inside the eye.

Section 29.5

Choroideremia

What is choroideremia?

Choroideremia is a rare inherited disorder that causes progressive loss of vision due to degeneration of the choroid and retina.

What are the symptoms?

Choroideremia, formerly called tapetochoroidal dystrophy, occurs almost exclusively in males. In childhood, night blindness is the most common first symptom. As the disease progresses, there is loss of peripheral vision or "tunnel vision," and later a loss of central vision. Progression of the disease continues throughout the individual's life, although both the rate and the degree of visual loss can vary, even within the same family.

Vision loss due to choroideremia is caused by degeneration of several layers of cells that are essential to sight. These layers, which line the inside of the back of the eye, are called the choroids, the retinal pigment epithelium, and the photoreceptors. The choroid consists of several blood vessel layers that are located between the retina and the sclera (the "white of the eye"). Choroidal vessels provide the retinal pigment epithelium and photoreceptors with oxygen and nutrients necessary for normal function. The retinal pigment epithelium and the photoreceptors are part of the retina. The epithelium is associated closely with the photoreceptors and is needed for normal function. The photoreceptors are responsible for converting light into the electrical impulses that transfer messages to the brain where "seeing" actually occurs.

The retinal pigment epithelium and the choroid initially deteriorate to cause choroideremia. Eventually, the photoreceptors break down as well. As the disease progresses, the clinical appearance of these cell layers changes in a characteristic manner and more vision is lost.

Is it an inherited disease?

Choroideremia is genetically passed through families by the X-linked pattern of inheritance. In this type of inheritance, the gene for the disease is located on the X chromosome. Females have two X chromosomes and can carry the disease gene on one of their X chromosomes. Because they have a healthy version of the gene on their other X chromosome, carrier females typically are not affected by X-linked diseases such as juvenile retinoschisis. Sometimes, however, when carrier females are examined, the retina shows minor signs of the disease.

Males have only one X chromosome (paired with one Y chromosome) and are therefore genetically susceptible to X-linked diseases. Males cannot be carriers of X-linked diseases. Males affected with an X-linked disease always pass the gene on the X chromosome to their daughters, who then become carriers. Affected males never pass an X-linked disease gene to their sons because fathers pass the Y chromosome to their sons.

Female carriers have a 50 percent chance (or one chance in two) of passing the X-linked disease gene to their daughters, who become carriers, and a 50 percent chance of passing the gene to their sons, who are then affected by the disease.

What treatment is available?

Recently, scientists discovered mutations on a gene on the X chromosome that causes choroideremia. New research based on these findings now drives the search for a treatment. Investigators are now developing a gene therapy for evaluation in animal studies. With success in an animal model, they will move the treatment into clinical studies.

Choroideremia is one of the few retinal degenerative diseases that might be detected prenatally in some cases; female carriers may want to seek information about this testing from a medical geneticist or a genetic counselor. All members of an affected family are encouraged to consult an ophthalmologist and to seek genetic counseling. These professionals can provide explanations of the disease and the recurrence risk for all family members and for future offspring.

Until a treatment is discovered, help is available through low vision aids, including optical, electronic, and computer-based devices. Personal, educational, and vocational counseling, as well as adaptive training skills, job placement, and income assistance, are available through community resources.

Are there any other related diseases?

Early in the course of the disease, choroideremia could be confused with X-linked retinitis pigmentosa. Both have symptoms of night blindness and tunnel vision. However, differences are clear in a complete medical eye examination, especially as the disease progresses. The disease most similar clinically to choroideremia is gyrate atrophy. It too can be distinguished based on its inheritance, as an autosomal recessive disorder, and based on its cause, known to be a defect in an unrelated gene.

Part Five

Eye Injuries and Disorders of the Surrounding Structures

Chapter 30

Eye Emergencies

Chapter Contents

Section 30.1

Recognizing Eye Emergencies

What Is an Eye Emergency?

An eye emergency is an event where eyesight is at risk. Events that risk eyesight require prompt treatment to prevent vision loss. Eye emergencies are common.

What Do I Do?

Contact your ophthalmologist immediately. If your ophthalmologist is not immediately available to assist or direct you, report to the nearest emergency room.

If you feel that you have an urgent problem that requires immediate attention, you may call 911 or proceed to an emergency room of your choice. If you have an emergent eye condition, you should try to go to a hospital with an ophthalmologist on staff and readily available.

Chemicals in the Eye

If you get an acidic or caustic chemical in your eye (e.g., chemical burn), please stop reading this and irrigate your eye with clean contact lens solution; if none is available, you may use clean tap water. Do this for fifteen minutes, and then go directly to the nearest emergency room.

Mechanical Injury to the Eye

If you mechanically injure your eye or something gets in your eye, *do not* push on your eye. *Do* cover your eye with a rigid shield, if one is available. However, do not put anything under the shield that would press on your eye. A rigid shield can be fashioned from the bottom of a paper cup. Alternatively, put your glasses or sunglasses on, which will also provide protection.

Minor Eye Injury

For minor or less urgent injuries, proceeding directly to an ophthalmology clinic is often the wisest choice. Remember that ophthalmology is a very specialized field that requires special equipment: the direct approach is the wisest, quickest, and, often, least expensive option.

What Are the Symptoms of an Eye Emergency?

The following symptoms require immediate consultation with an ophthalmologist:

- Chemical contact with eye or face
- Severe eye, head, or face injury
- Sudden loss of all or part of your vision
- Bulging eye
- Painful eye
- Onset of flashing lights, floaters, or a noticeable increase in the amount of flashes and floaters
- Appearance of a "veil," or curtain across the field of vision
- Sudden changes in pupil size
- Eye that is sensitive to light
- Foreign body in the eye
- Double vision
- Post-operative patients with pain in or around the eye, infectious discharge, increased redness, or decreased vision (in either eye)

The following symptoms require contacting an ophthalmologist as soon as possible:

- Red eye
- Sensation of a foreign body present
- Excessive tearing
- Presence of pus or crusting

Prevention of Eye Injuries

Protective Equipment

The good news is that most of these injuries can be prevented with protective eyewear. The best prevention of an eye injury is to use protective eye equipment as appropriate, such as when playing sports or working with caustic chemicals. For other eye emergencies, the best prevention is an immediate response to the symptoms of an eye emergency.

Sports Injuries

Each year, more than half a million people suffer eye injuries while playing basketball, baseball, racquetball, hockey, and other sports. Children are especially prone to sports-related eye injuries; they suffer more than 160,000 such injuries annually.

To reduce your risk of injury, wear certified protective eyewear whenever you play ball sports or hockey. Certified lenses display approval stickers from either the American Society for Testing and Materials (ASTM) or the Canadian Standards Association (CSA). Regular glasses, sunglasses, open-sided eye guards, and contact lenses do not provide adequate protection.

Adequate eye protection is especially important for people with low vision or a blind eye, as they may be at greater risk of going completely blind after suffering an eye injury.

If you do injure your eye, seek emergency medical attention if:

- your eye is hit at a high speed;

- you experience a change in your vision;

- you have double vision;

- you feel pain in your eye;

- your eye is black and blue.

With prompt medical attention, eyesight often can be preserved even after severe injuries.

Section 30.2

First Aid for Eye Emergencies

Knowing how to deal with an eye injury can mean the difference between a minor inconvenience and blindness. It is important to contact your eye doctor as soon after an eye injury occurs as possible. That said, here are some first aid suggestions.

If you have a foreign object in your eye, don't rub it. Lift your upper eyelid outward and gently pull down over the lower lashes. This causes tears to flow and often washes the object out of your eye. You may have to repeat this several times. If the object does not wash out, contact your optometric physician. Do not try to remove a particle that is embedded. You can cause more damage quite easily. If you are wearing contact lenses, remove the lens and clean it thoroughly before putting it back in your eye. If discomfort persists, remove, clean again, and reapply. If discomfort continues, remove the lens and call your doctor.

For chemicals splashed in your eyes, immediately flush your eyes with cool water for at least fifteen minutes. Chemical burns can cause permanent damage and blindness, so irrigating the eyes thoroughly is critical. If possible, hold your head under a slowly running faucet, or pour water slowly from a glass or clear container. Seek professional attention immediately. If you are wearing contact lenses, remove them immediately. Then flush your eyes and seek professional help as described.

A blow to your face resulting in a black eye can be treated with cold compresses for about fifteen minutes every hour. Your doctor should also check your eye for internal damage. If the blow breaks your contact lenses, try to remove pieces of the lens immediately. Rinsing with saline or approved contact lens solutions will help. Then call your optometric physician.

Do not try to treat a cut, laceration, or penetrating eye injury. Do not flush the eye with water or put any medicine in the eye. If you are wearing a contact lens, don't try to remove it. Gently cover the eye with a bandage or gauze pad and go directly to your eye doctor or a nearby hospital.

Remember, the best way to treat eye injuries is to prevent them from happening in the first place. Don't forget to be aware of potential eye hazards and wear appropriate eye protection.

Chapter 31

Preventing Eye Injuries

Chapter Contents

Section 31.1

Preventing Eye Injuries in Children

"On the Lookout: Preventing Eye Injuries in Children," by David A. Schlessinger, M.D., FAACS, reprinted with permission from www .parentguidenews.com. © 2011 PG Media Network Corp. All rights reserved. Reprinted with permission.

We should all carefully ensure the longevity and good health of our eyes. When eye injuries occur in children, they can have long-term effects that can be irreversible and significantly hinder quality of life. Where and when are children most susceptible to eye injuries? Let's start right in your home.

Computers

Children are becoming increasingly reliant on computers, spending excessive amounts of time online for school assignments and to interact with their friends. Ergonomically speaking, computers can be the cause of a variety of complaints, such as headaches, joint pain, backaches, and vision problems. To avoid or minimize these ailments, a few things can help:

- Make sure the computer screen is placed at a level that is comfortable and minimizes strain to a user's body.

- Check to see that glare is not an issue. There are screens and accessories that feature a minimized glare to reduce the strain on a person's eyes.

- Encourage your child to take periodic breaks at twenty-minute intervals where the child gets up, stretches, and walks around the room. Breaks can be short in duration; and the more frequent, the better.

- Tell children to avert their eyes from the screen whenever possible.

Hazardous Items

Keep cleaning agents and other hazardous materials away from your little ones so they are not ingested, and be mindful that bleach and other cleaning products can be extremely dangerous and cause a chemical burn. If your child endures a chemical burn, immediately take the child to a medical professional. Until the child is under a doctor's care, repeatedly flush the eyes with water. The best solution? Lock hazardous items in a place where your child cannot get to them.

Sports, Toys, and the Playground

Baseball, football, tennis—even a simple game of jacks—all sports and activities pose a problem if a child is on the receiving end of a ball impacting the eye or surrounding area. A good way to ensure eye injuries don't happen to your active little one is to prompt children to always wear protective glasses or headgear when participating in sports. When the eyes are not properly protected, common problems that can arise from an object's direct impact with the eyes include the following:

- **Hyphema:** A person can accumulate blood in the anterior chamber (front) of the eye upon direct impact of an object with the eye. Even a small hyphema can be a sign of major intraocular trauma. What are signs that your child has hyphema? Look for a gathering of blood at the base of the iris (the colored portion of the eye). This type of injury can potentially lead to loss of vision and result in glaucoma. If this should occur, seek out an ophthalmologist immediately. In the interim, apply cold compresses in twenty-minute intervals to the area to keep swelling to a minimum during the first twenty-four hours. Acetaminophen can also be administered in a dosage appropriate for your child's age and weight. And keep the child's head elevated.

- **Bruising:** An impact to the delicate area around the eye will likely result in a "black eye." Sometimes these bruises look worse than they are, but they should be checked by a physician to confirm no damage has been done to the orbit (see below).

- **Orbital fracture:** An orbital fracture can be caused by many kinds of impacts, including the ones listed as well as a hit to the eye area. Sometimes our children may experience a conflict in the playground where a dispute gets physical, or perhaps the swing of a bat went farther than intended. When the bones that surround the eye area are broken, it can have lasting adverse effects. Treat potential fractures immediately.

411

Foreign Bodies

Sometimes during play or even while performing routine tasks, a person can suffer as a foreign body, such as sand, fragments of glass (should a dish or glass be broken), or debris in the air enters the eye. This can cause redness and mild to severe irritation and corneal abrasions. To counteract the harm, repeatedly flush the eye with water until the irritation is gone. If pain or redness persists, call an ophthalmologist or take your child to an emergency room.

Lacerations and Cuts

The skin around the eyelids is extremely delicate. Even minor trauma can cause it to tear open. Lacerations of the eyelids should be cleaned, and an ice pack applied. These injuries should then be urgently addressed by an ophthalmologist or plastic surgeon. It is important that the wounds be repaired properly and quickly. When treated properly, the eyelids usually heal quickly without scarring. Keep any bruised or lacerated area out of the sun, as this can lead to permanent pigment changes.

With the use of protective eyewear and a little bit of caution and common sense, eye injuries are unlikely to occur in children. When they do happen, remember to have an ophthalmologist check your child immediately. Most emergency rooms have ophthalmologists on staff, enabling children to receive the treatment they may require even on holiday weekends or while traveling.

Section 31.2

Preventing Eye Injuries from Fireworks

"Prevent Eye Injuries from Fireworks!" © 2011 Prevent Blindness America (www.preventblindness.org). Reprinted with permission.

There is no safe way for nonprofessionals to use fireworks. It is only safe to enjoy the splendor and excitement of fireworks at a professional display.

According to the U.S. Consumer Product Safety Commission, fireworks are involved in thousands of injuries treated in U.S. hospital emergency rooms each year.

Most fireworks injuries occur during the one-month period surrounding the Fourth of July:

- Eyes are among the most commonly injured part of the body.
- Firecrackers, sparklers, and roman candles account for many of the injuries.
- Males suffer three times more injuries than females.
- About a third or more of injuries are to children under age fifteen.

Do Not Let Children Play with Fireworks

Fireworks and celebrations go together, especially during the Fourth of July, but there are precautions parents can take to prevent these injuries. The best defense against kids suffering severe eye injuries and burns is to not let kids play with any fireworks.

Do Not Purchase, Use, or Store Fireworks of Any Type

Protect yourself, your family, and your friends by avoiding fireworks. Attend only authorized public fireworks displays conducted by licensed operators, but be aware that even professional displays can be dangerous.

Prevent Blindness America supports the development and enforcement of bans on the importation, sale, and use of all fireworks, except those used in authorized public displays by licensed operators, as the only effective means of eliminating the social and economic impact of fireworks-related trauma and damage.

If an Accident Does Occur, Minimize the Damage to the Eye

These six steps can help save your child's sight:

- Do not rub the eye. Rubbing the eye may increase bleeding or make the injury worse.

- Do not attempt to rinse out the eye. This can be even more damaging than rubbing.

- Do not apply pressure to the eye itself. Holding or taping a foam cup or the bottom of a juice carton to the eye are just two tips. Protecting the eye from further contact with any item, including the child's hand, is the goal.

- Do not stop for medicine! Over-the-counter pain relievers will not do much to relieve pain. Aspirin should never be given to children and ibuprofen can thin the blood, increasing bleeding. Take the child to the emergency room at once—this is more important than stopping for a pain reliever.

- Do not apply ointment. Ointment, which may not be sterile, makes the area around the eye slippery and harder for the doctor to examine.

- Do not let your child play with fireworks, even if his or her friends are setting them off. Sparklers burn at 1,800 degrees Fahrenheit, and bottle rockets can stray off course or throw shrapnel when they explode.

Section 31.3

Preventing Eye Injuries at Home

"Preventing Eye Injuries at Home," reprinted with permission from *Indiana University News*, http://newsinfo.iu.edu. © 2010 Trustees of Indiana University.

More than half of all eye injuries occur in the home—so take time to safeguard your home to prevent injuries that could result in the loss of sight.

"Much of what we advise is common sense, but it bears repeating if it will save one individual from potential vision loss or damage to his or her eyes," says Louis B. Cantor, chairman of the Department of Ophthalmology at the Indiana University School of Medicine. "It's a good idea to secure loose railings, soften sharp edges, and eliminate slippery stairs in the home. The presence of any one of these can lead to falls and injuries for senior citizens—and other members of the household."

Nearly half of the country's annual 2.5 million eye injuries take place in the home, and 11 percent of those are caused by slips and falls. The American Academy of Ophthalmology (AAO) encourages seniors and adults of all ages to make certain their homes are safe and that injuries, particularly those to the eyes, are prevented.

As parents and grandparents age, people often make modifications to their homes, such as adding ramps to stairways and fitting bathrooms with nonslip surfaces and railings in tubs and showers, Cantor said. But loose railings, slippery surfaces, and sharp edges can lead to falls and eye injuries to people of all ages.

Slips and falls are not the only cause of home eye injuries. Individuals can be injured while doing yard work, home repair, or working with chemical cleaners, Cantor said. The AAO recommends that every household in American have at least one pair of American National Standards Institute (ANSI)–approved protective eyewear to be worn when doing projects in and around the home. Wearing protective eyewear can prevent up to 90 percent of all home eye injuries.

The AAO and the Department of Ophthalmology offer these tips to reduce the incidence of eye injuries in the home:

- Make sure that rugs and shower/bathtub mats are slip-proof.

- Secure railings so that they are not loose.

- Cushion sharp corners and edges of furnishings and home fixtures.

- Use caution while operating power tools—from nail guns to hedge trimmers—and always wear ANSI-approved safety glasses.

- Be careful when opening or preparing solvents or chemicals for use in the home. It's always best to wear protective eyewear.

- Don't allow children or other adults to play in the yard while mowing. Lawnmowers can throw stones or other projectiles that can cause eye injuries.

- Make sure protective eyewear is used while playing sports, even if it's just playing basketball in the driveway or tossing a football in the backyard.

More than one in five at-home eye injuries are caused by home repair or power tools. More than 40 percent of all home injuries take place in the yard or garden, while nearly 30 percent take place in the home's living areas. Accidents were reported as the cause of 80 percent of all eye injuries, according to the AAO's Eye Injury Snapshot conducted earlier this year.

If an eye injury is received, see an ophthalmologist or go to an emergency room immediately. Delaying medical attention can result in vision loss or blindness, said Dr. Cantor.

Section 31.4

Preventing Sports Eye Injuries

Reprinted from the following documents from the National Eye Institute, National Institutes of Health: "About Sports Eye Injury and Protective Eyewear," May 2011, and "Sport-Specific Risk," October 2008.

About Sports Eye Injury and Protective Eyewear

Eye injuries are the leading cause of blindness in children in the United States and most injuries occurring in school-aged children are sports-related.[1] These injuries account for an estimated one hundred thousand physician visits per year at a cost of more than $175 million.

Ninety percent of sports-related eye injuries can be avoided with the use of protective eyewear.[1] Protective eyewear includes safety glasses and goggles, safety shields, and eye guards designed for a particular sport. Ordinary prescription glasses, contact lenses, and sunglasses do not protect against eye injuries. Safety goggles should be worn over them.

Currently, most youth sports leagues do not require the use of eye protection. Parents and coaches must insist that children wear safety glasses or goggles whenever they play.

Protective eyewear, which is made of ultra-strong polycarbonate, is ten times more impact resistant than other plastics, and does not reduce vision. All children who play sports should use protective eyewear—not just those who wear eyeglasses or contact lenses. For children who do wear glasses or contact lenses, most protective eyewear can be made to match their prescriptions. It is especially important for student athletes who have vision in only one eye or a history of eye injury or eye surgery to use protective eyewear.

Whether you are a parent, teacher, or coach, you can encourage schools to adopt a policy on protective eyewear. Meanwhile, parents and coaches should insist that children wear protective eyewear whenever they play sports and be good role models and wear it themselves.

Note

1. Harrison, A., & Telander, D.G. (2002). Eye Injuries in the youth athlete: a case-based approach. *Sports Medicine*, 31(1), 33–40.

Sport-Specific Risk

Some sports carry a greater risk than others. For example, baseball is the leading cause of sports-related eye injury in children fourteen and under and is considered high risk. Football carries a moderate risk. Check the list below for the risk categories for eye injury for various sports.

High Risk

- Baseball
- Basketball
- Boxing
- Hockey
- Paintball
- Racquetball
- Softball
- Squash

Moderate Risk

- Football
- Golf
- Badminton
- Soccer
- Tennis
- Fishing

Low Risk

- Bicycling
- Diving
- Skiing
- Swimming
- Wrestling

Section 31.5

Preventing Eye Injuries from the Sun

"Prevent Eye Damage: Protect Yourself from UV Radiation,"
U.S. Environmental Protection Agency, August 2010.

Most Americans understand the link between ultraviolet (UV) radiation and skin cancer. Many are less aware of the connection between UV radiation and eye damage. With increased levels of UV radiation reaching the Earth's surface, largely due to stratospheric ozone layer depletion, it is important to take the necessary precautions to protect your eyes.

Potential Effects of UV Radiation on Eyes

UV radiation, whether from natural sunlight or artificial UV rays, can damage the eye, affecting surface tissues and internal structures, such as the cornea and lens.

Long-term exposure to UV radiation can lead to cataracts, skin cancer around the eyelids, and other eye disorders.

In the short term, excessive exposure to UV radiation from daily activities, including reflections off of snow, pavement, and other surfaces, can burn the front surface of the eye, similar to a sunburn on the skin.

The cumulative effects of spending long hours in the sun without adequate eye protection can increase the likelihood of developing the following eye disorders:

- **Cataract:** A clouding of the eye's lens that can blur vision.

- **Snow blindness (photokeratitis):** A temporary but painful burn to the cornea caused by a day at the beach without sunglasses; reflections off of snow, water, or concrete; or exposure to artificial light sources such as tanning beds.

- **Pterygium:** An abnormal, but usually noncancerous, growth in the corner of the eye. It can grow over the cornea, partially blocking vision, and may require surgery to be removed.

- **Skin cancer around the eyelids:** Basal cell carcinoma is the most common type of skin cancer to affect the eyelids. In most cases, lesions occur on the lower lid, but they can occur anywhere on the eyelids, in the corners of the eye, under the eyebrows, and on adjacent areas of the face.

Did You Know . . .

- 22.3 million Americans have cataracts.

- The direct medical costs of cataracts are $6.8 billion annually.

Choosing Sunglasses for Children

When choosing sunglasses for children, SunWise, in partnership with Prevent Blindness America, recommends that you do the following:

- Read the labels: Always look for labels that clearly state the sunglasses block 99–100 percent of UV-A and UV-B rays.

- Check often to make sure the sunglasses fit well and are not damaged.

- Choose sunglasses that fit your child's face and lifestyle but that are large enough to shield the eyes from most angles.

- Find a wide-brimmed hat to wear with the sunglasses. Wide-brimmed hats greatly reduce the amount of UV radiation that reaches the eyes.

Protect Your Eyes

The greatest amount of UV protection is achieved with a combination of: sunglasses that block 99–100 percent of both UV-A and UV-B rays; a wide-brimmed hat; and for those who wear contact lenses, UV-blocking contacts. Wrap-around sunglasses and wide-brimmed hats add extra protection because they help block UV rays from entering the eyes from the sides and above.

Frequently Asked Questions

Who is at risk for eye damage?

Everyone is at risk. Every person in every ethnic group is susceptible to eye damage from UV radiation.

When do I need to wear sunglasses?

Every day, even on cloudy days. Snow, water, sand, and pavement reflect UV rays, increasing the amount reaching your eyes and skin.

What should I look for when choosing a pair of sunglasses?

No matter what sunglass styles or options you choose, you should insist that your sunglasses block 99–100 percent of both UV-A and UV-B radiation.

Do I have to buy expensive sunglasses to ensure that I am being protected from UV radiation?

No. As long as the label says that the glasses provide 99–100 percent UV-A and UV-B protection, price should not be a deciding factor.

Do all contact lenses block UV rays?

No. Not all contact lenses offer UV protection and not all provide similar absorption levels. Ask your eye care professional for more information, and remember, a combination approach works best!

Section 31.6

Preventing Eye Injuries in the Workplace

"Eye Protection in the Workplace" is reprinted from the Occupational Safety and Health Administration, Fact Sheet No. OSHA93-03, January 1, 1993. Reviewed by David A. Cooke, MD, FACP, December 2011. "Eye Safety Checklist" is reprinted from the U.S. Centers for Disease Control and Prevention, May 27, 2009.

Eye Protection in the Workplace

Every day an estimated one thousand eye injuries occur in American workplaces. The financial cost of these injuries is enormous—more than $300 million per year in lost production time, medical expenses, and workers compensation. No dollar figure can adequately reflect the personal toll these accidents take on the injured workers.

The Occupational Safety and Health Administration (OSHA) and the twenty-five states and territories operating their own job safety and health programs are determined to help reduce eye injuries. In concert with efforts by concerned voluntary groups, OSHA has begun a nationwide information campaign to improve workplace eye protection.

Take a moment to think about possible eye hazards at your workplace. A 1980 survey by the Labor Department's Bureau of Labor Statistics (BLS) of about one thousand minor eye injuries reveals how and why many on-the-job accidents occur.

What contributes to eye injuries at work?

Not wearing eye protection. BLS reports that nearly three out of every five workers injured were not wearing eye protection at the time of the accident.

Wearing the wrong kind of eye protection for the job. About 40 percent of the injured workers were wearing some form of eye protection when the accident occurred. These workers were most likely to be wearing protective eyeglasses with no side shields, though injuries among employees wearing full-cup or flat-fold side shields occurred as well.

422

What causes eye injuries?

Flying particles. BLS found that almost 70 percent of the accidents studied resulted from flying or falling objects or sparks striking the eye. Injured workers estimated that nearly three-fifths of the objects were smaller than a pinhead. Most of the particles were said to be traveling faster than a hand-thrown object when the accident occurred.

Contact with chemicals. Contact with chemicals caused one-fifth of the injuries. Other accidents were caused by objects swinging from a fixed or attached position, like tree limbs, ropes, chains, or tools, which were pulled into the eye while the worker was using them.

Where do accidents occur most often?

Potential eye hazards can be found in nearly every industry, but BLS reported that more than 40 percent of injuries occurred among craft workers, like mechanics, repairers, carpenters, and plumbers. Over a third of the injured workers were operatives, such as assemblers, sanders, and grinding machine operators. Laborers suffered about one-fifth of the eye injuries. Almost half the injured workers were employed in manufacturing; slightly more than 20 percent were in construction.

How can eye injuries be prevented?

Always wear effective eye protection. OSHA standards require that employers provide workers with suitable eye protection. To be effective, the eyewear must be of the appropriate type for the hazard encountered and properly fitted. For example, the BLS survey showed that 94 percent of the injuries to workers wearing eye protection resulted from objects or chemicals going around or under the protector. Eye protective devices should allow for air to circulate between the eye and the lens. Only thirteen workers injured while wearing eye protection reported breakage.

Nearly one-fifth of the injured workers with eye protection wore face shields or welding helmets. However, only 6 percent of the workers injured while wearing eye protection wore goggles, which generally offer better protection for the eyes. Best protection is afforded when goggles are worn with face shields.

Better training and education. BLS reported that most workers were hurt while doing their regular jobs. Workers injured while not wearing protective eyewear most often said they believed it was not required by the situation. Even though the vast majority of employers furnished eye protection at no cost to employees, about 40 percent of the workers received no information on where and what kind of eyewear should be used.

Maintenance. Eye protection devices must be properly maintained. Scratched and dirty devices reduce vision, cause glare, and may contribute to accidents.

Where can I get more information?

Your nearest OSHA area office. Safety and health experts are available to explain mandatory requirements for effective eye protection and answer questions. They can also refer you to an on-site consultation service available in nearly every state through which you can get free, penalty-free advice for eliminating possible eye hazards, designing a training program, or other safety and health matters.

Don't know where the nearest federal or state office is? Call an OSHA regional office at the U.S. Department of Labor in Boston, New York, Philadelphia, Atlanta, Chicago, Dallas, Kansas City, Denver, San Francisco, or Seattle.

Eye Protection Works!

BLS reported that more than 50 percent of workers injured while wearing eye protection thought the eyewear had minimized their injuries. But nearly half the workers also felt that another type of protection could have better prevented or reduced the injuries they suffered.

It is estimated that 90 percent of eye injuries can be prevented through the use of proper protective eyewear. That is our goal and, by working together, OSHA, employers, workers, and health organizations can make it happen.

Eye Safety Checklist

Create a safe work environment:

- Minimize hazards from falling or unstable debris.
- Make sure that tools work and safety features (machine guards) are in place.
- Make sure that workers (particularly volunteers) know how to use tools properly.
- Keep bystanders out of the hazard area.

Evaluate safety hazards:

- Identify the primary hazards at the site.

- Identify hazards posed by nearby workers, large machinery, and falling/shifting debris.

Wear the proper eye and face protection:

- Select the appropriate eye protection for the hazard.

- Make sure the eye protection is in good condition.

- Make sure the eye protection fits properly and will stay in place.

Use good work practices:

- Caution—Brush, shake, or vacuum dust and debris from hard-hats, hair, forehead, or the top of the eye protection before removing the protection.

- Do not rub eyes with dirty hands or clothing.

- Clean eyewear regularly.

Prepare for eye injuries and first aid needs. Have an eye wash or sterile solution on hand.

Chapter 32

Protective Equipment for Eyes at Risk

Chapter Contents

Section 32.1

Sports Eye Protection

Each year, more than forty thousand people are treated for eye injuries related to sports activities. Using the right kind of eye protection while playing sports can help prevent serious eye injuries and even blindness.

For sports use, polycarbonate lenses must be used with protectors that meet or exceed the requirements of the American Society for Testing and Materials (ASTM). Each sport has a specific ASTM code, so look for the ASTM label on the product before making a purchase.

Baseball

Type of eye protection:

- Faceguard (attached to helmet) made of polycarbonate material
- Sports eye guards

Eye injuries prevented:

- Scratches on the cornea
- Inflamed iris
- Blood spilling into the eye's anterior chamber
- Traumatic cataract
- Swollen retina

Basketball

Type of eye protection:

- Sports eye guards

Eye injuries prevented:

- Fracture of the eye socket

- Scratches on the cornea
- Inflamed iris
- Blood spilling into the eye's anterior chamber
- Swollen retina

Soccer

Type of eye protection:

- Sports eye guards

Eye injuries prevented:

- Inflamed iris
- Blood spilling into the eye's anterior chamber
- Swollen retina

Football

Type of eye protection:

- Polycarbonate shield attached to faceguard
- Sports eye guards

Eye injuries prevented:

- Scratches on the cornea
- Inflamed iris
- Blood spilling into the eye's anterior chamber
- Swollen retina

Hockey

Type of eye protection:

- Wire or polycarbonate mask
- Sports eye guards

Eye injuries prevented:

- Scratches on the cornea
- Inflamed iris
- Blood spilling into the eye's anterior chamber

- Traumatic cataract
- Swollen retina

Section 32.2

Workplace Eye Protection

Excerpted from "Personal Protective Equipment," Occupational
Safety and Health Administration, 2003. Reviewed by David A.
Cooke, MD, FACP, December 2011.

Employees can be exposed to a large number of hazards that pose
danger to their eyes and face. The Occupational Safety and Health
Administration (OSHA) requires employers to ensure that employees
have appropriate eye or face protection if they are exposed to eye or
face hazards from flying particles, molten metal, liquid chemicals,
acids or caustic liquids, chemical gases or vapors, potentially infected
material, or potentially harmful light radiation.

Many occupational eye injuries occur because workers are not wearing any eye protection, while others result from wearing improper
or poorly fitting eye protection. Employers must be sure that their
employees wear appropriate eye and face protection and that the selected form of protection is appropriate to the work being performed
and properly fits each worker exposed to the hazard.

Prescription Lenses

Everyday use of prescription corrective lenses will not provide adequate protection against most occupational eye and face hazards, so
employers must make sure that employees with corrective lenses either wear eye protection that incorporates the prescription into the
design or wear additional eye protection over their prescription lenses.
It is important to ensure that the protective eyewear does not disturb
the proper positioning of the prescription lenses so that the employee's
vision will not be inhibited or limited. Also, employees who wear contact lenses must wear eye or face personal protective equipment (PPE)
when working in hazardous conditions.

Eye Protection for Exposed Workers

OSHA suggests that eye protection be routinely considered for use by carpenters, electricians, machinists, mechanics, millwrights, plumbers and pipe fitters, sheet metal workers and tinsmiths, assemblers, sanders, grinding machine operators, sawyers, welders, laborers, chemical process operators and handlers, and timber cutting and logging workers. Employers of workers in other job categories should decide whether there is a need for eye and face PPE through a hazard assessment.

Examples of potential eye or face injuries include the following:

- Dust, dirt, metal, or wood chips entering the eye from activities such as chipping, grinding, sawing, hammering, the use of power tools, or even strong wind forces.

- Chemical splashes from corrosive substances, hot liquids, solvents, or other hazardous solutions.

- Objects swinging into the eye or face, such as tree limbs, chains, tools, or ropes.

- Radiant energy from welding, harmful rays from the use of lasers or other radiant light (as well as heat, glare, sparks, splash, and flying particles).

Types of Eye Protection

Selecting the most suitable eye and face protection for employees should take into consideration the following elements:

- Ability to protect against specific workplace hazards.

- Protection should fit properly and be reasonably comfortable to wear.

- Protection should provide unrestricted vision and movement.

- Protection should be durable and cleanable.

- Protection should allow unrestricted functioning of any other required PPE.

The eye and face protection selected for employee use must clearly identify the manufacturer. Any new eye and face protective devices must comply with ANSI Z87.1-1989 or be at least as effective as this standard requires. Any equipment purchased before this requirement took effect on July 5, 1994, must comply with the earlier ANSI Standard (ANSI Z87.1-1968) or be shown to be equally effective.

An employer may choose to provide one pair of protective eyewear for each position rather than individual eyewear for each employee. If this is done, the employer must make sure that employees disinfect shared protective eyewear after each use. Protective eyewear with corrective lenses may be used only by the employee for whom the corrective prescription was issued and may not be shared among employees.

Some of the most common types of eye and face protection include the following:

- **Safety spectacles:** These protective eyeglasses have safety frames constructed of metal or plastic and impact-resistant lenses. Side shields are available on some models.

- **Goggles:** These are tight-fitting eye protection that completely cover the eyes, eye sockets, and the facial area immediately surrounding the eyes and provide protection from impact, dust, and splashes. Some goggles will fit over corrective lenses.

- **Welding shields:** Constructed of vulcanized fiber or fiberglass and fitted with a filtered lens, welding shields protect eyes from burns caused by infrared or intense radiant light; they also protect both the eyes and face from flying sparks, metal spatter, and slag chips produced during welding, brazing, soldering, and cutting operations. OSHA requires filter lenses to have a shade number appropriate to protect against the specific hazards of the work being performed in order to protect against harmful light radiation.

- **Laser safety goggles:** These specialty goggles protect against intense concentrations of light produced by lasers. The type of laser safety goggles an employer chooses will depend upon the equipment and operating conditions in the workplace.

- **Face shields:** These transparent sheets of plastic extend from the eyebrows to below the chin and across the entire width of the employee's head. Some are polarized for glare protection. Face shields protect against nuisance dusts and potential splashes or sprays of hazardous liquids but will not provide adequate protection against impact hazards. Face shields used in combination with goggles or safety spectacles will provide additional protection against impact hazards.

Each type of protective eyewear is designed to protect against specific hazards. Employers can identify the specific workplace hazards that threaten employees' eyes and faces by completing a hazard assessment

Chapter 33

Eye Injuries

Chapter Contents

Section 33.1

Black Eye

What Causes a Black Eye?

A black eye is not uncommon after an injury to the face or the head. Even a minor impact to the face can result in a large, angry-looking "shiner." The swelling and trademark black-and-blue color occurs when small blood vessels in the face and head break, and blood and other fluids collect in the space around the eye.

The majority of black eyes are relatively minor bruises that heal on their own in a about three to five days. As the bruise heals, the swelling around the eye decreases, and the skin color often goes from black and blue to green and yellow.

Sometimes, a black eye is a warning sign of a more serious head, face, or eye injury. Two black eyes after an impact to the head shouldn't be taken lightly; it may indicate a severe head injury such as a skull fracture. While rare, a black eye may also indicate damage to the eyeball itself.

Black Eye Signs and Symptoms

- Pain and swelling around the eyelid and eye socket. In some cases the eye may actually swell shut.

- Discoloration around the eyelid and eye socket. This may begin as simple redness and progress to black and blue bruising.

- Blurring of the vision may also occur for a short time.

- Mild headaches or neck pain may also occur after a blow to the head.

When to Seek Medical Treatment for a Black Eye

If you have any of the following conditions along with a black eye, you should get medical attention to rule out a serious eye or head injury:

- Changes or loss of vision that don't clear up quickly
- Severe or persistent pain
- Swelling that continues beyond forty-eight hours
- Any injury caused by an object in the eye
- Blood pooling in the eye
- Cuts or lacerations in or near the eye
- Any deformity in the eye socket, face, or jaw that may indicate a fracture
- Broken or missing teeth
- Behavior changes or confusion
- Fluid draining from the nose, mouth, ears, or eye
- Signs of concussion or other serious head injuries that may have occurred from head trauma

Home Treatment for a Black Eye

Most black eyes will heal on their own within a few days, but you can help speed healing and reduce pain by taking the following actions:

- Stop any activity and apply ice wrapped in a thin cloth (or a cold compress or a bag of frozen vegetables) to the area around the eye.
- Avoid putting direct pressure on the eyeball itself.
- Keep the ice on the area for fifteen minutes at a time every waking hour for the first twenty-four hours.
- Keep your head elevated while sleeping. Using two pillows may help reduce swelling throughout the night.
- Pain medications may help reduce swelling and inflammation and decrease pain, but stay away from aspirin, which may increase bleeding.
- Continue to apply ice several times a day until the swelling subsides.
- Continue to check for any warning signs of a serious head injury for up to forty-eight hours.
- Allow the eye to heal before returning to sports

Should I Put Raw Steak on My Black Eye?

You've seen it in the movies, but there is no evidence that putting raw steak on a black eye helps it heal any faster. In fact, putting raw meat on any contusion or open wound is a good way to wind up with an infection. Stick with ice.

Section 33.2

Blowout Fracture

What is a "blowout" fracture?

A blowout fracture is a fracture of one or more of the bones surrounding the eye and is commonly referred to as an orbital floor fracture.

What is the orbit?

The orbit consists of the bones surrounding the eye. When looking at a skull, the orbit is the hole in the skull encompassing the eye.

What is the "floor" of the orbit?

The bones on the bottom of the orbit are the floor. The bones on the top are the roof and the bones on the side are the walls.

What is the function of the orbit?

The orbit holds the eye in the correct position. The orbit also protects the eye. Because the bones surrounding the eye "stick out" further than the eye, objects tend to hit the orbit and not the eye.

What causes a blowout fracture?

Blowout fractures result from trauma to the orbital bones. When an object hits the orbital bones (usually the eye brow and upper cheek bone) the force is transmitted to the bones. If the force is great enough the bones buckle and break.

What are common causes of blowout fractures?

Any large object with force or speed can cause a blowout fracture. Typical causes include motor vehicle accidents, balls used in sports, fists, and elbows.

What are the symptoms of an orbital blowout fracture?

The most common symptoms are bruising, tenderness, and swelling around the eye; redness of the eye; double vision (diplopia); numbness of the cheek, nose, or teeth; and nose bleeds (epistaxis).

Symptoms that typically indicate a more serious injury are pain on eye movement, double vision, air under the skin around the eye, and numbness of the cheek/mouth/nose on the side of the injury. Severe trauma may cause facial bone fractures, injury to the eye itself, and injuries to the skull/brain.

How do you know if there is a fracture?

X-rays and computed tomography (CT) scans of the orbit and face are used to make the diagnosis.

Are there different types of blowout fractures?

Blowout fractures are classified on several features including:

- size (big or small);
- location (front or back);
- bone in place or displaced;
- tissue/muscle entrapped in fracture;
- accompanying symptoms (double vision, pain, eye position).

A "simple" fracture is one with minimal or no double vision, minimal or no interference with eye movements, and minimal fracture size.

What can be done for a simple blowout fracture?

Most simple blowout fractures usually heal without lasting problems. Treatment consists of:

- ice to decrease swelling;

- decongestants to aid in the drainage of blood and fluid accumulating in the sinuses;

- avoidance of nose blowing to prevent pressure from propelling the sinus contents into the orbit;

- oral steroids in some cases to decrease swelling and scarring;

- sometimes oral antibiotics.

When should surgical repair of blowout fractures be considered?

Fractures with persistent symptoms, usually double vision or pain, are usually candidates for surgical repair. Timing of the repair varies, but usually is within two weeks of the injury. Initial repair may consist of any of the following:

- exploration of fracture site and repositioning of bone;

- release of trapped tissue from fracture site;

- covering of fracture site with synthetic material.

What long-term problems may develop following blowout fractures?

Most fractures heal without long-term effects. However, strabismus surgery (eye muscle surgery) is sometimes necessary for persistent double vision. Occasionally persistent double vision can be treated with nonsurgical methods (prism glasses or botulinum toxin injections).

Section 33.3

Chemical Burns

Overview

It can happen in the blink of an eye. While pouring liquid drain cleaner down a sink, some of the chemical splashes up in your face, hitting you squarely in the eye. Chemical injuries don't just happen in the workplace. Most homes have dozens of everyday products that pose tremendous danger to vision if they contact the eye.

The severity of the injury is related to whether the chemical is alkali or acid based.

Alkali-Based Chemicals

- Lime (cement, plaster, whitewash)

- Drain cleaners

- Lye

- Metal polishes

- Ammonia

- Oven cleaners

Acid-Based Chemicals

- Swimming pool acid (muriatic acid)

- Battery (sulfuric) acid

Alkali chemicals are more destructive then acidic chemicals because of their ability to adhere to the eye and penetrate tissues. However, acid burns may be compounded by glass injuries caused by an explosion.

Often, the difference between a serious but treatable injury and losing vision is a matter of understanding a few principles of ocular first aid.

Emergency Care and Prevention

After chemical exposure, the first step is to immediately (within seconds) begin flushing the eye with water. If the accident occurs in an industrial setting, special irrigating facilities should be available. If the injury happens at home, begin flushing the eye with water right away, call for help immediately, and contact your local ophthalmologist.

First Aid at Home

- Help the patient hold his or her head over a sink.

- Gently hold the lids apart with a cotton swab or dry cloth.

- Pour water over the eye, making sure to rinse inside the eyelids.

- Call your ophthalmologist.

The easiest way to irrigate at home is for the patient to hold his or her head over a sink while the helper continuously pours water over the eye with a glass or cup. It is important to gently hold the lids apart while irrigating in order to rinse underneath the lids and wash away as much of the chemical as possible. Using a dry cloth is helpful because the lids are difficult to hold back when they are wet. Continue flushing the eye for approximately twenty minutes.

Secondary Care at the Ophthalmologist's Office

If possible, bring the chemical used at the time of the accident to the doctor's office. The type of chemical, concentration, and key ingredients may give the doctor valuable information needed for treatment. The doctor may continue irrigation to insure that the chemical is diluted as much as possible. The eye will be carefully examined under magnification to determine the extent of the injury and whether there are any foreign particles imbedded in the eye.

An Ounce of Prevention . . .

Taking care to prevent chemical injuries is the best first aid. Follow these simple steps to reduce your risk:

- Follow package directions and warnings before using chemicals.

- When using chemicals, always wear safety glasses.

- Never put your face over a drain after applying chemicals.

The chance of regaining useful vision following a chemical accident is dependent on the nature and type of injury. However, knowing how to initiate treatment at home greatly increases the odds of recovery and saving vision.

Section 33.4

Foreign Objects in the Eye

Overview

Anyone who has felt as if there was a grain of sand in his or her eye has probably had a foreign body. Foreign bodies might be superficial, or in more serious injuries, they may penetrate the eye. Fortunately, the cornea has such an incredible reflex tearing system that most superficial foreign bodies are naturally flushed out with our natural tears. But if the object is more deeply embedded, medical attention is required.

Signs and Symptoms

- Mild to extreme irritation
- Scratching
- Burning
- Soreness
- Intense pain
- Redness
- Tearing
- Light sensitivity
- Decreased vision
- Difficulty opening the eye

The symptoms of a foreign body may range from irritation to intense, excruciating pain. This is dependent on the location, material, and type of injury.

In rare situations where an object penetrates the eye, there may be few or no symptoms. If you have no symptoms, but suspect an object may have penetrated your eye, it's always best to seek medical attention. The entry point of an intraocular foreign body is sometimes nearly invisible. Depending on their location, foreign bodies inside the eye may or may not cause pain or decreased vision.

Detection and Diagnosis

The evaluation includes vision testing along with careful examination of the surface of the eye with a slit lamp microscope. When a superficial foreign body is suspected, the upper lid should be gently turned up to check underneath for trapped particles. If the foreign body is difficult to see even with a microscope, the doctor may instill a drop of fluorescein dye to highlight the area.

An examination inside the eye with ophthalmoscopy may also be indicated, depending on the severity of the injury.

Treatment

If a foreign object becomes embedded within the cornea, conjunctiva, or sclera, a medical professional must remove it. Attempting to remove it yourself is dangerous and could result in a permanent scar that could affect your vision.

Superficial foreign bodies are usually treated in the office. After numbing the eye with topical anesthetic, the particle is carefully removed using a microscope. Afterward, antibiotic medications are generally prescribed to prevent infection. In some cases, foreign bodies become trapped underneath the eyelid. It is extremely important to examine under the eyelid for any remnant particles.

Intraocular foreign bodies typically must be removed in the operating room using a microscope and special instruments designed for working inside the eye. These injuries are often vision threatening and should be treated quickly.

Wearing appropriate safety glasses is the best way to prevent this type of injury. Protecting the eyes is especially important when working with machinery that could cause chips of wood or metal to splinter, as well as lawn equipment such as hedge and line trimmers.

If a particle of wood, glass, metal, or any other foreign substance becomes trapped in your eye, here are some tips:

- Do not touch or rub your eye! This can embed the object more deeply, making it more difficult to remove.

- Keep your eye closed as much as possible. Blinking only increases the irritation.

- Do not try to remove the object yourself. This is very dangerous and may make the problem worse.

- Seek professional help immediately.

- Tell your doctor what you were doing at the time of the injury, or what materials you may have been working with.

Section 33.5

Hyphema

"Hyphema," © 2011 A.D.A.M., Inc.
Reprinted with permission.

Hyphema is blood in the front area of the eye.

Causes

Hyphema is usually caused by trauma to the eye. Other causes of bleeding in the front chamber of the eye include:

- blood vessel abnormality;
- cancer of the eye;
- severe inflammation of the iris.

Symptoms

- Bleeding in the front portion of the eye
- Eye pain
- Light sensitivity
- Vision abnormalities

Exams and Tests

- Eye examination

- Intraocular pressure measurement (tonometry)
- Ultrasound testing

Treatment

In some mild cases, no treatment is needed. The blood is absorbed in a few days.

The healthcare provider may recommend bed rest, eye patching, and sedation to reduce the likelihood of recurrent bleeding.

Eye drops to decrease the inflammation or lower the intraocular pressure may be used if needed.

The ophthalmologist may need to remove the blood, especially if the intraocular pressure is severely increased or the blood is slow to absorb again. You may need to stay in a hospital.

Outlook (Prognosis)

The outcome depends upon the amount of injury to the eye. Patients with sickle cell disease are more likely to have eye complications and must be monitored more carefully.

Severe vision loss can occur.

Possible Complications

- Acute glaucoma
- Recurring bleeding
- Impaired vision

When to Contact a Medical Professional

Call your healthcare provider if you notice blood in the front of the eye or you have a traumatic eye injury. You will need prompt diagnosis and treatment by an ophthalmologist.

Prevention

Many eye injuries can be prevented by wearing safety goggles or other protective eyewear. Always wear eye protection while playing sports such as racquetball, or contact sports such as basketball.

References

Tingey DP, Shingleton BJ. Glaucoma associated with ocular trauma. In: Yanoff M, Duker JS, eds. *Ophthalmology. 3rd ed.* St. Louis, Mo: Mosby Elsevier; 2008:chap 10.17.

Chapter 34

Eyelid Disorders

Chapter Contents

Section 34.1

Blepharitis

"Facts about Blepharitis," National Eye Institute,
National Institutes of Health, August 2009.

Blepharitis Defined

What is blepharitis?

Blepharitis is a common condition that causes inflammation of the eyelids. The condition can be difficult to manage because it tends to recur.

Frequently Asked Questions about Blepharitis

What other conditions are associated with blepharitis?

Complications from blepharitis include:

- **Stye:** A red tender bump on the eyelid that is caused by an acute infection of the oil glands of the eyelid.

- **Chalazion:** This condition can follow the development of a stye. It is a usually painless firm lump caused by inflammation of the oil glands of the eyelid. Chalazion can be painful and red if there is also an infection.

- **Problems with the tear film:** Abnormal or decreased oil secretions that are part of the tear film can result in excess tearing or dry eye. Because tears are necessary to keep the cornea healthy, tear film problems can make people more at risk for corneal infections.

Causes

What causes blepharitis?

Blepharitis occurs in two forms:

- Anterior blepharitis affects the outside front of the eyelid, where the eyelashes are attached. The two most common causes of anterior blepharitis are bacteria (*Staphylococcus*) and scalp dandruff.

- Posterior blepharitis affects the inner eyelid (the moist part that makes contact with the eye) and is caused by problems with the oil (meibomian) glands in this part of the eyelid. Two skin disorders can cause this form of blepharitis: acne rosacea, which leads to red and inflamed skin, and scalp dandruff (seborrheic dermatitis).

Symptoms

What are the symptoms of blepharitis?

Symptoms of either form of blepharitis include a foreign body or burning sensation, excessive tearing, itching, sensitivity to light (photophobia), red and swollen eyelids, redness of the eye, blurred vision, frothy tears, dry eye, or crusting of the eyelashes on awakening.

Treatment

How is blepharitis treated?

Treatment for both forms of blepharitis involves keeping the lids clean and free of crusts. Warm compresses should be applied to the lid to loosen the crusts, followed by a light scrubbing of the eyelid with a cotton swab and a mixture of water and baby shampoo. Because blepharitis rarely goes away completely, most patients must maintain an eyelid hygiene routine for life. If the blepharitis is severe, an eye care professional may also prescribe antibiotics or steroid eye drops.

When scalp dandruff is present, a dandruff shampoo for the hair is recommended as well. In addition to the warm compresses, patients with posterior blepharitis will need to massage their eyelids to clean the oil accumulated in the glands. Patients who also have acne rosacea should have that condition treated at the same time.

Section 34.2

Blepharospasm

"Facts about Blepharospasm," National Eye Institute,
National Institutes of Health, August 2009.

Blepharospasm Defined

What is blepharospasm?

Blepharospasm is an abnormal, involuntary blinking or spasm of the eyelids.

Causes

What causes blepharospasm?

Blepharospasm is associated with an abnormal function of the basal ganglion from an unknown cause. The basal ganglion is the part of the brain responsible for controlling the muscles. In rare cases, heredity may play a role in the development of blepharospasm.

Symptoms

What are the symptoms of blepharospasm?

Most people develop blepharospasm without any warning symptoms. It may begin with a gradual increase in blinking or eye irritation. Some people may also experience fatigue, emotional tension, or sensitivity to bright light. As the condition progresses, the symptoms become more frequent, and facial spasms may develop. Blepharospasm may decrease or cease while a person is sleeping or concentrating on a specific task.

Treatment

How is blepharospasm treated?

To date, there is no successful cure for blepharospasm, although several treatment options can reduce its severity.

In the United States and Canada, the injection of Oculinum (botulinum toxin, or Botox) into the muscles of the eyelids is an approved treatment for blepharospasm. Botulinum toxin, produced by the bacterium *Clostridium botulinum*, paralyzes the muscles of the eyelids.

Medications taken by mouth for blepharospasm are available but usually produce unpredictable results. Any symptom relief is usually short term and tends to be helpful in only 15 percent of the cases.

Myectomy, a surgical procedure to remove some of the muscles and nerves of the eyelids, is also a possible treatment option. This surgery has improved symptoms in 75 to 85 percent of people with blepharospasm.

Alternative treatments may include biofeedback, acupuncture, hypnosis, chiropractic, and nutritional therapy. The benefits of these alternative therapies have not been proven.

Section 34.3

Chalazion

What is a chalazion?

A chalazion is a bump in the eyelid that is usually about the size of a small pea although it is occasionally smaller or larger. More than one chalazion can occur in an eyelid at the same time.

What causes a chalazion?

Small glands lining the edge of the eyelids produce oil that helps lubricate the surface of the eye. When one of these glands becomes blocked, oil backs up inside the gland and forms a bump in the eyelid. Sometimes there is a reaction to the deposit, causing the chalazion to become red, swollen, and painful.

Is a chalazion the same thing as a stye?

Not really, although the terms are often used interchangeably. A stye (hordeolum) is a bump in the eyelid that occurs when an oil gland becomes infected. In effect, it is like a small boil on the edge of the eyelid. A chalazion is an accumulation of material in the eyelid as a result of a blocked oil gland.

Why do chalazia occur?

Usually there is no known underlying cause. However, chronic inflammation of the oil gland openings (blepharitis) predisposes to the development of a chalazion. This situation may result in recurrent chalazia. Blepharitis may be aggravated by poor eyelid hygiene, which includes eye rubbing in children.

What are the treatment options for chalazia?

Most chalazia resolve spontaneously within several days to months. Warm soaks of the affected area can promote drainage of the blocked gland. Anti-inflammatory eye drops, ointments, or an injection into the bump may be indicated. A large swollen or persistent chalazion may necessitate oral antibiotics and/or surgical drainage. Children may require deep sedation or general anesthesia for the surgical procedure.

For those with a recurrent problem, a daily regimen of eyelid scrubs or washes can reduce the chances of developing new chalazia. This is especially useful when blepharitis is present.

Section 34.4

Eyelid Tumors

The eyelid skin is the thinnest and most sensitive skin on your body. As a result, this is often the first area on your face to show change from sun damage and aging. Unfortunately, sun damage and other environmental toxins not only cause the skin to age but can cause serious damage. Skin cancer of the eyelids is relatively common and several types exist. The presence of a nodule or lesion on the eyelid that grows, bleeds, or ulcerates should be evaluated. This involves examination and sometimes a biopsy.

Basal Cell Carcinoma

Basal cell tumors represent 90 percent of eyelid tumors. These skin cancers grow slowly over months and years. They most often appear as a pearly nodule that eventually starts to break down and ulcerate. Despite being a cancer, these tumors don't spread to distant areas but rather just continue to grow and infiltrate the surrounding tissue. They typically can be cured by simple excision followed by reconstruction of the defect left behind after the tumor removal.

Squamous Cell Carcinoma and Melanoma

These types of tumors occur much less commonly but are more aggressive and require more involved care to ensure complete treatment. Again, primary treatment involves removing the tumor, but care must also be taken to ensure the tumor has not spread anywhere, causing larger health problems. Your surgeon will help coordinate this as part of your treatment, depending on the size and circumstances of the tumor at presentation.

451

Treatment

Skin cancer needs to be removed surgically by a skilled individual who can not only remove the tumor but reconstruct the eyelid or area where the tumor was removed. Sometimes surgeons will do this themselves at a surgical facility with an on-site pathologist who can immediately examine the specimen to ensure the whole tumor was removed. Other times, the help of a dermatologic surgeon specializing in Mohs surgical excision will be utilized. This procedure is completed in two steps, the first in the dermatologist's office with immediate examination of the tumor to ensure its complete removal followed by the reconstructive surgery by your surgeon. Oculofacial plastic surgeons are the optimal person to repair these defects as the eyelid is quite delicate. Members of the American Society of Ophthalmic and Plastic and Reconstructive Surgery (ASOPRS) are well versed in the intricacies of the eyelid anatomy and the pitfalls associated with reconstructing this area.

Section 34.5

Ptosis

"Ptosis," reprinted with permission from the Scheie Eye Institute of the University of Pennsylvania Health System, www.pennmedicine .org/ophth. © 2011 The Trustees of the University of Pennsylvania. All rights reserved.

What is ptosis? What are its symptoms?

"Ptosis" refers to a drooping eyelid, and means that an upper eyelid falls to a position that is lower than normal. Because the involved eyelid may sag to the extent that it covers the pupil of the eye, it may interfere with normal vision by obscuring the upper aspect of the field of vision. In addition to the visual consequences, some patients find that a drooping eyelid has an undesirable effect on their appearance, and elect to have their eyelids raised to address the cosmetic issues associated with this problem. Ptosis may affect one or both eyes.

What are the types of ptosis? How are these causes treated?

In cases of levator dehiscence ptosis, the tendon of the muscle that lifts the eyelid (the levator palpebrae) may loosen or detach from its point of insertion. As a result, the muscle's natural effect is weakened. The risk of this type of ptosis increases with age, although cases of trauma, prior eye surgery, and contact lens use may result in levator dehiscence. When this problem occurs, surgery can be performed to reattach this tendon or to shorten this muscle to increase its strength. This surgery is generally performed under local anesthetic, except in children, and carries an excellent success rate.

Congenital ptosis is usually due to a developmental problem with the levator muscle. This problem is generally present from birth, although it may be diagnosed slightly later in life. Congenital ptosis may also be treated by shortening the levator muscle, although certain patients require suspension of the eyelid from the eyebrow.

Weaknesses of the muscles of the eyelid or malfunction of the nerves that control these muscles may result in ptosis. A careful examination by an ophthalmologist is critical to assess these situations and to look for specific underlying causes. Consequently, these patients generally require medical treatment and may not need surgery.

Other cases of ptosis are due to masses that increase the weight of the eyelid, such as a cyst, tumor, or swelling. In these cases, the muscles of the eyelid function normally, but they are required to lift a heavier weight and the eyelid subsequently droops. These cases are best dealt with on a case-by-case basis, as the treatment for these disorders varies considerably.

While excess skin around the eyelids (dermatochalasis) and drooping of the eyebrows (brow ptosis) are not truly causes of ptosis, they may create situations by which it appears that the patient's eyelids are lower than normal. Excess skin can generally be addressed by removal (blepharoplasty). Eyebrows can be elevated surgically (brow lift).

Regardless of the age of the patient or the degree of ptosis, each patient requires a careful examination. With proper evaluation and intervention, the prognosis is excellent for this problem.

Chapter 35

Disorders of the Tear Duct

Chapter Contents

Section 35.1

Blocked Tear Duct (Dacryostenosis)

"Tear-Duct Obstruction and Surgery," July 2011, reprinted with permission from www.kidshealth.org. Copyright © 2011 The Nemours Foundation. This information was provided by KidsHealth, one of the largest resources online for medically reviewed health information written for parents, kids, and teens. For more articles like this one, visit www.KidsHealth.org, or www.TeensHealth.org.

Many children are born with an underdeveloped tear-duct system, a problem that can lead to tear-duct blockage, excess tearing, and infection.

Blocked tear ducts are common in infants; as many as one-third may be born with this condition. Fortunately, more than 90 percent of all cases resolve by the time kids are one year old with little or no treatment.

The earlier that blocked tear ducts are discovered, the less likely it is that infection will result or that surgery will be necessary.

About Tear Ducts

Our eyes are continually exposed to dust, bacteria, viruses, and other objects that could cause damage, and the eyelids and eyelashes play a key role in preventing that.

Besides serving as protective barriers, the lids and lashes also help the eyes stay moist. Without moisture, the corneas would dry out and could become cloudy or injured.

Working with the lids and lashes, the protective system of glands and ducts (called the lacrimal system) keeps eyes from drying out. Small glands at the edge of the eyelid produce an oily film that mixes with the liquid part of tears and keeps them from evaporating.

Lacrimal (or tear-producing) glands secrete the watery part of tears. These glands are located under the brow bone behind the upper eyelid, at the edge of the eye socket, and in the lids.

Eyelids move tears across the eyes. Tears keep the eyes lubricated and clean and contain antibodies that protect against infection. They drain out of the eyes through two openings (puncta, or lacrimal ducts), one on each of the upper and lower lids.

From these puncta, tears enter small tubes called canaliculi or ducts, located at the inner corner of the eyelids, then pass into the lacrimal sac, which is next to the inner corner of the eyes (between the eyes and the nose).

From the lacrimal sacs, tears move down through the nasolacrimal duct and drain into the back of the nose. (That's why you usually get a runny nose when you cry—your eyes are producing excess tears, and your nose can't handle the additional flow.) When you blink, the motion forces the lacrimal sacs to compress, squeezing tears out of them, away from the eyes, and into the nasolacrimal duct.

The nasolacrimal duct and the lacrimal ducts are also known as tear ducts. However, it's the nasolacrimal duct that's involved in tear-duct blockage.

Causes of Blocked Tear Ducts

Many kids are born without a fully developed nasolacrimal duct. This is called congenital nasolacrimal duct obstruction or dacryostenosis. Most commonly, an infant is born with a duct that is too narrow or has a web of tissue blocking the duct and therefore doesn't drain properly or becomes blocked easily. Most kids outgrow this by the first birthday.

Other causes of blockage, especially in older kids, are rare. Some kids have nasal polyps, which are cysts or growths of extra tissue in the nose at the end of the tear duct. A blockage also can be caused by a cyst or tumor in the nose, but again, this is unusual in children.

Trauma to the eye area or an eye injury that lacerates (cuts through) the tear ducts also could block a duct, but reconstructive surgery at the time of the accident or injury may prevent this.

Signs of Blocked Tear Ducts

Kids with blocked tear ducts usually develop symptoms between birth and twelve weeks of age, although the problem might not be apparent until an eye becomes infected. The most common signs are excessive tearing, even when a child is not crying (this is called epiphora). You also may notice pus in the corner of the eye, or that your child wakes up with a crust over the eyelid or in the eyelashes.

Kids with blocked tear ducts can develop an infection in the lacrimal sac called dacryocystitis. Signs include redness at the inner corner of the eye and a slight tenderness and swelling or bump at the side of the nose.

Some infants are born with a swollen lacrimal sac, causing a blue bump called a dacryocystocele to appear next to the inside corner of the eye.

Although this condition should be monitored closely by your doctor, it doesn't always lead to infection and can be treated at home with firm massage and observation. If it becomes infected, sometimes topical antibiotics are required. However, with some infections, the child may need to be admitted to the hospital for intravenous antibiotics, followed by surgical probing of the duct.

When to Call the Doctor

If your child's eyes tear excessively but show no sign of infection, consult with your doctor or a pediatric ophthalmologist (eye specialist). Early treatment of a blocked duct may prevent the need for surgery.

If there are signs of infection (such as redness, pus, or swelling) or if a mass or bump is felt on the inside corner of the eye, call your doctor immediately because the infection can spread to other parts of the face and the blockage can lead to an abscess if not treated.

Treating Blocked Tear Ducts

Kids with blocked tear ducts often can be treated at home. Your doctor or pediatric ophthalmologist may recommend that you massage the eye several times daily for a couple of months. Before massaging the tear duct, wash your hands. Place your index finger on the side of your child's nose and firmly massage down toward the corner of the nose. You may also want to apply warm compresses to the eye to help promote drainage and ease discomfort.

If your child develops an infection as a result of the tear-duct blockage, the doctor will prescribe antibiotic eye drops or ointment to treat the infection. It's important to remember that antibiotics will not get rid of the obstruction. Once the infection has cleared, you can continue massaging the tear duct as the doctor recommends.

Surgical Treatments

If your child still has excess tearing after six to eight months, develops a serious infection, or has repeated infections, the doctor may recommend that the tear duct be opened surgically. This has an 85 to 95 percent success rate for kids who are one year old or younger; the success rate drops as children get older. Surgical probing may be repeated if it's not initially successful.

The probe should be performed by an ophthalmologist—your doctor can refer you to one. Probes are done on an outpatient surgery basis (unless your child is suffering from a severe infection and has already been admitted to the hospital) under general anesthesia.

The ophthalmologist first will do a complete eye exam to rule out other eye problems or types of inflammation that could cause similar symptoms. A dye disappearance test may help determine the cause of the problem. This involves placing fluorescein dye in the eye and then examining the tear film (the amount of tear in the eye) to see if it's greater than it should be. Or the doctor will wait to see if dye has drained properly by having the child blow his or her nose and then checking to see if any of the dye exited through the nose.

A surgical probe takes about ten minutes. A thin, blunt metal wire is gently passed through the tear duct to open any obstruction. Sterile saline is then irrigated through the duct into the nose to make sure that there is now an open path. There's very little discomfort after the probing.

If surgical probing is unsuccessful, your doctor may recommend further surgical treatment. The more traditional form of treatment is called silicone tube intubation, in which silicone tubes are placed in tear ducts to stretch them. The tubes are left in place for as long as six months and then removed in another short surgical procedure or in the office, depending upon the stent used.

A newer form of treatment is balloon catheter dilation (DCP), in which a balloon is inserted through an opening in the corner of the eye and into the tear duct. The balloon is inflated with a sterile solution to expand the tear duct. It is then deflated and removed.

Both of these procedures are fairly short but require that a child be put under anesthesia. Both are considered to be generally successful, with an 80 to 90 percent success rate in younger kids.

It may take up to a week after surgery before symptoms improve. Your doctor will give you antibiotic ointment or drops along with specific instructions on how to care for your child.

Section 35.2

Dacryocystitis

Overview

Dacryocystitis is an infection of the tear sac that lies between the inner corner of the eyelids and the nose. It usually results from blockage of the duct that carries tears from the tear sac to the nose. The blocked duct harbors bacteria and becomes infected. Dacryocystitis may be acute (sudden onset) or chronic (frequently recurs). It may be related to a malformation of the tear duct, injury, eye infection, or trauma.

This problem is most common in infants because their tear ducts are often underdeveloped and clog easily. Babies often have recurrent episodes of infection; however, in most cases, the problem resolves as the child grows. In adults, the infection may originate from an injury or inflammation of the nasal passages. In many cases, however, the cause is unknown.

Signs and Symptoms

- Generally affects one eye
- Excessive tearing
- Tenderness, redness, and swelling
- Discharge
- Red, inflamed bump on the inner corner of the lower lid

Detection and Diagnosis

During the exam, the doctor will determine the extent of the blockage. Cultures may be taken of the discharge to identify the type of infection. The doctor will also determine whether the infection has affected the eye.

Treatment

The treatment for dacryocystitis is dependent on the person's age, whether the problem is chronic or acute, and the cause of the infection.

Infants are usually treated first by gently massaging the area between the eye and nose to help open the obstruction along with antibiotic drops or ointments for the infection. Surgery may be necessary to clear the obstruction if medical treatment is not effective and the problem persists over several months.

Before surgery, the doctor may treat the child with antibiotics to make sure the infection is cleared. The operation is performed under general anesthesia. The tear duct is gently probed to open the passage.

For adults, the doctor may clear the obstruction by irrigating the tear duct with saline. Surgery is sometimes necessary for adults if irrigation or antibiotics fail to resolve the infection or if the infection becomes chronic. In these cases, dacryocystorhinostomy (DCR) is performed under general anesthesia to create a new passage for the tear flow.

Part Six

Congenital and Other Disorders That Affect Vision

Chapter 36

Hereditary Disorders Affecting Vision

Chapter Contents

Section 36.1

Achromatopsia

What is achromatopsia?

Two kinds of nerves are in the back of the eye. The nerves get the light through the pupil. They send visual messages to the brain. One kind of nerves is called rods. The other is called cones. The cones can send messages about still objects, details, and color. The cones let us read and look at pictures. Sometimes the cones do not work. That is called achromatopsia. "A" means "no" in Latin and "choma" means "color." "Opsia" means "eye." This eye problem is also called stationary cone dystrophy and rod monochromatism.

Some people who have achromatopsia also have nystagmus. Their eyes move back and forth without them wanting them to.

What causes achromatopsia?

Achromatopsia is an inherited eye condition. That means that a baby is born with it. When people have a baby, the baby's body has many things that the parents' bodies have. For example, a mother may have curly hair, and her baby may have curly hair just like hers. The father may have brown eyes, and his child will probably have brown eyes, too. But it is possible that two parents who have curly hair could have a baby with straight hair. Two parents who have brown eyes could have a baby who has blue eyes. They have the gene that makes straight hair and blue eyes hidden in their bodies.

Parents who have children who have achromatopsia may not have known that they have achromatopsia in their bodies. It was hidden. They may not know that achromatopsia is in their body cells until they have a child who has achromatopsia. Or they may remember that someone else in the family had achromatopsia.

What kind of vision do people have who have achromatopsia?

People who have achromatopsia see less clearly than people who are fully sighted. They see best when things are moving or when they are moving themselves. They see best in dim light. They may like to look, then close their eyes and see the image that stays in their eyes after they close them. They cannot tell the difference between some colors. Often they are farsighted. If they are farsighted, glasses may help them. Hyperopia is the medical word for farsighted.

What will help you if you have achromatopsia?

- Glasses may help you see things that are close to you.

- Sunglasses will help you in bright light. Try out some sunglasses with red tint. Many people who have achromatopsia like glasses with a dark red tint. You may like another color better. Try sunglasses that wrap around your face and that have a frame that shades your eyes from above.

- Wearing a hat with a dark brim may also help when the sun is bright. It can also help when the lights in class are too bright.

- Try to get lights that you can make bright or dim yourself. Sit and stand so that light is behind you or next to you.

- Before you turn on the computer or the TV, see if there is light glaring on the dark screen. Move the screen so light does not reflect on it before you turn it on.

- You may want to learn Braille if it is too hard to read print or if the print you read is too big for most books.

- You may want to use a white cane when the sun is very bright. It may help you not bump into things or trip.

Section 36.2

Albinism

The word "albinism" refers to a group of inherited conditions. People
with albinism have little or no pigment in their eyes, skin, or hair. They
have inherited altered genes that do not make the usual amounts of
a pigment called melanin. One person in seventeen thousand in the
United States has some type of albinism. Albinism affects people from
all races. Most children with albinism are born to parents who have
normal hair and eye color for their ethnic backgrounds. Sometimes
people do not recognize that they have albinism. A common myth
is that people with albinism have red eyes. In fact there are different types of albinism and the amount of pigment in the eyes varies.
Although some individuals with albinism have reddish or violet eyes,
most have blue eyes. Some have hazel or brown eyes. However, all
forms of albinism are associated with vision problems.

Vision Problems

People with albinism always have problems with vision (not correctable with eyeglasses) and many have low vision. The degree of vision impairment varies with the different types of albinism and many
people with albinism are "legally blind," but most use their vision for
many tasks including reading and do not use Braille. Some people
with albinism have sufficient vision to drive a car. Vision problems in
albinism result from abnormal development of the retina and abnormal
patterns of nerve connections between the eye and the brain. It is the
presence of these eye problems that defines the diagnosis of albinism.
Therefore the main test for albinism is simply an eye examination.

Skin Problems

While most people with albinism are fair in complexion, skin or hair
color is not diagnostic of albinism. People with many types of albinism

need to take precautions to avoid damage to the skin caused by the sun such as wearing sunscreen lotions, hats, and sun-protective clothing.

Types of Albinism

While most people with albinism have very light skin and hair, not all do. Oculocutaneous (pronounced ock-you-low-kew-TAIN-ee-us) albinism (OCA) involves the eyes, hair, and skin. Ocular albinism (OA), which is much less common, involves primarily the eyes, while skin and hair may appear similar or slightly lighter than that of other family members.

Over the years, researchers have used various systems for classifying oculocutaneous albinism. In general, these systems contrasted types of albinism having almost no pigmentation with types having slight pigmentation. In less pigmented types of albinism, hair and skin are cream-colored and vision is often in the range of 20/200. In types with slight pigmentation, hair appears more yellow or red-tinged and vision may be better. Early descriptions of albinism called these main categories of albinism "complete" and "incomplete" albinism. Later researchers used a test that involved plucking a hair root and seeing if it would make pigment in a test tube. This test separated "ty-neg" (no pigment) from "ty-pos" (some pigment). Further research showed that this test was inconsistent and added little information to the clinical exam.

Recent research has used analysis of deoxyribonucleic acid (DNA), the chemical that encodes genetic information, to arrive at a more precise classification system for albinism. Four forms of OCA are now recognized—OCA1, OCA2, OCA3, and OCA4; some are further divided into subtypes:

- Oculocutaneous albinism type 1 (OCA1 or tyrosinase-related albinism) results from a genetic defect in an enzyme called tyrosinase (hence "ty" above). This enzyme helps the body to change the amino acid tyrosine into pigment. (An amino acid is a "building block" of protein.) There are two subtypes of OCA1. In OCA1A, the enzyme is inactive and no melanin is produced, leading to white hair and very light skin. In OCA1B, the enzyme is minimally active and a small amount of melanin is produced, leading to hair that may darken to blond, yellow/orange, or even light brown, as well as slightly more pigment in the skin.

- Oculocutaneous albinism type 2 (OCA2 or P gene albinism) results from a genetic defect in the P protein that helps the tyrosinase enzyme to function. Individuals with OCA2 make a minimal amount of melanin pigment and can have hair color ranging from very light blond to brown.

- Oculocutaneous albinism type 3 (OCA3) is rarely described and results from a genetic defect in TYRP1, a protein related to tyrosinase. Individuals with OCA3 can have substantial pigment.

- Oculocutaneous albinism type 4 (OCA4) results from a genetic defect in the SLC45A2 protein that helps the tyrosinase enzyme to function. Individuals with OCA4 make a minimal amount of melanin pigment similar to persons with OCA2.

Researchers have also identified several other genes that result in albinism with other features. One group of these includes at least eight genes leading to Hermansky-Pudlak syndrome (HPS). In addition to albinism, HPS is associated with bleeding problems and bruising. Some forms are also associated with lung and bowel disease. HPS is a less common form of albinism but should be suspected if a person with albinism shows unusual bruising or bleeding.

Genetics of Albinism

The genes for OCA are located on "autosomal" chromosomes. Autosomes are the chromosomes that contain genes for our general body characteristics, contrasted to the sex chromosomes. We normally have two copies of these chromosomes and the genes on them—one inherited from our father, the other inherited from our mother. Neither of these gene copies is functional in people with albinism. However, albinism is a "recessive trait," so even if only one of the two copies of the OCA gene is functional, a person can make pigment, but will carry the albinism trait. Both parents must carry a defective OCA gene to have a child with albinism. When both parents carry the defective gene (and neither parent has albinism) there is a one in four chance at each pregnancy that the baby will be born with albinism. This type of inheritance is called "autosomal recessive" inheritance.

Ocular albinism (OA1) is caused by a genetic defect of the GPR143 gene that plays a signaling role that is especially important to pigmentation in the eye. OA1 follows a simpler pattern of inheritance because the gene for OA1 is on the X chromosome. Females have two copies of the X chromosome while males have only one copy (and a Y chromosome that makes them male). To have ocular albinism, a male only needs to inherit one defective copy of the gene for ocular albinism from his carrier mother. Therefore almost all of the people with OA1 are males. Indeed, parents should be suspicious if a female child is said to have ocular albinism.

For couples who have not had a child with albinism, there is no simple test to determine whether a person carries a defective gene for albinism. Researchers have analyzed the DNA of many people with albinism and found the changes that cause albinism, but these changes are not always in exactly the same place, even for a given type of albinism. Moreover, many of the tests do not find all possible changes. Therefore, the tests for the defective gene may be inconclusive.

If parents have had a child with albinism previously, and if that affected child has had a confirmed diagnosis by DNA analysis, there is a way to test in subsequent pregnancies to see if the fetus has albinism. The test uses either amniocentesis (placing a needle into the uterus to draw off fluid) or chorionic villous sampling (CVS). Cells in the fluid are examined to see if they have an albinism gene from each parent.

For specific information and genetic testing, seek the advice of a qualified geneticist or genetic counselor. The American College of Medical Genetics and the National Society of Genetic Counselors maintain a referral list. Those considering prenatal testing should be made aware that people with albinism usually adapt quite well to their disabilities and lead very fulfilling lives.

Vision Rehabilitation

Eye problems in albinism result from abnormal development of the eye because of lack of pigment and often include:

- Nystagmus: regular horizontal back and forth movement of the eyes.

- Strabismus: muscle imbalance of the eyes, "crossed eyes" (esotropia), "lazy eye" or an eye that deviates out (exotropia).

- Photophobia: sensitivity to bright light and glare.

- People with albinism may be either far-sighted or near-sighted and usually have astigmatism.

- Foveal hypoplasia: the retina, the surface inside the eye that receives light, does not develop normally before birth and in infancy.

- Optic nerve misrouting: the nerve signals from the retina to the brain do not follow the usual nerve routes.

- The iris, the colored area in the center of the eye, has little to no pigment to screen out stray light coming into the eye.

(Light normally enters the eye only through the pupil, the dark opening in the center of the iris, but in albinism light can pass through the iris as well.)

For the most part, treatment of the eye conditions consists of visual rehabilitation. Surgery to correct strabismus may improve the appearance of the eyes. However, since surgery will not correct the misrouting of nerves from the eyes to the brain, surgery will not improve eyesight or fine binocular vision. In the case of esotropia or "crossed eyes," surgery may help vision by expanding the visual field (the area that the eyes can see while looking at one point).

People with albinism are sensitive to glare, but they do not prefer to be in the dark, and they need light to see just like anyone else. Sunglasses or tinted contact lenses help outdoors. Indoors, it is important to place lights for reading or close work over a shoulder rather than in front.

Various optical aids are helpful to people with albinism and the choice of an optical aid depends on how a person uses his or her eyes in jobs, hobbies, or other usual activities. Some people do well using bifocals which have a strong reading lens, prescription reading glasses, or contact lenses. Others use hand-held magnifiers or special small telescopes and some prefer to use screen magnification products on computers.

Some people with albinism use bioptics, glasses which have small telescopes mounted on, in, or behind their regular lenses, so that one can look through either the regular lens or the telescope. Newer designs of bioptics use smaller lightweight lenses. Some states allow the use of bioptic telescopes for driving.

Optometrists or ophthalmologists who are experienced in working with low-vision patients can recommend various optical aids. Clinics should provide aids on trial loan and provide instruction in their use. The American Foundation for the Blind maintains a directory of low vision clinics. In Canada, support is available from the Canadian National Institute for the Blind.

Medical Problems

In the United States, most people with albinism live normal life spans and have the same types of general medical problems as the rest of the population. The lives of people with Hermansky-Pudlak syndrome can be shortened by lung disease or other problems. Other conditions include Chédiak-Higashi and Griscelli syndrome.

In tropical countries, those who do not use skin protection may develop life-threatening skin cancers. If they use appropriate skin protection, such as sunscreen lotions rated 20 sun protection factor (SPF) or higher and opaque clothing, people with albinism can enjoy outdoor activities even in summer.

People with albinism are at risk of isolation because the condition is often misunderstood. Social stigmatization can occur, especially within communities of color, where the race or paternity of a person with albinism may be questioned. Families and schools must make an effort not to exclude children with albinism from group activities. Contact with others with albinism or who have albinism in their families or communities is most helpful.

Section 36.3

Alström Syndrome

"What Is Alstrom Syndrome?" © 2008 Alstrom Syndrome International (www.alstrom.org). Reprinted with permission.

What Is Alström Syndrome?

It is a rare genetic disease. It affects several parts of the body. Alström syndrome is named for a Swedish doctor, Carl-Henry Alström, who first described it in 1959.

Cause

Alström syndrome is caused by a mutated gene, called ALMS1, which is passed on through families. The mutated gene may be present without causing the disease if a person received a mutated gene from one parent and a gene that was not mutated from the other. If a mother and a father both have the hidden, mutated gene, however, there is a 25 percent chance that their children will inherit one mutated gene from each of them. The offspring who receive mutated ALMS1 genes from both parents have Alström syndrome.

Below are some explanations of the symptoms that people with Alström syndrome can have. It is important to know that *not all* people have all of these symptoms and Alström syndrome is extremely variable!

Eyes

The first symptoms of Alström syndrome which are usually noticed are extra sensitivity to light and rapid movement of the eyes, called "photophobia" and "nystagmus." These are caused by the slow degeneration of the retina. The retina is composed of layers of film in the back of the eye that hold the photoreceptors. The photoreceptors capture light and send visual information to the brain via the optic nerve. The photoreceptors that are used for seeing in well-lit situations are called "cones." Typically the cones deteriorate first in the eyes of children who have Alström syndrome. The photoreceptors that remain are called "rods." They work best in dimly lit situations. The rods may also stop working as the person who has Alström syndrome gets older.

This eye condition is called cone-rod dystrophy. Sometimes it is diagnosed as retinitis pigmentosa. Children who have it can usually benefit from enlarged print, tinted glasses, which may include a corrective prescription, and devices such as magnifiers, monocular telescopes, and electronic magnifiers. By late teen years people who have Alström syndrome are left with very little or no vision.

Ears

Children who have Alström syndrome can begin to lose hearing. This can happen in childhood or in adulthood. If your child has Alström syndrome or a suspected diagnosis, it is important to have regular hearing tests so that any hearing loss can be identified and dealt with. The hearing loss is called "sensorineural," which means there is a loss of nerve function in the hearing system, and auditory information is not getting to the brain for processing. People who have Alström syndrome usually benefit from using hearing aids.

Stature

People who have Alström syndrome are often more overweight as children than their family members and are shorter as adults than their family members.

Heart

In some cases, the heart muscle of people who have Alström syndrome can be enlarged, a condition called "dilated cardiomyopathy."

This condition shows up sometimes in infancy and sometimes in adolescence. It leads to the heart having difficulty pumping blood efficiently to all parts of the body. Fluid and blood may build up in the lungs, causing shortness of breath. The feet, ankles, and legs may swell with fluid. This is called "congestive heart failure," although the heart does not stop; it just does not work well. This condition can be helped by medications that remove extra fluid from the tissues and others that help the heart to function better.

Intelligence

People who have Alström syndrome typically have a similar level of intelligence to their family members. They may have learning difficulties related to their poor vision and hearing loss.

Other Symptoms

Other organs are affected in various ways by Alström syndrome. Type 2 diabetes mellitus may develop in childhood or teenage years because the body does not process insulin the way it should. Children who have Alström syndrome are "insulin resistant." People with Alström syndrome who have type 2 diabetes do not always need to take insulin, but need to follow a careful diet which is low in calories and refined carbohydrates. It is important to try to increase the amount of exercise for all people with Alström syndrome.

People who have Alström syndrome often have higher than normal levels of fats, called cholesterol and triglycerides, in the blood. Your physician may prescribe a medication to control this.

The liver and the kidneys of people who have Alström syndrome are usually affected. Problems in the functions of these organs typically show up when the children are in their late teens, but your physician should monitor this with at least yearly blood tests. Kidney or liver failure in adulthood is often the cause of severe problems for people who have Alström syndrome.

There are several other conditions which may result from Alström syndrome, including curvature of the spine (scoliosis), digestive disturbances, respiratory problems, high blood pressure, and thyroid problems. It is important to get regular medical care to make sure all of the symptoms of Alström syndrome are managed as well as possible.

Section 36.4

Bardet-Biedl Syndrome

What is Bardet-Biedl syndrome?

Bardet-Biedl syndrome is a complex disorder that affects many parts of the body including the retina. Individuals with this syndrome have a retinal degeneration similar to retinitis pigmentosa (RP).

What are the symptoms?

The diagnosis of Bardet-Biedl syndrome is usually confirmed in childhood when visual problems due to RP are discovered. The first symptom of RP is night blindness. Night blindness makes it difficult to see in low light levels. RP then causes a progressive loss of peripheral (side) vision. Peripheral vision loss is often referred to as tunnel vision. Individuals with Bardet-Biedl also experience central vision loss during childhood or adolescence. RP symptoms progress rapidly and usually lead to severe visual impairment by early adulthood.

In addition to RP, polydactyly (extra fingers and/or toes) and obesity are defining characteristics of Bardet-Biedl syndrome. A diagnosis of Bardet-Biedl syndrome is usually first suspected when a child is born with polydactyly. Subsequent RP symptoms and obesity confirm the diagnosis. Extra fingers and toes are usually removed in infancy or early childhood. Slight webbing (extra skin) between fingers and between toes is also common. Most individuals have short, broad feet as well. Obesity may be present by childhood and is usually limited to the trunk of the body. Many individuals are also shorter than average.

Approximately half of all individuals with Bardet-Biedl syndrome experience developmental disabilities ranging from mild impairment or delayed emotional development to mental retardation. The degree of mental retardation can range from mild cognitive disability to severe mental retardation. Individuals may also experience renal (kidney) disease. Renal abnormalities can affect the structure and the function of the kidneys and can lead to severe renal impairment.

Upon reaching adulthood, males with Bardet-Biedl syndrome can have small genitalia (testes and penis). Because female sexual organ size is more difficult to assess, it is not known how many women have this characteristic. Females with Bardet-Biedl can experience irregular menstrual cycles.

Is it an inherited disease?

Bardet-Biedl syndrome is genetically passed through families by the autosomal recessive pattern of inheritance. In this type of inheritance both parents, called carriers, have one gene for the syndrome paired with one normal gene. Each of their children then has a 25 percent chance (or one chance in four) of inheriting the two Bardet-Biedl genes (one from each parent) needed to cause the disorder. Carriers are unaffected because they have only one copy of the gene. At this time, it is impossible to determine who is a carrier for Bardet-Biedl syndrome until after the birth of an affected child.

What treatment is available?

There are no treatments for all of the characteristics associated with Bardet-Biedl syndrome. As vision worsens, individuals will benefit from the use of low-vision aids and orientation as well as from mobility training. Researchers have identified twelve genes that are linked to Bardet-Biedl syndrome, giving them clear targets for treatment development.

To manage the complications of renal disease associated with Bardet-Biedl syndrome, every individual with the disorder should be examined by a nephrologist, a physician who specializes in kidney diseases.

Are there other related syndromes?

Bardet-Biedl syndrome is often confused with Laurence-Moon syndrome. Individuals with Laurence-Moon syndrome almost always experience neurologic problems but rarely polydactyly. Polydactyly is a defining feature of Bardet-Biedl syndrome, while neurologic problems almost never occur. Laurence-Moon syndrome is extremely rare; only a few cases have been documented. Because of the similarity of these syndromes, Bardet-Biedl syndrome is often referred to as Laurence-Moon/Bardet-Biedl syndrome or Laurence-Moon/Biedl syndrome.

Section 36.5

Bietti Crystalline Disorder

"Facts about Bietti's Crystalline Dystrophy,"
National Eye Institute, National Institutes of
Health, August 2009.

Bietti crystalline dystrophy (BCD) is an inherited eye disease named for Dr. G. B. Bietti, an Italian ophthalmologist, who described three patients with similar symptoms in 1937.

This diseased is also known as Bietti crystalline corneoretinal dystrophy.

Cause

What causes Bietti crystalline dystrophy?

From family studies, we know that BCD is inherited primarily in an autosomal recessive fashion. This means that an affected person receives one nonworking gene from each of his or her parents. A person who inherits a nonworking gene from only one parent will be a carrier, but will not develop the disease. A person with BCD syndrome will pass on one gene to each of his or her children. However, unless the person has children with another carrier of BCD genes, the individual's children are not at risk for developing the disease.

In September 2000, National Eye Institute (NEI) researchers reported that the BCD gene had been localized to chromosome 4. In this region of chromosome 4 there are hundreds of genes. Researchers are now looking for which of the genes in this region of chromosome 4 causes BCD. Finding the gene may shed light on the composition of the crystals found in the corneas of patients with BCD and on what causes the condition.

In March 2004, NEI researchers identified the BCD gene, now named CYP4V2. Researchers believe that this gene has a role in fatty acid and steroid metabolism. This is consistent with findings from biochemical studies of patients with BCD.

Symptoms

What are the symptoms of BCD?

The symptoms of BCD include: crystals in the cornea (the clear covering of the eye); yellow, shiny deposits on the retina; and progressive atrophy of the retina, choriocapillaries, and choroid (the back layers of the eye). This tends to lead to progressive night blindness and visual field constriction. BCD is a rare disease and appears to be more common in people with Asian ancestry.

People with BCD have crystals in some of their white blood cells (lymphocytes) that can be seen by using an electron microscope. Researchers have been unable to determine exactly what substance makes up these crystalline deposits. Their presence does not appear to harm the patient in any other way except to affect vision.

Treatment

Can Bietti crystalline dystrophy be treated?

At this time, there is no treatment for BCD. Scientists hope that findings from gene research will be helpful in finding treatments for patients with BCD.

Reference

Li, A, Jiao, X, Munier, FL, Schorderet, DF, Yao, W, Iwata, F, Hayakawa, M, Kanai, A, Shy Chen, M, Lewis, R, Heckenlively, J, Weleber, RG, Traboulsi, EI, Zhang, Z, Xiao, X, Kaiser-Kupfer, M, Sergeev, Y, Hejtmancik, JF. Bietti crystalline corneoretinal dystrophy is caused by mutations in the novel gene CYP4V2. *American Journal of Human Genetics.* 74(5): 817–26.

Section 36.6

Fuchs Corneal Dystrophy

Overview

Fuchs dystrophy is an inherited condition that affects the delicate inner layer (endothelium) of the cornea. The endothelium functions as a pump mechanism, constantly removing fluids from the cornea to maintain its clarity. Patients gradually lose these endothelial cells as the dystrophy progresses. Once lost, the endothelial cells do not grow back, but instead spread out to fill the empty spaces. The pump system becomes less efficient, causing corneal clouding, swelling, and eventually, reduced vision.

In the early stages, Fuchs patients notice glare and light sensitivity. As the dystrophy progresses, the vision may seem blurred in the morning and sharper later in the day. This happens because the internal layers of the cornea tend to retain more moisture during sleep that evaporates when the eyes are open. As the dystrophy worsens, the vision becomes continuously blurred.

Fuchs affects both eyes and is slightly more common among women then men. It generally begins at thirty to forty years of age and gradually progresses. If the vision becomes significantly impaired, a corneal transplant may be indicated. Sometimes corneal transplant (also known as penetrating keratoplasty or PKP) is performed along with cataract and intraocular lens implant surgery.

Signs and Symptoms

- Hazy vision that is often most pronounced in the morning
- Fluctuating vision
- Glare when looking at lights
- Light sensitivity
- Sandy, gritty sensation

Detection and Diagnosis

Fuchs is detected by examining the cornea with a slit lamp microscope that magnifies the endothelial cells thousands of times. The health of the endothelium is evaluated and monitored with pachymetry and specular microscopy.

Treatment

Fuchs cannot be cured; however, with certain medications, blurred vision resulting from the corneal swelling can be controlled. Salt solutions such as sodium chloride drops or ointment are often prescribed to draw fluid from the cornea and reduce swelling. Another simple technique that reduces moisture in the cornea is to hold a hair dryer at arm's length, blowing air into the face with the eyes closed. This technique draws moisture from the cornea, temporarily decreases swelling, and improves the vision.

Corneal transplant is indicated when the vision deteriorates to the point that it impairs the patient's ability to function normally.

Section 36.7

Stargardt Disease

What is Stargardt disease?

Stargardt disease is the most common form of inherited juvenile macular degeneration. The progressive vision loss associated with Stargardt disease is caused by the death of photoreceptor cells in the central portion of the retina called the macula.

The retina is the delicate light-sensing tissue lining the back inside wall of the eye. Photoreceptor cells in the retina provide vision by conveying information from the visual field to the brain. The macula is responsible for sharp central vision—for tasks like reading, watching television, and looking at faces.

Decreased central vision is a hallmark of Stargardt disease. Side vision is usually preserved. Stargardt disease typically develops during childhood and adolescence. Also involved in Stargardt disease is a region beneath the macula called the retinal pigment epithelium.

What are the symptoms?

The symptom that brings most people to an eye doctor is a change in central vision. A doctor looking at the retina of a person with Stargardt disease will see characteristic yellowish flecks in and under the macula. The flecks might extend outward in a ring-like fashion.

The flecks are deposits of lipofuscin, a fatty byproduct of normal cell activity. In Stargardt disease, lipofuscin accumulates abnormally. The Foundation Fighting Blindness supports research studying lipofuscin build up and ways to prevent it.

A decrease in color perception also occurs in Stargardt disease. This is because photoreceptor cells involved in color perception are concentrated in the macula.

How quickly does vision fade?

The progression of symptoms in Stargardt disease is variable. Visual acuity (the ability to distinguish details and shape) may decrease slowly at first, accelerate, and then level off.

A study of ninety-five people with Stargardt disease showed that once a visual acuity of 20/40 is reached, there is often rapid progression of additional vision loss until it reaches 20/200. (Normal vision is 20/20. A person with 20/40 vision sees at twenty feet what someone with normal vision sees at forty feet.) By age fifty, approximately 50 percent of people in the study had visual acuities of 20/200 or worse.

Eventually, almost everyone with Stargardt disease has a visual acuity in the range of 20/200 to 20/400. The vision loss is not correctable with prescription eyeglasses, contact lenses, or refractive surgery.

Is it an inherited disease?

Stargardt disease is almost always inherited as an autosomal recessive trait. It is inherited when both parents, called carriers, have one gene for the disease paired with one normal gene. Each offspring has a 25 percent chance of inheriting two copies of the Stargardt gene (one from each parent) needed to cause the disease. Carrier parents are unaffected because they have only one copy of the gene.

Genetic counselors are an excellent resource for discussing inheritability, family planning, career choices, and other issues related to living with Stargardt disease.

In 1997, Foundation Fighting Blindness (FFB)–funded researchers found the gene for Stargardt disease, ABCA4, which normally causes the production of a protein involved in the visual cycle. Lipofuscin buildup appears to be related to a mutation in this gene, and the resulting production of a dysfunctional protein.

What treatment is available?

FFB is supporting several promising avenues of research, including gene and drug therapies. Researchers are planning a clinical study of a treatment that involves delivery of a healthy version of the ABCA4 gene into retinal cells to restore production of the normal protein. They are also optimistic about several drugs that may slow vision loss by reducing the buildup of lipofuscin.

Because there is some evidence that sunlight may influence lipofuscin accumulation in the retina, ultraviolet (UV)–blocking sunglasses

483

are generally recommended for outdoors. For people who already have significant vision loss, low vision aides are available.

Are there any related diseases?

Stargardt disease is also known as Stargardt macular dystrophy or fundus flavimaculatus. In addition to recessive Stargardt disease, there are other rarer forms inherited as dominant rather than recessive traits.

Section 36.8

Usher Syndrome

"Facts about Usher Syndrome," National Eye Institute,
National Institutes of Health, October 2010.

Usher Syndrome Defined

What is Usher syndrome?

Usher syndrome is the most common condition that affects both hearing and vision. A syndrome is a disease or disorder that has more than one feature or symptom. The major symptoms of Usher syndrome are hearing loss and an eye disorder called retinitis pigmentosa, or RP. Retinitis pigmentosa causes night blindness and a loss of peripheral vision (side vision) through the progressive degeneration of the retina. The retina is a light-sensitive tissue at the back of the eye and is crucial for vision. As retinitis pigmentosa progresses, the field of vision narrows, a condition known as "tunnel vision," until only central vision (the ability to see straight ahead) remains. Many people with Usher syndrome also have severe balance problems.

What are the types of Usher syndrome?

There are three clinical types of Usher syndrome: type 1, type 2, and type 3. In the United States, types 1 and 2 are the most common types. Together, they account for approximately 90 to 95 percent of all cases of children who have Usher syndrome.

Type 1: Children with type 1 Usher syndrome are profoundly deaf at birth and have severe balance problems. Many of these individuals obtain little or no benefit from hearing aids. Parents should consult their doctor and other hearing health professionals as early as possible to determine the best communication method for their child. Intervention should be introduced early, during the first few years of life, so that the child can take advantage of the unique window of time during which the brain is most receptive to learning language, whether spoken or signed. If a child is diagnosed with type 1 Usher syndrome early on, before he or she loses the ability to see, that child is more likely to benefit from the full spectrum of intervention strategies that can help him or her participate more fully in life's activities.

Because of the balance problems associated with type 1 Usher syndrome, children with this disorder are slow to sit without support and typically don't walk independently before they are eighteen months of age. These children usually begin to develop vision problems in early childhood, almost always by the time they reach ten years of age. Visual problems most often begin with difficulty seeing at night, but tend to progress rapidly until the individual is completely blind.

Type 2: Children with type 2 Usher syndrome are born with moderate to severe hearing loss and normal balance. Although the severity of hearing loss varies, most of these children can benefit from hearing aids and communicate orally. The visual problems in type 2 Usher syndrome tend to progress more slowly than those in type 1, with the onset of retinitis pigmentosa often not apparent until the teens.

Type 3: Children with type 3 Usher syndrome have normal hearing at birth. Although most children with the disorder have normal to near-normal balance, some may develop balance problems later on. Hearing and sight worsen over time, but the rate at which they decline can vary from person to person, even within the same family. A person with type 3 Usher syndrome may develop hearing loss by the teens, and he or she will usually require hearing aids by mid- to late adulthood. Night blindness usually begins sometime during puberty. Blind spots appear by the late teens to early adulthood, and, by mid-adulthood, the individual is usually legally blind.

Cause and Risks

What causes Usher syndrome?

Usher syndrome is inherited, which means that it is passed from parents to their children through genes. Genes are located in almost every cell of the body. Genes contain instructions that tell cells what to do. Each person inherits two copies of each gene, one from each parent. Sometimes genes are altered, or mutated. Mutated genes may cause cells to act differently than expected.

Table 36.1. Types of Usher Syndrome

	Type 1	**Type 2**	**Type 3**
Hearing	Profound deafness in both ears from birth	Moderate to severe hearing loss from birth	Normal at birth; progressive loss in childhood or early teens
Vision	Decreased night vision before age ten	Decreased night vision begins in late childhood or teens	Varies in severity; night vision problems often begin in teens
Vestibular function (balance)	Balance problems from birth	Normal	Normal to near-normal, chance of later problems

Usher syndrome is inherited as an autosomal recessive trait. The term autosomal means that the mutated gene is not located on either of the chromosomes that determine a person's sex; in other words, both males and females can have the disorder and can pass along the disorder to a child. The word *recessive* means that to have Usher syndrome, an individual must receive a mutated form of the Usher syndrome gene from each parent. If a child has a mutation in one Usher syndrome gene but the other gene is normal, he or she is predicted to have normal vision and hearing. Individuals with a mutation in a gene that can cause an autosomal recessive disorder are called carriers, because they "carry" the gene with a mutation but show no symptoms of the disorder. If both parents are carriers of a mutated gene for Usher syndrome, they will have a one-in-four chance of having a child with Usher syndrome with each birth.

Usually, parents who have normal hearing and vision do not know if they are carriers of an Usher syndrome gene mutation. Currently, it is not possible to determine whether an individual who does not have a family history of Usher syndrome is a carrier. National Institute on Deafness and Other Communication Disorders (NIDCD) scientists are hoping to change this, however, as they learn more about the genes responsible for Usher syndrome.

What are the risks of Usher syndrome?

Genetic disorders can be caused by a change(s) in a gene. Every individual has two copies of the same gene. Genetic disorders are inherited in different ways. Usher syndrome is a recessive disorder. Recessive means:

- a person must inherit a change in the same gene from each parent in order to have the disorder;

- a person with one changed gene does not have the disorder, but can pass either the changed or the unchanged gene on to his or her child.

An individual with Usher syndrome usually has inherited a change in the same gene from each parent.

An individual who has one changed Usher syndrome gene is called a carrier. When two carriers of the same Usher syndrome gene have a child together, with each birth there is a:

- 1 in 4 chance of having a child with Usher syndrome;

- 2 in 4 chance of having a child who is a carrier;

- 1 in 4 chance of having a child who neither has Usher syndrome nor is a carrier.

Who is affected by Usher syndrome?

Approximately 3 to 6 percent of all children who are deaf and another 3 to 6 percent of children who are hard of hearing have Usher syndrome. In developed countries such as the United States, about four babies in every one hundred thousand births have Usher syndrome.

Symptoms and Detection

What are Usher syndrome symptoms?

Usher syndrome has two major symptoms—hearing loss and an eye disorder called retinitis pigmentosa, or RP. Retinitis pigmentosa causes night blindness and a loss of peripheral vision (side vision) through the progressive degeneration of the retina. The retina is a light-sensitive tissue at the back of the eye and is crucial for vision. As retinitis pigmentosa progresses, the field of vision narrows, a condition known as "tunnel vision," until only central vision (the ability to see straight ahead) remains.

How is Usher syndrome diagnosed?

Because Usher syndrome affects hearing, balance, and vision, diagnosis of the disorder usually includes the evaluation of all three senses. Evaluation of the eyes may include a visual field test to measure a person's peripheral vision, an electroretinogram (ERG) to measure the electrical response of the eye's light-sensitive cells, and a retinal examination to observe the retina and other structures in the back of the eye. A hearing (audiologic) evaluation measures how loud sounds at a range of frequencies need to be before a person can hear them. An electronystagmogram (ENG) measures involuntary eye movements that could signify a balance problem. Early diagnosis of Usher syndrome is very important. The earlier that parents know if their child has Usher syndrome, the sooner that child can begin special educational training programs to manage the loss of hearing and vision.

Treatment

How is Usher syndrome treated?

Currently, there is no cure for Usher syndrome. The best treatment involves early identification so that educational programs can begin as soon as possible. The exact nature of these programs will depend on the severity of the hearing and vision loss as well as the age and abilities of the individual. Typically, treatment will include hearing aids, assistive listening devices, cochlear implants, or other communication methods such as American Sign Language; orientation and mobility training; and communication services and independent-living training that may include Braille instruction, low-vision services, or auditory training.

Some ophthalmologists believe that a high dose of vitamin A palmitate may slow, but not halt, the progression of retinitis pigmentosa. This belief stems from the results of a long-term clinical trial supported by the National Eye Institute and the Foundation for Fighting Blindness. Based on these findings, the researchers recommend that most adult patients with the common forms of RP take a daily supplement of 15,000 IU (international units) of vitamin A in the palmitate form under the supervision of their eye care professional. (Because people with type 1 Usher syndrome did not take part in the study, high-dose vitamin A is not recommended for these patients.) People who are considering taking vitamin A should discuss this treatment option with their healthcare provider before proceeding. Other guidelines regarding this treatment option include the following:

- Do not substitute vitamin A palmitate with a beta-carotene supplement.

- Avoid using supplements of more than 400 IU of vitamin E per day.

- Do not take vitamin A supplements greater than the recommended dose of 15,000 IU or modify your diet to select foods with high levels of vitamin A.

- Women who are considering pregnancy should stop taking the high-dose supplement of vitamin A three months before trying to conceive due to the increased risk of birth defects.

- Women who are pregnant should stop taking the high-dose supplement of vitamin A due to the increased risk of birth defects.

In addition, according to the same study, people with RP should avoid using supplements of more than 400 IU of vitamin E per day.

Current Research

What research is being done?

Researchers are currently trying to identify all of the genes that cause Usher syndrome and determine the function of those genes. This research will lead to improved genetic counseling and early diagnosis, and may eventually expand treatment options.

Scientists also are developing mouse models that have the same characteristics as the human types of Usher syndrome. Mouse models will make it easier to determine the function of the genes involved in Usher syndrome. Other areas of study include the early identification of children with Usher syndrome, treatment strategies such as the use of cochlear implants for hearing loss, and intervention strategies to help slow or stop the progression of retinitis pigmentosa.

NIDCD researchers, along with collaborators from universities in New York and Israel, pinpointed a mutation, named R245X, of the PCHD15 gene that accounts for a large percentage of type 1 Usher syndrome in today's Ashkenazi Jewish population. (The term Ashkenazi describes Jewish people who originate from Eastern Europe.) Based on this finding, the researchers conclude that Ashkenazi Jewish infants with bilateral, profound hearing loss who lack another known mutation that causes hearing loss should be screened for the R245X mutation.

Is genetic testing for Usher syndrome available?

So far, eleven genetic loci (a segment of chromosome on which a certain gene is located) have been found to cause Usher syndrome, and nine genes have been pinpointed that cause the disorder. They are as follows:

- **Type 1 Usher syndrome:** MYO7A, USH1C, CDH23, PCHD15, SANS

- **Type 2 Usher syndrome:** USH2A, VLGR1, WHRN

- **Type 3 Usher syndrome:** USH3A

With so many possible genes involved in Usher syndrome, genetic tests for the disorder are not conducted on a widespread basis. Diagnosis of Usher syndrome is usually performed through hearing, balance, and vision tests. Genetic testing for a few of the identified genes is clinically available. Genetic testing for additional Usher syndrome genes may be available through clinical research studies.

What are some of the latest research findings?

NIDCD researchers, along with collaborators from universities in New York and Israel, pinpointed a mutation, named R245X, of the PCHD15 gene that accounts for a large percentage of type 1 Usher syndrome in today's Ashkenazi Jewish population. (The term Ashkenazi describes Jewish people who originate from Eastern Europe.) Based on this finding, the researchers conclude that Ashkenazi Jewish infants with bilateral, profound hearing loss who lack another known mutation that causes hearing loss should be screened for the R245X mutation.

Chapter 37

Other Congenital Disorders Affecting Vision

Chapter Contents

Section 37.1

Aniridia

What is aniridia?

Simply put, aniridia is a genetic condition where there is little or no iris.

Are people with aniridia blind?

No. Their vision may vary from 20/40 to 20/400. People with aniridia may be "legally blind," which is defined as vision that is not correctable to better than 20/200. However, this is quite different from total blindness. With 20/200 vision, one can still see colors, lights, and the outline of large objects.

What can aniridics see?

It is difficult to say. Because the range of vision is different for each aniridic, there is not one good description to explain what all aniridics can see. All aniridics will have challenges with seeing detail, due to the underdeveloped retina (foveal hypoplasia). Most pediatric ophthalmologists will tell parents of an aniridic child, "we will have to wait until he/she can tell us what he/she can see." This can be very scary and frustrating. An aniridic child's sight can develop and get better over time.

Will their vision get worse over time?

It can. The nondegenerative parts of this condition are the lack of iris (it will never grow) and the foveal hypoplasia (the underdeveloped retina). These conditions will not worsen with time (other than the "normal" changes that occur with age and are correctable with glasses).

However, the impact of the secondary conditions such as glaucoma, corneal pannus, and cataracts can worsen one's sight.

What causes the irregular eye movements?

This is a condition called nystagmus. The involuntary eye movements may be from side to side, up and down, or rotary. Nystagmus is present to varying degrees in people with aniridia and typically declines with age. It tends to increase when the person is upset, excited, or tired.

Does nystagmus affect vision?

Although people with nystagmus are not aware that their eyes are moving, it does make it more difficult for them to focus clearly on details. In fact, they often will find a "null point" which is the point where their nystagmus is the least apparent (see below).

What is the "null point"?

People with aniridia have a poorly developed fovea. In normal-sighted people, the fovea is in the center of the macula and an image will land there when the person is looking straight ahead. Their fovea is where they focus for their best detail vision—such as seeing a freckle on a person's face. Because a person with aniridia has an underdeveloped fovea, they must find their best area of focus which may be anywhere on their retina. Typically, they will move their head to the position necessary to focus on this spot, consequently slowing their nystagmus and allowing for their best vision. This is their null point.

Is any of this correctable?

With the technology that is currently available, there are many treatment options for the secondary eye complications. First, there are instruments to measure eye pressure to keep glaucoma under control. If glaucoma is diagnosed, there are eye drops and/or surgeries to correct it. Also, there are surgical remedies for the corneal pannus such as stem cell transplants. Additionally, there are iris implants available (in all colors) to help decrease the amount of light that flows into the eye. However, this is not yet U.S. Food and Drug Association (FDA) approved.

How does someone get aniridia?

Aniridia is a genetic condition caused by an anomaly in the 11p13 section of the PAX6 gene. The genetic problem can be sporadic (happens first time within either the egg or sperm) or familial (passed on from one parent). Unlike most genetic conditions, this is autosomal dominant, meaning it takes only one mutated gene to cause this condition. Aniridia is not contagious. There is a 50 percent chance of an aniridic passing it on to one's offspring.

How can two people without aniridia produce a child with aniridia?

Both parents of an aniridic can be "normal," having *no* genetic mutation or deletion of the PAX 6 gene. If these two people have an aniridic child, the aniridia is called "sporadic." The child obtained this genetic mutation or deletion from a spontaneous change in the egg or sperm. The condition existed *before* conception. So, there was *nothing* done during the pregnancy that caused this problem. If these two parents should have another child, the chance of aniridia occurring in the next pregnancy is the same chance as any one else in the general population—very slim.

If an aniridic has a child, what are the chances of that newborn child having aniridia?

Unlike most genetic conditions, aniridia is dominant. It only takes one parent to have the mutation or deletion to pass on this condition. Therefore, the chance of an aniridic man or aniridic woman having an aniridic child is fifty (50) percent. If an aniridic should have a child with aniridia, the condition is called "familial" aniridia, because it was passed on by an aniridic parent. Currently, there is the possibility of identifying the mutation or deletion in the PAX 6 gene and using egg or sperm sorting to try to stop the aniridia from being passed on. This technology is very new and not much is known about its success rate.

How is aniridia diagnosed?

Aniridia can be diagnosed by an experienced ophthalmologist with a simple eye exam. There are genetic tests available as well but they are not yet perfected. For more information on genetic testing, contact a qualified genetic counselor. Genetic counselors are generally affiliated with universities and/or children's hospitals. Since aniridia is also associated with glaucoma, it is important that the ophthalmologist check an infant's eye pressure.

What is foveal hypoplasia?

The fovea is the part of the retina in the center of the macula where one would normally focus for the sharpest, most detailed vision. In people with aniridia, this area is poorly formed or, in some cases, not present. This is known as foveal hypoplasia.

Is aniridia associated with mental retardation?

In most cases, aniridia is caused by a mutation in the PAX6 gene, and is not associated with mental retardation. However, in about 30 percent of cases, sporadic (noninherited) aniridia is caused by a missing or deleted PAX6 gene, rather than a mutation. In these cases, deletion of other genes in the same area results in WAGR syndrome (WAGR is an acronym for: Wilms tumor, aniridia, genitourinary abnormalities, and mental retardation). Although mental retardation is common in individuals with WAGR syndrome, neither mental retardation nor any of the other conditions is always present. For this reason, genetic testing is recommended for all infants born with sporadic aniridia.

Should aniridics have ultrasounds to test for Wilms tumors?

Most pediatricians recommend that aniridic children with a deleted PAX 6 be tested for Wilms tumors every three months, as the possibility is high if there is a deletion. There is debate as to whether children with only a mutated PAX 6 gene undergo ultrasounds. Many pediatricians believe that this noninvasive ultrasound is a safeguard for catching tumors early. Early detection is *key* in fighting these cancerous tumors. Therefore, the consensus is that "it can't hurt" to get the ultrasounds. As to how often, the safest procedure is to have the ultrasound every three months until the child is eight years of age, when the probability of the Wilms tumors decreases significantly. At that time, the monitoring is decreased to every six months or even annually. There has been a case of Wilms tumors being detected in a twenty-four-year-old aniridic patient, so the annual monitoring is a good idea.

Do people with aniridia have to go to special schools?

No. Most children with aniridia function well in a mainstream classroom, with proper accommodations.

Can people with aniridia read books?

Yes! Although Braille is typically not necessary for people with aniridia, a few may learn to use it in order to give their eyes a rest. Depending on the degree of visual impairment, other accommodations may be necessary. These include large-print books, a closed-circuit television (CCTV), magnifiers, and high-contrast materials.

Do people with aniridia spend a lot of time going to doctors?

Yes! It is very important for aniridia patients to closely monitor each eye and to see the correct specialist for each problem (glaucoma ophthalmologists, cornea ophthalmologists, pediatric ophthalmologists, etc).

How does the sun affect the eyes of people with aniridia?

Most people with aniridia are sensitive to light. Imagine a "normal" person with their eyes dilated at an eye doctor appointment. This is how the eye of an aniridic is at all times. Therefore, it is very important for them to wear sunglasses: (a) for comfort; and (b) to protect the retina. One of the purposes of the iris is to protect the retina from too much sun. The retina can be damaged from too much sun exposure if the aniridic does not wear sunglasses.

Can people with aniridia go outside?

Absolutely. With proper sunglasses, they can go anywhere, including the beach!

Are there other medical problems associated with aniridia?

Yes. Recent research indicates that other medical problems may be associated with aniridia (all types). These include: glucose intolerance (thought to be a precursor to diabetes in some individuals), central auditory processing disorder (difficulty with discriminating and interpreting sounds), decreased or absent sense of smell, and subtle abnormalities in the structure of the brain, such as decreased size or absence of the anterior commissure and/or the pineal gland. When aniridia occurs as part of WAGR syndrome, there may be medical problems in addition to those listed above.

Can people with aniridia drive a car?

Sometimes. The requirements vary by country and by state. They may be required to wear a bioptic device to drive.

Section 37.2

Anophthalmia and Microphthalmia

"Facts about Anophthalmia and Microphthalmia," National Eye
Institute, National Institutes of Health, August 2009.

Anophthalmia and Microphthalmia Defined

What are anophthalmia and microphthalmia?

Anophthalmia and microphthalmia are often used interchangeably.
Microphthalmia is a disorder in which one or both eyes are abnormally
small, while anophthalmia is the absence of one or both eyes. These
rare disorders develop during pregnancy and can be associated with
other birth defects.

Causes and Risk Factors

What causes anophthalmia and microphthalmia?

Causes of these conditions may include genetic mutations and
abnormal chromosomes. Researchers also believe that environmental factors, such as exposure to x-rays, chemicals, drugs, pesticides,
toxins, radiation, or viruses, increase the risk of anophthalmia and
microphthalmia, but research is not conclusive. Sometimes the cause
in an individual patient cannot be determined.

Treatment

Can anophthalmia and microphthalmia be treated?

There is no treatment for severe anophthalmia or microphthalmia that will create a new eye or restore vision. However, some less
severe forms of microphthalmia may benefit from medical or surgical
treatments. In almost all cases improvements to a child's appearance
are possible. Children can be fitted for a prosthetic (artificial) eye for
cosmetic purposes and to promote socket growth. A newborn with
anophthalmia or microphthalmia will need to visit several eye care

497

professionals, including those who specialize in pediatrics, vitreoretinal disease, orbital and oculoplastic surgery, ophthalmic genetics, and prosthetic devices for the eye. Each specialist can provide information and possible treatments resulting in the best care for the child and family. The specialist in prosthetic devices for the eye will make conformers, plastic structures that help support the face and encourage the eye socket to grow. As the face develops, new conformers will need to be made. A child with anophthalmia may also need to use expanders in addition to conformers to further enlarge the eye socket. Once the face is fully developed, prosthetic eyes can be made and placed. Prosthetic eyes will not restore vision.

How do conformers and prosthetic eyes look?

A painted prosthesis that looks like a normal eye is usually fitted between ages one and two. Until then, clear conformers are used. When the conformers are in place the eye socket will look black. These conformers are not painted to look like a normal eye because they are changed too frequently. Every few weeks a child will progress to a larger size conformer until about two years of age. If a child needs to wear conformers after age two, the conformers will be painted like a regular prosthesis, giving the appearance of a normal but smaller eye. The average child will need three to four new painted prostheses before the age of ten.

How is microphthalmia managed if there is residual vision in the eye?

Children with microphthalmia may have some residual vision (limited sight). In these cases, the good eye can be patched to strengthen vision in the microphthalmic eye. A prosthesis can be made to cap the microphthalmic eye to help with cosmetic appearance, while preserving the remaining sight.

Section 37.3

Color Blindness

Color vision deficiency, also called color blindness, affects 8 percent of boys and 0.5 percent of girls, or about one in twenty-five children. An affected child sees colors differently than most of his or her classmates or family members. Depending upon the type of color vision deficiency, a child's view may vary subtly or dramatically.

A child with color vision deficiency may have difficulties when his or her perceptions clash with normal color perceptions. No medical treatment can cure the color vision deficiency, but greater awareness of the condition can minimize any difficulties.

Possible Signs of Color Vision Deficiency

A child with a color vision deficiency might:

- give alternate names to colors, particularly nonprimary shades.
- draw with an alternate color scheme. The drawings might include green skin or hair, black tree trunks, or brown grass.
- call things white that others call light pink or light green.
- describe as similar some shades of reddish and greenish colors (i.e., peach and light green, or evergreen and cranberry).

In most cases, a child with color vision deficiency has a maternal grandfather with the condition.

For a definitive diagnosis, see your eye care professional.

Testing

Some states and/ or school districts require color vision screening; your child may undergo testing at school, often in kindergarten. School screenings alert parents and teachers that there may be a color perception issue, yet do not replace an examination by an eye care professional.

Your doctor will administer a color vision test by having the child view a set of diagrams called plates. Most plates have a number, letter, or symbol hidden in a circle of dots. The most common test is the Ishihara, though there are many others. After a child views and responds to a set of plates, the doctor will diagnose the particular type of color vision deficiency.

Parents with normal color vision may be startled by watching their child take a test. Symbols that appear obvious to the parents may be undetectable to their child. Parents should remember that the carefully calibrated plates do not reproduce the everyday world.

Many online tests reproduce the Ishihara or other color vision tests. While these tests may be informative and convenient, they are not diagnostic tools.

Causes

Color vision deficiency runs in families, and is carried on the X chromosome. Males are XY, and females are XX.

A boy with color vision deficiency inherited the affected X from his mother, who inherited it from her father, the boy's grandfather. A woman who carries the gene usually has normal color vision. When she has children, she passes on either her affected X or her normal X chromosome. Her boys each have a 50 percent chance of inheriting the affected X, so each has a 50 percent chance of having color vision deficiency. Since the Y from the boys' father does not alter the inheritance, boys have color vision deficiency in far greater numbers than girls.

A girl with color vision deficiency has two affected X chromosomes, and so has both a father with a deficiency and a mother who is a carrier (or also has a deficiency). Many girls carry one affected X and have normal color vision. If a woman with color vision deficiency has children, all of her boys will have the condition.

The altered gene on the X chromosome affects the cones in the back of the retina. The millions of cones detect light and color and enable our vision.

People with normal color vision have trichromatic vision, with three types of cones sensitive to different wavelengths of light. People with mild color vision deficiencies have three types of cones with the sensitivity of one cone set shifted from the normal. Those with more significant color vision deficiencies lack one cone set. People with dichromatic (two-cone) vision see far fewer hues than people with trichromatic (three-cone) vision.

Types

Most people with color vision deficiency (95 percent) have a red-green type. Only 5 percent of people with color vision deficiency have a blue-yellow type. Both the red-green and the blue-yellow types have subtypes, depending upon how the cones are affected.

Most people identified as color blind are actually only partially color blind. Total color blindness, called achromatopsia, is an extremely rare disorder with additional vision impairments.

Treatment and Coping Strategies

Color vision deficiency is not curable or treatable. No glasses, contact lenses, medication, or instruction will alter how affected individuals see colors. The best treatment is awareness.

Since children cannot change how they see, the adults around them should make adjustments. The following strategies may be useful for parents:

- Explain to the child and his or her siblings that he or she sees colors differently than most people.

- In most cases, accept the color names the child chooses. Only he knows what he sees.

- When you ask the child to retrieve something, use attributes other than color; have her get the shirt with wide stripes or the fuzzy pillow.

- If it is helpful to the child and siblings, adopt a color-relative vocabulary in your household. "It's blue to me, but it might be purple to him."

- Be sensitive about wardrobe color choices. Your child's idea of matching is different than yours.

- Discuss the condition with the child's teachers and coaches.

- When the child considers future occupations, explain that some professions have color vision requirements. Assist the child with research into potential occupations when he or she is in middle and high school.

- Parents should realize that most people with color vision deficiency do not view it as a handicap or limitation, but rather as an individual characteristic.

School and Color Vision Deficiency

Inform your child's teachers about the color vision deficiency. Your child may color a different way and may have difficulty with certain tasks. Putting toys away by color, distinguishing colors on maps, or reading certain colors of lettering could be problematic. The child cannot change how he or she perceives color; more time or further instruction will not overcome the problem. Teachers and parents should modify assigned tasks so that the child can succeed.

Teachers should be prepared to deal with any negative peer reaction to the child's work. A simple explanation to the children that not everyone sees things the same way and an example of acceptance should alleviate any teasing.

Disadvantages and an Advantage

The most obvious limitation for people with color vision deficiency is reduced occupational choice. Operators of public or commercial transportation must have normal color vision, as must police officers, firefighters, and most pilots. Some occupations do not have formal requirements but the nature of the work may put people with color vision deficiency at a disadvantage. Before pursuing a career as a designer, geologist, chemist, printer, or another profession where distinguishing colors is important, young people with color vision deficiency and their parents should research the occupation.

Traffic lights generally look different to people with color vision deficiency. Most drivers with the condition rely on the position of the lights and rarely have problems.

There may be an advantage to having color vision deficiency. Because of their practice at detecting subtle differences in shading, affected individuals may be able to detect camouflage more easily than people with normal color vision. An animal surrounded by vegetation or a camouflage net might be in plain view to their practiced eyes.

Section 37.4

Down Syndrome

Excerpted from "Vision and Down Syndrome," © 2011 National Down Syndrome Society. Reprinted with permission. To view this document and other information, including a resource list, visit www.ndsss.org.

Trisomy 21 has effects on the developing eye, which could impact the proper development of vision. Eye disease is reported in over half of patients with Down syndrome, from less severe problems such as tear duct abnormalities to vision-threatening diagnoses, such as early-age cataracts. Particular attention should be given to vision in people with Down syndrome.

The National Down Syndrome Society (NDSS) interviews Danielle Ledoux, MD assistant in ophthalmology at Children's Hospital, Boston, and instructor in ophthalmology at Harvard Medical School.

What is different about the eyes in Down syndrome?

As any family member of a person with Down syndrome knows, there are characteristic features about the eyes. This includes upward slanting of the eyelids, prominent folds of skin between the eye and the nose, and small white spots present on the iris (the colored part of the eye) called Brushfield spots. These spots are harmless, and can be seen in people without Down syndrome as well.

Do most children with Down syndrome need glasses?

Refractive error (the need for glasses) is much more common in children with Down syndrome than in the general population. This refractive error can be hyperopia (farsightedness), astigmatism, or myopia (nearsightedness). Another problem is weak accommodation (difficulty changing the focusing power of the eye from distance to near). We can test this easily in the office, and if detected, we will prescribe glasses that have bifocals. Some of my patients have difficulty adjusting to glasses, but once they get accustomed to having the glasses on their face, their vision is significantly better and often their eye alignment improves as well.

503

What are common, but less serious, eye abnormalities affecting Down syndrome patients?

In addition to the need for eyeglasses, many children with Down syndrome have tear duct abnormalities. Family members will notice this as frequent discharge and tearing from the eyes, worsened by colds. We generally recommend firm massage over the space between the eye and the nose (tear sac region) two to three times a day to attempt to open the tear duct. If this continues beyond a year of age, the tear ducts may need to be opened by a surgical procedure. Strabismus (eye misalignment) is also more common. Family members may notice that the eyes do not line up well with each other, but often the strabismus can be subtle, even to the pediatrician. The folds of skin I mentioned between the eyes and the nose can also cover up the underlying strabismus, or make the eyes appear as if they are crossing even if they are not. It is important to diagnose strabismus as a child, as crossed eyes can result in amblyopia (loss of vision also known as lazy eye) and loss of stereopsis (the use of the two eyes together, or depth perception).

How can the strabismus be treated?

Sometimes, simply glasses alone are enough to straighten eyes with strabismus. If glasses are needed, we always start there. If the eyes continue to have strabismus despite the correct pair of eyeglasses, then we recommend strabismus surgery (eye muscle surgery). This is a one- to two-hour procedure, which can often be done as an outpatient unless there are other reasons the person would need to be admitted, such as a serious heart condition. Unfortunately, our patients with Down syndrome are more likely to require more than one surgery to align their eyes, as they don't always respond as predictably to strabismus surgery as the general population with strabismus would.

What are the more severe eye problems that might develop?

My greatest concern is congenital cataracts (lack of clearness to the lens of the eye). If visually significant cataracts are present early in a child's eye, then a clear image is not delivered to the brain and therefore the brain can never "learn" to see. This is a severe form of amblyopia known as deprivational amblyopia. While we can take our time removing a cataract in an adult patient, significant cataracts present very early in a child's life that are not removed can result in lifelong poor vision. In that situation, even if the cataract is removed when the child is older, the vision never improves significantly. This is what makes early detection of cataracts in infants and children so important. A child with Down syndrome will be evaluated by the pediatrician at birth, and referred to an ophthalmologist if something abnormal is detected. There is also a unique form of cataract in Down syndrome patients that we have found in our research. However, depending on how developmentally delayed the person is, they may not be able to communicate that they can't see. For this reason, I recommend any patient with Down syndrome, no matter what age, have a complete eye examination if they are starting to show reduced cognitive function, or changes in their normal activities.

Are there other eye conditions in Down syndrome that can cause loss of eyesight?

I mentioned amblyopia (commonly called "lazy eye," which is decreased vision), which can be caused by multiple different eye problems such as strabismus, severe ptosis (eyelid droop), cataracts, or even uncorrected refractive error, especially if one eye needs a much stronger eyeglass prescription than the other. Ptosis is usually easier to appreciate but strabismus and significant refractive error can be very difficult for the pediatrician to diagnose. There are other more rare problems which can occur with the optic nerve or retina of the eye which can sometimes cause vision loss and unfortunately are generally not treatable. Nystagmus (a rhythmic shaking of the eyes) can also occur.

What is the recommended eye care for children with Down syndrome?

The American Academy of Pediatrics (AAP) and the United States Down Syndrome Medical Interest Group (DSMIG) recommend evaluation of the red reflex of the eyes at birth to look for cataracts, as well as to assess the eyes for strabismus or nystagmus. The red reflex is essentially the "red eye" seen in photography, which is the normal reflex of the retina when struck by direct light. If the eyes don't look normal, then the infant will be referred to a pediatric ophthalmologist—a physician who has completed specialty training in medical and surgical management of the child's eye. We, along with the AAP and the DSMIG, recommend a child with Down syndrome has their first eye exam by an ophthalmologist experienced in patients with special disabilities (for example, a pediatric ophthalmologist) by six months of age. After that, children with Down syndrome, even if they are without symptoms, should see an ophthalmologist every one to two years. If any eye problems are detected, they will be followed more frequently.

What sort of symptoms might we see if a child has an eye problem?

Unfortunately, children with Down syndrome often do not complain about their eye problems, either because they don't notice the problem or because they can't communicate the problem well enough. Signs to look for include squinting or closing one eye shut, an unusual head tilt, crossing or wandering of one or both eyes, or light sensitivity. In some severe cases, the sign of vision problems may be a regression in overall function or loss of developmental milestones. Ptosis will be seen as a lid droop, and a blocked tear duct will result in daily tearing and discharge.

Any thoughts for parents of a child with Down syndrome who are concerned about the eye or vision?

Getting regular eye exams is very important in children with Down syndrome because eye disorders are so common and are difficult for the pediatrician to diagnose. Because the examination can be difficult for both the child and the doctor, it is best to have the examination done by an ophthalmologist skilled in dealing with children with developmental delays. Don't be surprised to find out your child needs glasses; if needed, the glasses will help the vision, and possibly the eye alignment, as well as help in the development of normal vision pathways in the brain. This will help with your child's learning and functioning. Our research is looking at just how common eye problems are in Down syndrome, as well as the development of cataracts in these patients.

Section 37.5

Duane Syndrome

"Learning about Duane Syndrome," National Human
Genome Research Institute, June 28, 2010.

What is Duane syndrome?

Duane syndrome (DS) is a rare, congenital (present from birth) eye movement disorder. Most patients are diagnosed by the age of ten years and DS is more common in girls (60 percent of the cases) than boys (40 percent of the cases).

DS is a miswiring of the eye muscles, causing some eye muscles to contract when they shouldn't and other eye muscles not to contract when they should. People with DS have a limited (and sometimes absent) ability to move the eye outward toward the ear (abduction) and, in most cases, a limited ability to move the eye inward toward the nose (adduction).

Often, when the eye moves toward the nose, the eyeball also pulls into the socket (retraction), the eye opening narrows, and, in some cases, the eye will move upward or downward. Many patients with DS develop a face turn to maintain binocular vision and compensate for improper turning of the eyes.

In about 80 percent of cases of DS, only one eye is affected, most often the left. However, in some cases, both eyes are affected, with one eye usually more affected than the other.

Other names for this condition include: Duane retraction syndrome (or DR syndrome), eye retraction syndrome, retraction syndrome, congenital retraction syndrome, and Stilling-Turk-Duane syndrome.

In 70 percent of DS cases, this is the only disorder the individual has. However, other conditions and syndromes have been found in association with DS. These include malformation of the skeleton, ears, eyes, kidneys, and nervous system, as well as the following:

- Okihiro syndrome, an association of DS with forearm malformation and hearing loss

- Wildervanck syndrome, fusion of neck vertebrae and hearing loss

- Holt-Oram syndrome, abnormalities of the upper limbs and heart

- Morning glory syndrome, abnormalities of the optic disc or "blind spot,"

- Goldenhar syndrome, malformation of the jaw, cheek, and ear, usually on one side of the face

What are the symptoms of Duane syndrome?

Clinically, Duane syndrome is often subdivided into three types, each with associated symptoms:

- **Type 1:** The affected eye, or eyes, has limited ability to move outward toward the ear, but the ability to move inward toward the nose is normal or nearly so. The eye opening narrows and the eyeball pulls in when looking inward toward the nose, however the reverse occurs when looking outward toward the ear. About 78 percent of all DS cases are Type 1.

- **Type 2:** The affected eye, or eyes, has limited ability to move inward toward the nose, but the ability to move outward toward the ear is normal or nearly so. The eye opening narrows and the eyeball pulls in when looking inward toward the nose. About 7 percent of all DS cases are Type 2.

- **Type 3:** The affected eye, or eyes, has limited ability to move both inward toward the nose and outward toward the ears. The eye opening narrows and the eyeball pulls in when looking inward toward the nose. About 15 percent of all DS cases are Type 3.

Each of these three types can be further classified into three subgroups, depending on where the eyes are when the individual looks straight (the primary gaze):

- **Subgroup A:** The affected eye is turned inward toward the nose (esotropia).

- **Subgroup B:** The affected eye is turned outward toward the ear (exotropia).

- **Subgroup C:** The eyes are in a straight, primary position.

What causes Duane syndrome?

Common thought is that Duane syndrome (DS) is a miswiring of the medial and the lateral rectus muscles, the muscles that move the eyes. Also, patients with DS lack the abducens nerve, the sixth cranial nerve, which is involved in eye movement. However, the etiology or origin of these malfunctions is, at present, a mystery.

Many researchers believe that DS results from a disturbance—either by genetic or environmental factors—during embryonic development. Since the cranial nerves and ocular muscles are developing between the third and eighth week of pregnancy, this is most likely when the disturbance happens.

Presently, it appears that several factors may be involved in causing DS. Therefore it is doubtful that a single mechanism is responsible for this condition.

How is Duane syndrome diagnosed?

The diagnosis of Duane syndrome is based on clinical findings. Mutations in the CHN1 gene are associated with familial isolated Duane syndrome. Direct sequencing of the CHN1 gene is available as a clinical test, and has to date detected missense mutations in seven patients and affected family members. The CHN1 mutations have not been found to be a common cause of simplex Duane retraction syndrome.

What do we know about heredity and Duane syndrome?

Most likely, both genetic and environmental factors play a role in the development of Duane syndrome (DS). For those cases that show evidence of having a genetic cause, both dominant and recessive forms of DS have been found. (When a gene is dominant, only one gene from one parent is needed for the individual to express it physically. However, when a gene is recessive, a copy of the gene from both parents is needed for expression.)

The chromosomal location of the proposed gene for this syndrome is currently unknown. Some research shows that more than one gene may be involved. There is evidence that a gene involved in the development of DS is located on chromosome 2. Also, deletions of chromosomal material from chromosomes 4 and 8, as well as the presence of an extra marker chromosome thought to be derived from chromosome 22, have been linked to DS.

Section 37.6

WAGR Syndrome

Excerpted from "Learning about WAGR Syndrome," National
Human Genome Research Institute, November 3, 2010.

What is WAGR syndrome?

WAGR syndrome is a rare genetic condition that can affect both
boys and girls. Babies born with WAGR syndrome often have eye problems, and are at high risk for developing certain types of cancer, and
mental retardation. The term "WAGR" stands for the first letters of the
physical and mental problems associated with the condition:

- (W)ilms tumor, the most common form of kidney cancer in children

- (A)niridia, some or complete absence of the colored part of the
  eye, called the iris (singular), or irises/irides (plural)

- (G)enitourinary problems, such as testicles that are not descended
  or hypospadias (abnormal location of the opening for urination) in
  boys, or genital or urinary problems inside the body in girls

- Mental (R)etardation

Most people who have WAGR syndrome have two or more of these
conditions. Also, people can have WAGR syndrome, but not have all of
the above conditions.

Other names for WAGR syndrome that are used are:

- WAGR complex

- Wilms tumor-aniridia-genitourinary anomalies-mental retardation syndrome

- Wilms tumor-aniridia-gonadoblastoma-mental retardation syndrome

- Chromosome 11p deletion syndrome

- 11p deletion syndrome

The cause of WAGR syndrome is deletion of a group of genes located on chromosome number 11 (11p13 - the "p13" refers to the specific place on chromosome 11 that is affected). Chromosomes are packages of genetic characteristics. There are twenty-two pairs of chromosomes that are the same in males and females. The twenty-third pair determines a person's sex, with males having an X and a Y chromosome and females having two X chromosomes.

What are the symptoms of WAGR syndrome?

WAGR is called a genetic syndrome. The symptoms of WAGR syndrome are usually seen after the baby is born. The mother's pregnancy and the baby's birth history are not unusual. Enlargement of the baby's kidneys may be seen on a prenatal ultrasound. The eye problems (aniridia) are usually noticed in the newborn period, and for infant boys, the problems with the genitals and urinary systems are also usually obvious in the newborn period.

Individuals born with WAGR syndrome are at higher risk for developing other problems during infancy, childhood, and adulthood. These problems can affect the kidneys, eyes, testes, or ovaries. The specific symptoms that happen in a person who has WAGR syndrome depend on the combination of disorders that are present.

Wilms tumor: About one half of individuals who have WAGR syndrome develop a type of kidney cancer called Wilms tumor. In the early stages of Wilms tumor there are usually no symptoms. The first signs of this cancer may be blood in the urine, a low-grade fever, loss of appetite, weight loss, lack of energy, or swelling of the abdomen.

Aniridia: In infants who are born with aniridia that is associated with WAGR syndrome, the irises of the eyes fail to develop normally before birth. This causes partial or complete absence of the round colored part of the eye (iris). Aniridia is almost always present in babies born with WAGR syndrome. Other eye problems are often present or can develop as the child grows older. These include: clouding of the lens of the eye (cataract); rapid, involuntary movements of the eye (nystagmus); and all or partial loss of vision due to high pressure of the fluid in the eye (glaucoma).

Genital and urinary (GU) problems: A range of GU problems may be present in a baby born with WAGR syndrome. For boys, these may involve the urinary tract opening somewhere along the shaft of the penis rather than at the tip (hypospadias) or undescended testes (cryptorchism). In girls, these problems may include underdeveloped (streak) ovaries, and malformations of the uterus, fallopian tubes, or vagina. In some people with WAGR syndrome, problems with the development of the genitals may make their sexual assignment at birth (male or female) uncertain. Individuals with WAGR syndrome may have a higher risk for a type of cancer called gonadoblastoma, a cancer of the cells that form the testes in males and the ovaries in females.

Mental retardation: Mental retardation and developmental delay are common in children with WAGR syndrome. The severity of mental retardation varies from person to person, ranging from severe to mild mental retardation. Some children who have WAGR syndrome may have normal intelligence.

Other symptoms of WAGR syndrome may also include the following:

- Developmental, behavioral, and/or psychiatric disorders including autism, attention deficit disorder, obsessive compulsive disorder, anxiety disorders, and depression

- Early-onset overweight (obesity) and high blood cholesterol levels

- Excessive food intake (polyphagia/hyperphagia)

- Chronic kidney failure, most often after age twelve years

- Breathing problems, asthma, and pneumonia, and breathing problems during sleep (sleep apnea)

- Frequent infections of the ears, nose, and throat, especially during infancy and early childhood

- Teeth problems—crowded or uneven teeth

- Problems with muscle tone and strength, especially during infancy and childhood

- Seizure disorder (epilepsy)

- Inflammation of the pancreas (pancreatitis)

How is WAGR syndrome diagnosed?

Symptoms that suggest WAGR syndrome, like aniridia, are usually noted shortly after birth, and genetic testing for the 11p13 deletion is done. A genetic test called a chromosome analysis or karyotype is done to look for the deleted area (11p13) on chromosome number 11. A more specific genetic test called FISH (fluorescent in situ hybridization) is sometimes done to look for the deletion of specific genes on chromosome number 11.

How is WAGR syndrome treated?

Treatment of WAGR syndrome is aimed at the specific symptoms present in the individual. Monitoring to look for problems is also important to catch problems early so that treatment can be given as soon as possible.

Wilms tumor: Wilms tumor happens in about half of children with WAGR syndrome. The tumor usually develops between the ages of one and three years. Most cases of Wilms tumor have been detected by age eight years, but in rare cases may occur later. Babies who are suspected to have WAGR syndrome should have ultrasounds of their abdomen at birth. They then need to have abdominal ultrasounds every three months until they reach age eight years. Feeling the abdomen for signs of swelling and masses can be done by both the baby's doctor and the parents, when they are taught how to do this. After age eight years, watching for signs of Wilms tumor may be done by ultrasound and/or by watching for symptoms such as a low-grade fever, loss of appetite, weight loss, lack of energy, or swelling of the abdomen.

Wilms tumor can often be treated successfully. The overall survival rate of patients with Wilms tumor is excellent and is related to the features of the tumor and the stage of the disease. Treatment may include surgery to remove the kidney, radiation therapy, and chemotherapy.

Aniridia: The treatment of aniridia is aimed at keeping the person's vision. Drugs or surgery may help when there is glaucoma or cataracts. Contact lenses can harm the cornea and should be avoided.

Genital and urinary problems: Children with WAGR syndrome should have regular evaluations to detect abnormal development of their ovaries or testes. Surgery may be needed to remove abnormal gonads or to prevent cancer of the gonads (gonadoblastoma). When both gonads are removed, the individual is given hormone replacement treatment. Surgery may also be done when a boy with WAGR syndrome has undescended testes. When girls with WAGR syndrome have abnormal ovaries, they have routine pelvic ultrasounds or MRI's (magnetic resonance imaging) to watch for the development of gonadoblastoma.

Mental Retardation/developmental delays: Individuals with WAGR syndrome may have mental retardation ranging from severe to mild. Some individuals with WAGR syndrome have normal intelligence.

Children with WAGR syndrome should be referred for early intervention services soon after they are born, or when the diagnosis is made. Treatments include vision therapy and physical, occupational, and speech therapies. Special education services are also used to help children with WAGR syndrome develop to their fullest ability.

Kidney (renal) failure: The renal failure that can happen in WAGR syndrome often causes the person to have high blood pressure, high cholesterol, and leakage of protein from the blood into the urine (called proteinuria). All individuals with WAGR syndrome should be routinely screened for high blood pressure and urinary protein. These problems are treated with medications called "angiotensin-converting enzyme (ACE) inhibitors" or "angiotensin receptor blockers (ARBs)." Some people with WAGR syndrome and renal failure are treated with dialysis or kidney transplant.

Is WAGR syndrome inherited?

WAGR syndrome is called a "contiguous gene deletion syndrome." This means that it is caused by the loss of a section of genes on chromosome 11 (11p13). Most of the time the changes on chromosome 11p13 happen by chance when the egg or sperm are being formed or during the very early stages of the baby's development in the womb. More rarely, the gene changes are inherited because one of the parents carries a rearrangement (called a translocation) between two chromosomes that can cause the loss of some genes when he or she has a baby. A baby can also have a mixture of normal cells and cells that have the 11p13 changes in his or her body. This is called mosaic WAGR syndrome.

Genetic counseling is helpful for determining whether there may be an increased risk of having another child with WAGR syndrome.

Chapter 38

Infectious Diseases Affecting Vision

Chapter Contents

Section 38.1

Acanthamoeba

"Acanthamoeba Keratitis FAQs," U.S. Centers for Disease
Control and Prevention, November 2, 2010.

What is Acanthamoeba keratitis?

Acanthamoeba keratitis is a rare but serious infection of the eye
that can result in permanent visual impairment or blindness. This
infection is caused by a microscopic, free-living ameba (single-celled
living organism) called *Acanthamoeba. Acanthamoeba* causes Acanthamoeba keratitis when it infects the transparent outer covering of
the eye called the cornea. *Acanthamoeba* amebas are very common in
nature and can be found in bodies of water (for example, lakes and
oceans), soil, and air.

What are the symptoms of infection?

The symptoms of Acanthamoeba keratitis can be very similar to the
symptoms of other eye infections. These symptoms, which can last for
several weeks or months, may include the following:

- Eye pain
- Eye redness
- Blurred vision
- Sensitivity to light
- Sensation of something in the eye
- Excessive tearing

Patients should consult with their eye doctor if they have any of the
above symptoms. Acanthamoeba keratitis will eventually cause severe
pain and possible vision loss or blindness if untreated.

Who is at risk for infection?

Acanthamoeba keratitis is most common in people who wear contact lenses, but anyone can develop the infection. For people who wear

contact lenses, certain practices can increase the risk of getting Acanthamoeba keratitis:

- Storing and handling lenses improperly

- Disinfecting lenses improperly (such as using tap water or homemade solutions to clean the lenses)

- Swimming, using a hot tub, or showering while wearing lenses

- Coming into contact with contaminated water

- Having a history of trauma to the cornea

How is Acanthamoeba keratitis diagnosed and treated?

Early diagnosis is essential for effective treatment of Acanthamoeba keratitis.

The infection is usually diagnosed by an eye care provider based on symptoms, growth of the Acanthamoeba ameba from a scraping of the eye, and/or seeing the ameba by a process called confocal microscopy.

The infection is treated with one or more prescription medications. An eye care provider can determine the best treatment option for each patient.

What can I do to reduce my risk of developing Acanthamoeba keratitis?

These guidelines should be followed by all contact lens users to help reduce the risk of eye infections, including Acanthamoeba keratitis:

- Visit your eye care provider for regular eye examinations.

- Wear and replace contact lenses according to the schedule prescribed by your eye care provider.

- Remove contact lenses before any activity involving contact with water, including showering, using a hot tub, or swimming. For people who have difficulty seeing without their contacts, prescription goggles could be helpful. Extended-wear contact lens users should discuss concerns with their eye care provider.

- Wash hands with soap and water and dry them before handling contact lenses.

- Clean contact lenses according to the manufacturer's guidelines and instructions from your eye care provider:

- Use fresh cleaning or disinfecting solution each time lenses are cleaned and stored. Never reuse or top off old solution.

- Never use saline solution and rewetting drops to disinfect lenses.

- Store reusable lenses in the proper storage case:

  - Storage cases should be rinsed with sterile contact lens solution (never use tap water) and left open to dry after each use.

  - Replace storage cases at least once every three months.

Section 38.2

Herpes Eye Disease

What is herpes?

Herpes is a family of viruses with many different subtypes. Eye infections and mouth cold sores are most commonly caused by herpes simplex virus (HSV) type I.

What are the symptoms of herpes in the eye?

Herpes infections cause many ocular problems. A rash with vesicles or blisters can form on the eyelids which typically crusts over in three to seven days. When the ocular surface is involved, the eye may develop redness, tearing, light sensitivity, foreign body sensation, and even headache may occur. Decreased vision is possible.

Who gets herpes?

All age groups are affected by herpes. Neonatal herpetic infection can affect the eyes, central nervous system, and other organs and can be life threatening. An initial ocular herpes infection typically occurs during childhood. Recurrences throughout life are possible.

Why do herpes infections recur?

The virus may remain dormant inside nerves near the face when the body's immune system deactivates but does not kill the virus. Reactivation of the virus is associated with systemic illness, stress, and trauma.

What parts of the eye are affected by herpes?

The herpes virus can affect almost any part of the eye. The eyelids can develop a rash of vesicles, the conjunctiva become inflamed, and the cornea infected. The classic superficial cornea lesion (dendrite) and deep cornea infections can lead to permanent scarring and loss of vision. Iritis (inflammation of the uvea) and retinitis (inflammation of the retina) can also cause serious vision problems.

What is herpes zoster?

Herpes zoster virus (HZV) causes shingles and is the same virus that causes chicken pox. The virus remains dormant in the body after a chicken pox infection and can reactivate later. Herpes zoster infection involving the eye can appear very similar to a HSV infection. A rash usually develops on the forehead and around one eye and can eventually involve the conjunctiva, cornea, uvea, and retina.

How is herpes eye disease diagnosed?

The diagnosis of herpes eye disease is primarily made by clinical signs and symptoms. A culture may be obtained in questionable cases.

How is herpes eye disease treated?

Treatment of herpes eye disease depends upon the part of the eye that is involved. If the eyelid is the only site of involvement, treatment includes a topical antiviral ointment such as acyclovir. Oral acyclovir may also be used, especially for an initial infection. Antibiotic ointment may be used to prevent bacterial infection. If the conjunctiva or cornea is involved, topical antiviral drops (trifluridine) are typically utilized. Oral antivirals may be substituted for the topical therapy. If the uvea or deep layer of the cornea is involved, a topical anti-inflammatory steroid drop is typically prescribed.

Can herpes eye disease be prevented?

The herpes virus is contagious, but only few people who come in contact with the virus develop an ocular infection. Recurrence of ocular herpes infection is unfortunately common—upwards of one third of those involved. Studies by the HEDS (Herpes Eye Disease Study Group) have shown that the rate of recurrence can be significantly reduced by oral acyclovir. The medication is taken daily and has very few side effects.

Section 38.3

Histoplasmosis

"Facts about Histoplasmosis," National Eye Institute,
National Institutes of Health, August 2009.

Histoplasmosis Defined

What is histoplasmosis?

Histoplasmosis is a disease caused when airborne spores of the fungus *Histoplasma capsulatum* are inhaled into the lungs, the primary infection site. This microscopic fungus, which is found throughout the world in river valleys and soil where bird or bat droppings accumulate, is released into the air when soil is disturbed by plowing fields, sweeping chicken coops, or digging holes.

Histoplasmosis is often so mild that it produces no apparent symptoms. Any symptoms that might occur are often similar to those from a common cold. In fact, if you had histoplasmosis symptoms, you might dismiss them as those from a cold or flu, since the body's immune system normally overcomes the infection in a few days without treatment.

However, histoplasmosis, even mild cases, can later cause a serious eye disease called ocular histoplasmosis syndrome (OHS), a leading cause of vision loss in Americans ages twenty to forty.

Cause and Risk Factors

How does histoplasmosis cause ocular histoplasmosis syndrome?

Scientists believe that *Histoplasma capsulatum* (histo) spores spread from the lungs to the eye, lodging in the choroid, a layer of blood vessels that provides blood and nutrients to the retina. The retina is the light-sensitive layer of tissue that lines the back of the eye. Scientists have not yet been able to detect any trace of the histo fungus in the eyes of patients with ocular histoplasmosis syndrome. Nevertheless, there is good reason to suspect the histo organism as the cause of OHS.

How does OHS develop?

OHS develops when fragile, abnormal blood vessels grow underneath the retina. These abnormal blood vessels form a lesion known as choroidal neovascularization (CNV). If left untreated, the CNV lesion can turn into scar tissue and replace the normal retinal tissue in the macula. The macula is the central part of the retina that provides the sharp, central vision that allows us to read a newspaper or drive a car. When this scar tissue forms, visual messages from the retina to the brain are affected, and vision loss results.

Vision is also impaired when these abnormal blood vessels leak fluid and blood into the macula. If these abnormal blood vessels grow toward the center of the macula, they may affect a tiny depression called the fovea. The fovea is the region of the retina with the highest concentration of special retinal nerve cells, called cones, that produce sharp, daytime vision. Damage to the fovea and the cones can severely impair, and even destroy, this straight-ahead vision. Early treatment of OHS is essential; if the abnormal blood vessels have affected the fovea, controlling the disease will be more difficult. Since OHS rarely affects side, or peripheral vision, the disease does not cause total blindness.

Who is at risk for OHS?

Although only a tiny fraction of the people infected with the histo fungus ever develops OHS, any person who has had histoplasmosis should be alert for any changes in vision similar to those described above. Studies have shown the OHS patients usually test positive for previous exposure to histoplasmosis.

In the United States, the highest incidence of histoplasmosis occurs in a region often referred to as the "Histo Belt," where up to 90 percent of the adult population has been infected by histoplasmosis. This region includes all of Arkansas, Kentucky, Missouri, Tennessee, and West Virginia, as well as large portions of Alabama, Illinois, Indiana, Iowa, Kansas, Louisiana, Maryland, Mississippi, Nebraska, Ohio, Oklahoma, Texas, and Virginia. Since most cases of histoplasmosis are undiagnosed, anyone who has ever lived in an area known to have a high rate of histoplasmosis should consider having their eyes examined for histo spots.

Symptoms and Detlection

What are the symptoms of OHS?

OHS usually has no symptoms in its early stages; the initial OHS infection usually subsides without the need for treatment. This is true for other histo infections; in fact, often the only evidence that the inflammation ever occurred are tiny scars called "histo spots," which remain at the infection sites. Histo spots do not generally affect vision, but for reasons that are still not well understood, they can result in complications years—sometimes even decades—after the original eye infection. Histo spots have been associated with the growth of the abnormal blood vessels underneath the retina.

In later stages, OHS symptoms may appear if the abnormal blood vessels cause changes in vision. For example, straight lines may appear crooked or wavy, or a blind spot may appear in the field of vision. Because these symptoms indicate that OHS has already progressed enough to affect vision, anyone who has been exposed to histoplasmosis and perceives even slight changes in vision should consult an eye care professional.

How is OHS diagnosed?

An eye care professional will usually diagnose OHS if a careful eye examination reveals two conditions: (1) The presence of histo spots, which indicate previous exposure to the histo fungus spores; and (2) Swelling of the retina, which signals the growth of new, abnormal blood vessels. To confirm the diagnosis, a dilated eye examination must be performed. This means that the pupils are enlarged temporarily with special drops, allowing the eye care professional to better examine the retina.

If fluid, blood, or abnormal blood vessels are present, an eye care professional may want to perform a diagnostic procedure called fluorescein angiography. In this procedure, a dye, injected into the patient's arm, travels to the blood vessels of the retina. The dye allows a better view of the CNV lesion, and photographs can document the location and extent to which it has spread. Particular attention is paid to how close the abnormal blood vessels are to the fovea.

Treatment

How is OHS treated?

The only proven treatment for OHS is a form of laser surgery called photocoagulation. A small, powerful beam of light destroys the fragile, abnormal blood vessels, as well as a small amount of the overlying retinal tissue. Although the destruction of retinal tissue during the procedure can itself cause some loss of vision, this is done in the hope of protecting the fovea and preserving the finely tuned vision it provides.

How effective is laser surgery?

Controlled clinical trials, sponsored by the National Eye Institute, have shown that photocoagulation can reduce future vision loss from OHS by more than half. The treatment is most effective when:

- the CNV has not grown into the center of the fovea, where it can affect vision;
- the eye care professional is able to identify and destroy the entire area of CNV.

Does laser surgery restore lost vision?

Laser photocoagulation usually does not restore lost vision. However, it does reduce the chance of further CNV growth and any resulting vision loss.

Does laser surgery cure OHS?

No. OHS cannot be cured. Once contracted, OHS remains a threat to a person's sight for their lifetime.

People with OHS who experience one bout of abnormal blood vessel growth may have recurrent CNV. Each recurrence can damage vision and may require additional laser therapy. It is crucial to detect and treat OHS as early as possible before it causes significant visual impairment.

Is there a simple way to check for signs of OHS damage to the macula?

Yes. A person can check for signs of damage to the macula by looking at a printed pattern called an Amsler grid. If the macula has been damaged, the vertical and horizontal lines of the grid may appear curved, or a blank spot may seem to appear.

Many eye care professionals advise patients who have received treatment for OHS, as well as those with histo spots, to check their vision daily with the Amsler grid one eye at a time. Patients with OHS in one eye are likely to develop it in the other.

What help is available for people who have already lost significant vision from OHS?

Scientists and engineers have developed many useful devices to help people with severe visual impairment in both eyes. These devices, called low-vision aids, use special lenses or electronics to create enlarged visual images. An eye care professional can suggest sources that provide information on counseling, training, and special services for people with low vision. Many organizations for people who are blind also serve those with low vision.

Current Research

What research is being done?

The National Eye Institute (NEI) supports research aimed at learning more about the relationship between histoplasmosis and OHS and how to treat OHS effectively. One such multicenter clinical study is called the Submacular Surgery Trials (SST). This clinical study is examining whether CNV in the fovea, which cannot be treated by laser photocoagulation, can be successfully removed through traditional surgery.

Section 38.4

Toxoplasmosis

"Ocular Toxoplasmosis," National Institutes of Health,
Office of Rare Diseases, 2011.

Ocular toxoplasmosis is an infection in the eye caused by the parasite, *Toxoplasma gondii*. Toxoplasmosis is the most common cause of eye inflammation in the world. Toxoplamosis can be acquired or present at birth (congenital), having crossed the placenta from a newly infected mother to her fetus. Most humans acquire toxoplasmosis by eating raw or undercooked meat, vegetables, or milk products, or by coming into contact with infected cat litter boxes or sand boxes. In humans, the infection usually causes no symptoms, and resolves without treatment in a few months. In individuals with compromised immune systems, *Toxoplasma gondii* can reactivate to cause disease.[1]

Reactivation of a congenital infection was traditionally thought to be the most common cause of ocular toxoplasmosis, but an acquired infection is now considered to be more common.[2] A toxoplasmosis infection that affects the eye usually attacks the retina and initially resolves without symptoms. However, the inactive parasite may later reactivate, causing the ocular presentation of eye pain, blurred vision, and possibly permanent damage, including blindness. Although most cases of toxoplasmosis resolve on their own, for some, inflammation can be treated with antibiotics and steroids.[3]

References

1. Wu L, Roy H, et al. Ophthalmologic Manifestations of Toxoplasmosis. E-medicine. January 10, 2011 Available at: http://emedicine.medscape.com/article/1204441-overview#showall. Accessed July 25, 2011.

2. Gerwin B, Kimble J. Ophthalmic Pearls: Uveitis. American Academy Ophthalmology: *EyeNet Magazine*. 2011 Available at: http://www.aao.org/aao/publications/eyenet/200711/pearls.cfm. Accessed August 1, 2011.

3. Toxoplasmosis. American Association for Pediatric Ophthalmology and Strabismus. 2011 Available at: http://www.aapos .org/terms/conditions/106. Accessed July 28, 2011.

Section 38.5

Trachoma

Trachoma is an infection of the eyes that affects the inner upper eyelid and cornea. It is caused by the bacteria *Chlamydia trachomatis*. Repeated infections lead to scarring of the inner eyelid, thickening of the conjunctiva, and distortion of the eyelid. The eyelashes turn in and begin to rub against the eye, leading to corneal scarring and, if left untreated, blindness.

The World Health Organization (WHO) estimates that six million people worldwide are blind from trachoma and more than 150 million people are in need of treatment. Globally, the disease results in an estimated $2.9 billion in lost productivity each year.

Symptoms

- Conjunctivitis
- Discharge from the eye
- Swollen eyelids
- Turned-in eyelashes
- Swelling of lymph nodes just in front of the ears
- Cloudy cornea

Risk Factors

More than 10 percent of the world's population is at risk of blindness from trachoma, which is widespread in the poorest regions of Africa,

Asia, and the Middle East and in some parts of Latin American and Australia. Children are especially susceptible to the early, inflammatory stage of the disease, which generally occurs in overcrowded conditions where there is limited access to clean water and health care. Trachoma can easily spread from person to person by hands, clothing, or flies that have come in contact with discharge from the eyes or nose of an infected person. Women are two to three times more likely than men to become blind from trachoma.

Prevention

Primary interventions for preventing trachoma infection include improved sanitation, reduction of fly breeding sites, and increased facial cleanliness (with clean water). Good personal and environmental hygiene including the washing of faces, improved access to clean water, and proper disposal of human and animal waste has been shown to decrease the number of trachoma infections in communities.

Treatment

Early treatment with antibiotics can prevent long-term complications. Tetracycline eye ointment can be applied directly to the eye over a period of six weeks. Oral azithromycin is just as effective and is the treatment of choice. In cases where scarring of the lid has already occurred, a simple surgical procedure to reverse turned in lashes may be necessary to prevent chronic scarring of the cornea.

Chapter 39

Strokes and Vision Loss

What Is Stroke?

Stroke is a "brain attack" that occurs when the blood, which brings oxygen to your brain, stops flowing and brain cells die. Nearly 795,000 people in the United States will have a stroke each year.

How Does Vision Relate to the Brain?

Eyes receive signals from the outside, sending information to the brain where the process of "seeing" occurs. The brain identifies visual images and coordinates eye movement, ensuring eye alignment when the person or target is moving or not moving.

How Does Vision Loss Relate to Stroke?

Vision loss can be both a symptom and result of stroke. Temporary vision loss can be a sign of impending stroke, and requires immediate attention to determine if any blood vessels that supply the retina, the optic nerve, or the brain are blocked. Call 911 immediately if you develop sudden vision loss. A doctor or medical tests can determine whether your symptoms are life threatening.

Injury such as stroke can disturb the entire visual system. Vision complications depend on where the stroke occurs. The majority of visual processing occurs in the occipital lobe, which is located in the

"Stroke and Vision Loss," © 2011 National Stroke Association (www.stroke.org). All rights reserved. Reprinted with permission.

back of the brain. Most strokes affect one side of the brain. If the right occipital lobe is injured, the left vision field in each eye may be affected. A stroke of the left occipital lobe may disturb the right vision field in each eye. It is rare for both sides of the brain to be affected, but it can result in blindness.

Up to a quarter of stroke survivors may have vision loss, influencing quality of life and rehabilitation outcomes if not properly treated. While most stroke patients with vision loss do not fully recover their vision, partial recovery or natural vision improvement is possible.

Improvement usually takes place in the first months after a stroke. Proper diagnosis and a vision rehabilitation plan could help improve most daily activities, self-esteem, and feelings of independence.

What Are the Types of Vision Loss?

Many types of vision loss can occur, but the most common is loss of half of each eye's visual field (hemianopia). Other common types of vision loss include quadrantanopia (or quarter loss of the vision field) and scotoma (an island-like area of blindness). A visual field test will provide proper diagnosis.

What Are Other Possible Vision Problems Following a Stroke?

The brain stem is the originating point for three pairs of nerves that control eye movements. A stroke in this area can lead to one eye moving correctly, while the other will not. This can result in either double vision or the inability for both eyes to look in a particular direction.

The sensation that objects are moving originates in the brain stem or cerebellum. A stroke in this area may lead to reading difficulties.

Loss of feeling may occur on the eye's surface, making blinking difficult, not allowing an eyelid to properly close, or causing a droopy lid or blurry vision.

Stroke may also interfere with comprehending, understanding, or recognizing objects or faces visually. Such a condition, called visual agnosia, can be potentially hazardous.

What Are the Symptoms of Vision Loss?

- Bumping, tripping, or falling over objects
- Difficulty reading, such as missing words in a sentence
- Seeing only part of a television or movie screen

- Feeling unbalanced, startled, or uncomfortable in a normal environment

How Can Vision Loss Be Treated?

If you are experiencing vision loss after stroke, talk to your doctor and identify a neuro-ophthalmologist or neuro-optometrist that can diagnose your condition and recommend a vision rehabilitation plan for you. Vision rehabilitation includes compensatory and restorative therapies.

Compensatory Vision Rehabilitation

This therapy compensates for vision loss by shifting images from the nonseeing to the seeing visual field, thereby warning the patient of a potential obstacle. It includes prisms, visual field awareness systems, and scanning. Prism therapy involves the application of a prism to enhance the visual field. Prisms can shift images from one side of the visual field to the other side. There are different types of prism and visual field awareness systems. Patients can be fitted for and trained on a visual field awareness system.

Scanning training is another compensatory therapy, which helps improve use of the remaining visual field by training the eyes to scan more efficiently toward and away from the field loss.

Restorative Vision Therapy

Vision restoration therapy (VRT) was developed to increase the brain's ability to restore vision. It is a noninvasive therapy program customized specifically for the type of vision loss. Light dots are presented in a specific pattern while a patient fixates on a central point, targeting undamaged areas of the brain to take over visual function.

Everyday Activities to Improve Visual Skills

- Blinking and eyelid closure problems may require lubrication and adequate lid coverage to protect the surface of the eye. Discuss treatment options with your doctor.

- Blurry and/or double vision may be tied to dizziness. Discuss treatment options with your doctor.

- Place mealtime utensils, hygiene items, and furniture along the total visual field and cue when needed.

- Sort objects such as silverware or nuts as a method of enhancing form identification. Use touch or verbal cues to avoid discouragement.

Chapter 40

Traumatic Brain Injury and Vision Loss

Many individuals experience severe vision and eye problems as a result of stroke or closed head trauma. Vision disorders commonly encountered include double vision, blur, eyestrain, discomfort when reading, loss of part of the field of vision, dry eye, difficulty with visual judgments in space, and impaired visual memory.

Rehabilitation of eye and vision disorders is often neglected in patients with closed head trauma. Although they are extensively diagnosed, frequently little or nothing is done to treat the problems. This is unfortunate, since visual function can often be improved substantially, with significant relief from visual symptoms.

In recent years optometrists who specialize in vision therapy have become increasingly involved in the rehabilitation of these vision disorders. Optometric intervention plays an important role in the total rehabilitation effort, frequently allowing affected individuals to more adequately perform the varied activities of daily living, and thus to substantially improve their quality of life. We have found working in this area to be extremely gratifying, and are writing this chapter to share our experience and concepts with colleagues.

Double Vision

Many individuals suffer from double vision, which causes confusion and disorientation. Such individuals are often given an occluder. This

---

"Vision Disorders in Acquired Brain Injury," by Martin H. Birnbaum, O.D. and Michele R. Bessler, O.D. © 2011 VisionHelp. All rights reserved. Reprinted with permission. For additional information, visit www.visionhelp.com.

resolves the diplopia, but reduces the field of vision and interferes with daily function. Diplopia can often be eliminated without an eye patch, through the use of prisms and vision therapy. This approach not only eliminates double vision, but allows more normal visual judgments in space, and makes movement in space less hazardous.

Reading Difficulty

Many head trauma patients experience difficulty in reading. This may be caused by vergence and accommodative deficits that cause blurred or double vision, jerky eye movements, or visual field loss that makes it difficult to keep one's place. Depending on the specific cause, relief can usually be obtained with appropriate reading glasses, prisms, and vision therapy.

Moving a ruler down the page line by line frequently makes it easier to keep one's place when loses of place is caused by jerky eye movements or by visual field loss. Some individuals find it easier to read and keep place if the field is reduced to a single line of print through the use of a typoscope, a sheet of black cardboard or plastic with a cut-out the size of a line of print.

The typoscope makes it easier to keep place and to focus by isolating the line that is being read. The patient simply moves the typoscope across each line of print, and then down to the next line.

Visual Field Loss

Head injury often has severe effects on the field of vision, profoundly affecting the way we perceive the world around us. The field of vision can become impaired in many ways. The two most common are hemianopsia and unilateral neglect.

Hemianopsia is a condition in which one-half of the visual field is lost. Depending on whether it is a left or right hemianopsia, the affected individual sees nothing to the left or to the right of the object he or she is looking at. Individuals bump into walls and doorways, fail to see objects and people in the affected field, knock over cups and glasses, and suffer similar mishaps. Driving, as would be expected, is extremely hazardous.

Unilateral neglect is a condition that is in some ways similar, but in other ways quite different, from hemianopsia. It is caused by injury to the parietal lobe. Although either the left or the right visual field maybe affected, left field neglect (caused by injury to the right side of the brain) is much more common.

Individuals with unilateral neglect, like individuals with hemi-anopsia, do not see objects on one side, usually the left side in cases of neglect. They frequently bump into walls, doorways, and objects on the left side, and fail to see people and objects to the left. In addition, however, individuals with unilateral neglect may ignore one side of their own body, failing to dress the left side, or to shave or apply make-up to the left side of the face. They may even fail to see the left side of various objects, whether the objects are located in the left or the right visual field. When asked to draw a daisy or a clock, the individual with neglect may place all the petals on the right side of the daisy, or cram al twelve numbers of the clock dial onto the right side.

Much can be done to help individuals who suffer from hemianop-sia and unilateral neglect. Compensatory strategies are used to minimize the impact of the visual field loss. For example, a patient with a left fields loss should sit at the dinner table, in front of the television, and in other situations so that the majority of objects of interest in the visual field are situated to the right. When engaged in conversation with someone, the patient with left visual field loss should position themselves somewhat to the left of the person they are talking with, so that the major objects in the filed of vision are to their right. Similarly, the child or adult with left field loss should, in a classroom or theatre, position themselves on the left side of the room (when facing front), so that the bulk of the classroom or stage is in the right visual field.

Individuals with visual field loss should use eye movement scan strategies to look into the lost field to see what is there. For example, a person with a left visual field loss should get into the habit, whenever walking into a room, to scan and look around the left side of the room, to look for and notice objects and people that would otherwise not be seen. Eye movement exercises are frequently helpful in this regard, as are computer programs designed to foster rapid and accurate scanning into the affected field.

Visualization exercises in which the person looks into the affected field to see what is there, and then visualizes the objects in the lost visual field in the mind's eye, while looking straight ahead, help to expand awareness of objects in the lost visual field.

Yoked prisms and mirror devices are often helpful in cases of visual field loss. Yoked prisms, with their bases towards the affected field, are used to shift objects from the nonseeing to the seeing filed of vision. Such prisms also frequently redress mismatches between body image and perception of space, so that individuals feel more stable and secure moving through their visual space world. Tiny mirrors affixed to one's spectacles have also been used to aid in scanning into the affected field and expand visual field awareness.

We have found that most individuals with visual field loss do not suffer complete blindness in the affected field, but rather retain the ability to see and respond to objects that are sufficiently bright. Stimulatory exercises in which bright lights are flashed in the affected field are frequently effective in expanding awareness in the "blind" field. A typical sequence for such exercises is as follows:

1. Flash a penlight on and off in the affected field. The patient looks straight ahead at the therapist's or spouse's face. When the patient see the light go on in his peripheral field, he touches it with his index finger, while continuing to look straight ahead at the therapist's face. If the light cannot be seen in the affected field, use a brighter light, hold the light closer to the patient's eyes, and turn off the other lights in the room to increase contrast. Flash the light in various areas of the affected field, i.e., at eye level, above eye level, and below eye level.

2. Hold two flashlights, one in the normal and the other in the affected visual field. Flash them on and off, one at a time, in random sequence, while the patient looks straight ahead at the therapist's face. When the patient sees either light go on, he touches it with his index finger, while continuing to look at the therapist's face. It is important to flash the lights in a random, unpredictable sequence.

3. The therapist holds two flashlights, one in the normal and one in the affected visual field, and flashes sometimes one, sometimes the other, and sometimes both, in a random, unpredictable sequence, while the patient looks straight ahead at the therapist's face. The patient touches whichever light or lights he perceives as being on, while continuing to look at the therapist's face. The lights are sometimes flashed at eye level, sometimes above, and sometimes below.

These exercises are designed to increase awareness, sensitivity, and utilization of vision remaining in the affected field.

Low Vision

Some patients with acquired brain injury have a normal field of view, but are unable to read ordinary print or watch television with conventional glasses due to reduced visual acuity, or low vision. Optometric low vision care often allows such individuals to overcome this handicap so they can handle daily activities and maintain independence. Low vision aids include sophisticated telescopic lenses for distance vision, and simple magnifying lenses and more complex microscopic and electronic magnifiers for reading and other fine tasks.

Dry Eye

If the nerves or muscles of the eyelids are affected by stroke or head injury, the lids may not close fully on each blink or during sleep, causing the gritty, burning secretion associated with dry eye. Dry eye symptoms are typically relieved with the use of carefully selected lubricating drops and ointments. In severe cases, collagen plugs inserted into the tear ducts frequently work to increase lubrication of the eye and eliminate discomfort.

Visual-Perceptual-Motor Deficits

Individuals with acquired brain injury frequently experience unstable orientation in space, so that objects and even the walls and floor are perceived to move and shift about; difficulty with object localization and visual judgments in space; inability to sustain visual attention; and poor visual memory. These functions can often be improved through the use of prisms that restore one's ability to orient oneself in space, and rehabilitative vision therapy to improve visual perceptual, spatial, and information-processing functions.

Vision Rehabilitation

Vision problems resulting from acquired brain injury are often overlooked during initial treatment of the injury. Frequently the vision problems described above are neglected. This lengthens and impairs rehabilitation, results in incomplete treatment, and causes frustration for the patient, family, and treatment team.

Optometric rehabilitation can play an important role in the overall rehabilitation effort. Optometrists who specialize in vision therapy can provide needed treatment that allows patients with acquired brain injury to more easily and adequately perform the varied activities of daily living. Treatment regimens are designed to meet the needs of each individual patient, and frequently incorporate combinations of lenses, prisms, low-vision aids, and vision therapy activities to relieve symptoms and increase vision efficiency. Clinical experience and research studies each document the value of optometric rehabilitation for individuals who suffer from vision disorder as a result of acquired brain injury.

Chapter 41

Other Disorders with Eye-Related Complications

Chapter Contents

Section 41.1

The Eye in Systemic Disease

"The Eye in Systemic Disease," reprinted with permission from The University of Illinois Department of Ophthalmology and Visual Sciences, Eye Facts (http://www.uic.edu/com/eye/LearningAboutVision/EyeFacts/index.shtml), © 2011.

Systemic diseases are diseases that involve many organs or the whole body. Many of these diseases also affect the eyes. In fact, an eye exam sometimes leads to the first diagnosis of a systemic disease.

Why is the eye so important in systemic disease?

The eye is composed of many different types of tissue. This unique feature makes the eye susceptible to a wide variety of diseases as well as provides insights into many body systems. Almost any part of the eye can give important clues to the diagnosis of systemic diseases. Signs of a systemic disease may be evident on the outer surface of the eye (eyelids, conjunctiva, and cornea), middle of the eye, and at the back of the eye (retina).

The optic nerve and eye movements often reflect changes in the central nervous system. This is because a large part of the brain helps provide visual information and controls eye movements. Because the eye structures are uniquely transparent, a doctor can see inside the eye. The eye is the only organ in the body in which a doctor can directly see blood vessels. The health of the blood vessels in the eye often indicates the condition of the blood vessels (arteries and veins) throughout the body.

Which systemic diseases most commonly affect the eye?

The eye may be involved in these diseases, among others:

- **Diabetes mellitus:** An imbalance in blood glucose (sugar) levels

- **Acquired immunodeficiency syndrome (AIDS):** A life-threatening disease caused by a virus that cripples the body's immune defenses

- **Graves disease:** A thyroid disorder, most often in women, which can cause a goiter (swelling in the front part of the neck) and protruding eyes

- **Sarcoidosis:** A disease that mainly affects the lungs, brain, joints, and eyes, found most often in young African American women

- **Systemic lupus erythematosus:** A connective tissue disorder involving mainly the skin, joints, and kidneys

- **Rheumatoid arthritis**

- **Hypertension (high blood pressure)**

- **Atherosclerosis (hardening of the arteries)**

- **Sickle cell disease:** An inherited blood disorder that can block circulation throughout the body, primarily affecting African Americans

- **Multiple sclerosis:** A disease that damages nerve coverings, causing weakness, coordination and speech disturbances

How do systemic diseases affect the eye?

Various systemic diseases affect the eye differently.

Diabetes can cause severe eye complications, including swelling of the retina (macular edema), abnormal growth of new retinal blood vessels, and bleeding inside the eye. Changes in the blood vessels of the retina or fluctuations in vision sometimes lead to the first diagnosis of diabetes. Diabetic retinal disease is a leading cause of blindness in this country. In addition, people with diabetes develop cataracts earlier than other people. Therefore, it is important for them to have regular eye exams.

AIDS can cause infections in the eye, retinal detachment, eyelid tumors, and neuro-ophthalmic disorders. AIDS-related infections can often lead to blindness, but effective eye treatment is now available. Abnormal retinal circulation is another frequent complication of AIDS. Sometimes, the first signs of AIDS are abnormalities in the retina.

Graves disease can cause protruding eyes (proptosis), limitations of eye movement, double vision, and corneal disease. Severe cases may have damage to the optic nerve. Sometimes the eye symptoms in Graves disease can appear before other symptoms and signs.

Graves disease: The eye is prone to inflammation. A type of inflammation called uveitis is the most common eye problem caused by sarcoidosis. Uveitis can result in painful and red eyes, blurred vision, and glaucoma. Scleritis, an inflammation of the white part of the eye, can result from systemic lupus erythematosus and rheumatoid arthritis. Both of these conditions also can cause dry eyes. High blood pressure and atherosclerosis can damage the retinal blood vessels. Usually, this damage does not result in any visual symptoms at first. However, it can eventually lead to more severe complications in the retina as well as in the body. In persons with high blood pressure, the extent of damage in the eye can directly relate to damage that occurs in the kidneys. High blood pressure can be first diagnosed when changes in the blood vessels of the eye are found.

Sickle cell disease also can cause abnormal retinal vessels as well as bleeding inside the retina. Sickle cell eye disease can sometimes lead to blindness if not treated with laser therapy.

Multiple sclerosis can cause eye movement problems as well as optic nerve disease causing loss of vision. Neurologic diseases such as multiple sclerosis may be first suspected when an eye doctor finds changes in eye movement, vision, or the function of the optic nerve.

Cancer can start in the eye or can spread to the eye. Tumors of the eye are rare, however. Depending on its location, an eye tumor may or may not distort vision at an early stage. Early detection and treatment of cancer in the eye can be vision saving and, in some cases, life saving. Brain tumors also may affect vision by causing swelling of the optic nerve. Occasionally, a doctor may first suspect a brain tumor after finding optic nerve swelling on an eye exam.

Diseases other than those mentioned above also can affect the eye.

What about treatment?

For any of the eye problems mentioned above, it is important to have an examination by an ophthalmologist, who will confer with your primary care physician. The ophthalmologist, working with other healthcare specialists and your family physician, often plays an important role in treating systemic diseases. Depending on the condition, systemic treatment may be needed. Ophthalmic treatment can range from drugs for inflammatory diseases (e.g., uveitis) to laser therapy for retinal vascular diseases (e.g., diabetic retinopathy) to surgery for tumors.

Section 41.2

Acquired Immune Deficiency Syndrome (AIDS)

Any discussion of human immunodeficiency virus (HIV)/acquired immune deficiency syndrome (AIDS)–related illness reminds us of the astonishing volley of attacks our bodies continually fend off. Healthy bodies usually prevail in these daily skirmishes with invaders. But an immune system compromised by human immunodeficiency virus (HIV) may be unable to defend itself.

We call the resulting infections opportunistic because they exploit the body's weakened state. The development of such infections is what marks the transition from HIV-positive status to a diagnosis of active acquired immune deficiency syndrome (AIDS), sometimes called "full-blown" AIDS.

Pathogens of every description can ransack the body of a person with HIV. Each organ is vulnerable to a particular set of infections. The lung, for instance, may be assailed by tuberculosis, mycobacteriosis, candidiasis, or other infections. Likewise, the eye is subject to a wide range of infections that may damage its structure or function, causing low vision or blindness.

Types of Infections

Cytomegalovirus Retinopathy

Cytomegalovirus (CMV) retinitis is inflammation of the retina caused by infection with a virus from the herpes family—La Cosa Nostra of infectious diseases (see the sections below on herpes zoster and herpes simplex). Most people have been exposed to CMV, and a healthy body is able to fight it off, no sweat. But when the immune system is compromised by HIV infection, chemotherapy, an autoimmune disorder such as rheumatoid arthritis, or some other challenge, it's no match.

About 15 to 40 percent of patients with advanced HIV disease in the United States develop CMV retinitis. Since the initiation of effective antiretroviral therapy, however, the rate has fallen by about 75 percent. Symptoms are subtle and may consist only of floaters and a sensation of seeing flashing lights. Immediate treatment is necessary to preserve vision.

Patients who have CMV retinitis are at risk for immune recovery uveitis when they begin antiretroviral therapy. As the first two words of its name suggest, this syndrome is a kind of immune system backlash. A complex antibody reaction can occur during recovery that causes the middle layer of the eye to swell, a condition called uveitis. Patients who have a low T cell count when they begin therapy or who have a relatively large area of the retina affected by CMV are at greater risk of developing immune recovery uveitis.

Toxoplasmosis Retinitis

Toxoplasmosis is caused by a parasite transmitted to humans by eating contaminated, improperly cooked food. Transmission can also occur after direct contact with cat feces. HIV/AIDS patients with toxoplasmosis may develop inflammation of the choroid and retina that causes vision loss. Eye manifestations of toxoplasmosis include the following:

- Blurred vision
- Blind spots
- Pain
- Sensitivity to light

Ocular Tuberculosis

Most of us think of tuberculosis as a lung disease, but it's caused by a bacillus (*Mycobacterium tuberculosis*) that can affect the bones and joints, skin, gastrointestinal system, genitourinary system, and other body organs and systems. In the eye, it can cause uveitis, an inflammatory condition associated with retinal detachment, glaucoma, cataracts, and other causes of low vision. Early diagnosis may prevent vision loss.

The person with ocular tuberculosis can have a range of symptoms:

- Blurry vision
- Red-green color blindness

- Blind spots in the center of the visual field

- Eye pain and light sensitivity

- Excessive tear production

Ocular tuberculosis is treated with an onslaught of powerful antibiotics. These medicines are sometimes given as a preventive measure to those with compromised immune systems.

Other Common Pathogens

Many other pathogens (viruses, bacteria, fungi, and other organisms that can cause infection) normally associated with sites elsewhere in the body can also take hold in the eye:

- **Herpes zoster:** Herpes zoster is the virus that causes chickenpox. In older adults and in those with immune system compromise, the virus is sometimes reactivated as the painful neurological disease known as "shingles." In the eye, shingles can irritate the cornea, causing an infection. It may also cause inflammation of the optic nerve, retina, iris, and other structures. In addition, having a herpes zoster infection of the eye increases the risk of developing glaucoma.

- **Herpes simplex:** Herpes simplex is the virus that causes cold sores (type 1) and genital herpes (type 2). In the eye, the virus can stimulate inflammation of the cornea, eyelids, and conjunctiva. If the infection settles into the middle layers of the cornea, it can cause scarring that impairs vision. Symptoms include eye pain and redness, sensitivity to light, increased tear production, and a gritty sensation in the eye.

- **Syphilis:** Syphilis is a sexually transmitted infection (STI) cause by a parasite. The course of the disease is generally divided into three stages, and the ocular manifestations of syphilis usually occur during the second stage. The infected person may have a sore throat, fever, swollen lymph glands, or a rash, along with eye redness, blurred vision, and sensitivity to light. Inside the eye, the infection causes inflammation of the iris and other structures of the middle eye.

Ocular Toxic or Allergic Drug Reactions

Allergic reactions to medications taken to treat HIV/AIDS, particularly sulfa antibiotics, can cause a severe allergic reaction throughout the body. Such a reaction may lead to corneal scarring and consequent vision loss.

Late-Stage Infections

Some kinds of infections that can take up residence in the eye, such as the sinister-sounding *Cryptococcus neoformans*, tend not to take hold until the patient is already ill with other opportunistic infections. Thus the development of these late-stage eye infections may be a grave sign that the patient's immune system is failing.

Risk Factors and Treatment

The goal of therapy for HIV-positive patients is to keep the virus from replicating—that is, making copies of itself—in the body. Drugs that accomplish this are called antiretroviral agents. They reduce the viral load, or the amount of virus in the bloodstream, allowing the immune system to recover and T cell counts to increase.

The single most potent factor in reducing the risk of HIV/AIDS–related vision loss has been the introduction of highly active antiretroviral therapy (HAART) for the treatment of HIV/AIDS. HAART is a combination of antiretroviral agents that has markedly reduced the rate of visual complications, especially CMV, among HIV-positive patients, prompting some scientists to speculate that viral load and clinical stage correlate with the likelihood of vision loss.

Opportunistic infections in people with HIV/AIDS must be diagnosed and treated on an individual basis. They may have a common site—the eye—but each infection is as different as the specific pathogen that caused it.

Vision Rehabilitation

Vision rehabilitation services are available for people with HIV/AIDS–related low vision. Such programs help people adapt to visual impairment and make decisions about their care, and they teach friends and loved ones in caregiver roles how to help effectively. Teaching hospitals, community centers, senior centers, and government agencies often offer such services.

Section 41.3

Behçet Disease

"Facts about Behçet's Disease," National Eye Institute,
National Institutes of Health, September 2009.

Behçet Defined

What is Behçet disease?

Behçet disease is an autoimmune disease that results from damage to blood vessels throughout the body, particularly veins. In an autoimmune disease, the immune system attacks and harms the body's own tissues. This disease is also known as Adamantiades.

Causes

What causes Behçet disease?

The exact cause is unknown. It is believed that an autoimmune reaction may cause blood vessels to become inflamed, but it is not clear what triggers this reaction.

Symptoms

What are the symptoms of Behçet disease?

Behçet disease affects each person differently. The four most common symptoms are mouth sores, genital sores, inflammation inside of the eye, and skin problems. Inflammation inside of the eye (uveitis, retinitis, and iritis) occurs in more that half of those with Behçet disease and can cause blurred vision, pain, and redness.

Other symptoms may include arthritis, blood clots, and inflammation in the central nervous system and digestive organs.

Treatment

How is Behçet disease treated?

There is no cure for Behçet disease. Treatment typically focuses on reducing discomfort and preventing serious complications. Corticosteroids and other medications that suppress the immune system may be prescribed to treat inflammation.

What is the prognosis for someone with Behçet disease?

Behçet is a chronic disease that recurs. However, patients may have periods of time when symptoms go away temporarily (remission). How severe the disease is varies from patient to patient. Some patients may live normal lives, but others may become blind or severely disabled.

Section 41.4

Diabetes

Excerpted from "Facts about Diabetic Retinopathy," National Eye Institute, National Institutes of Health, October 2009.

Diabetic Retinopathy Defined
What is diabetic eye disease?

Diabetic eye disease refers to a group of eye problems that people with diabetes may face as a complication of diabetes. All can cause severe vision loss or even blindness.

Diabetic eye disease may include the following:

- **Diabetic retinopathy:** Damage to the blood vessels in the retina.

- **Cataract:** Clouding of the eye's lens. Cataracts develop at an earlier age in people with diabetes.

- **Glaucoma:** Increase in fluid pressure inside the eye that leads to optic nerve damage and loss of vision. A person with diabetes is nearly twice as likely to get glaucoma as other adults.

What is diabetic retinopathy?

Diabetic retinopathy is the most common diabetic eye disease and a leading cause of blindness in American adults. It is caused by changes in the blood vessels of the retina.

In some people with diabetic retinopathy, blood vessels may swell and leak fluid. In other people, abnormal new blood vessels grow on the surface of the retina. The retina is the light-sensitive tissue at the back of the eye. A healthy retina is necessary for good vision.

If you have diabetic retinopathy, at first you may not notice changes to your vision. But over time, diabetic retinopathy can get worse and cause vision loss. Diabetic retinopathy usually affects both eyes.

What are the sages of diabetic retinopathy?

Diabetic retinopathy has four stages:

- **Mild nonproliferative retinopathy:** At this earliest stage, microaneurysms occur. They are small areas of balloonlike swelling in the retina's tiny blood vessels.

- **Moderate nonproliferative retinopathy:** As the disease progresses, some blood vessels that nourish the retina are blocked.

- **Severe nonproliferative retinopathy:** Many more blood vessels are blocked, depriving several areas of the retina with their blood supply. These areas of the retina send signals to the body to grow new blood vessels for nourishment.

- **Proliferative retinopathy:** At this advanced stage, the signals sent by the retina for nourishment trigger the growth of new blood vessels. This condition is called proliferative retinopathy. These new blood vessels are abnormal and fragile. They grow along the retina and along the surface of the clear, vitreous gel that fills the inside of the eye. By themselves, these blood vessels do not cause symptoms or vision loss. However, they have thin, fragile walls. If they leak blood, severe vision loss and even blindness can result.

Causes and Risk Factors

How does diabetic retinopathy cause vision loss?

Blood vessels damaged from diabetic retinopathy can cause vision loss in two ways:

1. Fragile, abnormal blood vessels can develop and leak blood into the center of the eye, blurring vision. This is proliferative retinopathy and is the fourth and most advanced stage of the disease.

2. Fluid can leak into the center of the macula, the part of the eye where sharp, straight-ahead vision occurs. The fluid makes the macula swell, blurring vision. This condition is called macular edema. It can occur at any stage of diabetic retinopathy, although it is more likely to occur as the disease progresses. About half of the people with proliferative retinopathy also have macular edema.

Who is at risk for diabetic retinopathy?

All people with diabetes—both type 1 and type 2—are at risk. That's why everyone with diabetes should get a comprehensive dilated eye exam at least once a year. The longer someone has diabetes, the more likely he or she will get diabetic retinopathy. Between 40 and 45 percent of Americans diagnosed with diabetes have some stage of diabetic retinopathy. If you have diabetic retinopathy, your doctor can recommend treatment to help prevent its progression.

During pregnancy, diabetic retinopathy may be a problem for women with diabetes. To protect vision, every pregnant woman with diabetes should have a comprehensive dilated eye exam as soon as possible. Your doctor may recommend additional exams during your pregnancy.

What can I do to protect my vision?

If you have diabetes, get a comprehensive dilated eye exam at least once a year and remember the following things:

- Proliferative retinopathy can develop without symptoms. At this advanced stage, you are at high risk for vision loss.

- Macular edema can develop without symptoms at any of the four stages of diabetic retinopathy.

- You can develop both proliferative retinopathy and macular edema and still see fine. However, you are at high risk for vision loss.

- Your eye care professional can tell if you have macular edema or any stage of diabetic retinopathy. Whether or not you have symptoms, early detection and timely treatment can prevent vision loss.

If you have diabetic retinopathy, you may need an eye exam more often. People with proliferative retinopathy can reduce their risk of blindness by 95 percent with timely treatment and appropriate follow-up care.

Symptoms and Detection

Does diabetic retinopathy have any symptoms?

Often there are no symptoms in the early stages of the disease, nor is there any pain. Don't wait for symptoms. Be sure to have a comprehensive dilated eye exam at least once a year.

Blurred vision may occur when the macula—the part of the retina that provides sharp central vision—swells from leaking fluid. This condition is called macular edema.

If new blood vessels grow on the surface of the retina, they can bleed into the eye and block vision.

What are the symptoms of proliferative retinopathy if bleeding occurs?

At first, you will see a few specks of blood, or spots, "floating" in your vision. If spots occur, see your eye care professional as soon as possible. You may need treatment before more serious bleeding occurs. Hemorrhages tend to happen more than once, often during sleep.

Sometimes, without treatment, the spots clear, and you will see better. However, bleeding can reoccur and cause severely blurred vision. You need to be examined by your eye care professional at the first sign of blurred vision, before more bleeding occurs.

If left untreated, proliferative retinopathy can cause severe vision loss and even blindness. Also, the earlier you receive treatment, the more likely treatment will be effective.

How are diabetic retinopathy and macular edema detected?

Diabetic retinopathy and macular edema are detected during a comprehensive eye exam that includes the following:

- **Visual acuity test:** This eye chart test measures how well you see at various distances.

- **Dilated eye exam:** Drops are placed in your eyes to widen, or dilate, the pupils. This allows the eye care professional to see more of the inside of your eyes to check for signs of the disease. Your eye care professional uses a special magnifying lens to examine your retina and optic nerve for signs of damage and other eye problems. After the exam, your close-up vision may remain blurred for several hours.

- **Tonometry:** An instrument measures the pressure inside the eye. Numbing drops may be applied to your eye for this test.

Your eye care professional checks your retina for early signs of the disease, including the following:

- Leaking blood vessels

- Retinal swelling (macular edema)

- Pale, fatty deposits on the retina—signs of leaking blood vessels

- Damaged nerve tissue

- Any changes to the blood vessels

If your eye care professional believes you need treatment for macular edema, he or she may suggest a fluorescein angiogram. In this test, a special dye is injected into your arm. Pictures are taken as the dye passes through the blood vessels in your retina. The test allows your eye care professional to identify any leaking blood vessels and recommend treatment.

Treatment

How is diabetic retinopathy treated?

During the first three stages of diabetic retinopathy, no treatment is needed, unless you have macular edema. To prevent progression of diabetic retinopathy, people with diabetes should control their levels of blood sugar, blood pressure, and blood cholesterol.

Proliferative retinopathy is treated with laser surgery. This procedure is called scatter laser treatment. Scatter laser treatment helps to shrink the abnormal blood vessels. Your doctor places one thousand to two thousand laser burns in the areas of the retina away from the macula, causing the abnormal blood vessels to shrink. Because a high number of laser burns are necessary, two or more sessions usually are required to complete treatment. Although you may notice some loss of your side vision, scatter laser treatment can save the rest of your sight. Scatter laser treatment may slightly reduce your color vision and night vision.

Scatter laser treatment works better before the fragile, new blood vessels have started to bleed. That is why it is important to have regular, comprehensive dilated eye exams. Even if bleeding has started, scatter laser treatment may still be possible, depending on the amount of bleeding.

If the bleeding is severe, you may need a surgical procedure called a vitrectomy. During a vitrectomy, blood is removed from the center of your eye.

How is a macular edema treated?

Macular edema is treated with laser surgery. This procedure is called focal laser treatment. Your doctor places up to several hundred small laser burns in the areas of retinal leakage surrounding the macula. These burns slow the leakage of fluid and reduce the amount of fluid in the retina. The surgery is usually completed in one session. Further treatment may be needed.

A patient may need focal laser surgery more than once to control the leaking fluid. If you have macular edema in both eyes and require laser surgery, generally only one eye will be treated at a time, usually several weeks apart.

Focal laser treatment stabilizes vision. In fact, focal laser treatment reduces the risk of vision loss by 50 percent. In a small number of cases, if vision is lost, it can be improved. Contact your eye care professional if you have vision loss.

What happens during laser treatment?

Both focal and scatter laser treatment are performed in your doctor's office or eye clinic. Before the surgery, your doctor will dilate your pupil and apply drops to numb the eye. The area behind your eye also may be numbed to prevent discomfort.

The lights in the office will be dim. As you sit facing the laser machine, your doctor will hold a special lens to your eye. During the procedure, you may see flashes of light. These flashes eventually may create a stinging sensation that can be uncomfortable. You will need someone to drive you home after surgery. Because your pupil will remain dilated for a few hours, you should bring a pair of sunglasses.

For the rest of the day, your vision will probably be a little blurry. If your eye hurts, your doctor can suggest treatment.

Laser surgery and appropriate follow-up care can reduce the risk of blindness by 90 percent. However, laser surgery often cannot restore vision that has already been lost. That is why finding diabetic retinopathy early is the best way to prevent vision loss.

What is a vitrectomy?

If you have a lot of blood in the center of the eye (vitreous gel), you may need a vitrectomy to restore your sight. If you need vitrectomies in both eyes, they are usually done several weeks apart.

A vitrectomy is performed under either local or general anesthesia. Your doctor makes a tiny incision in your eye. Next, a small instrument is used to remove the vitreous gel that is clouded with blood. The vitreous gel is replaced with a salt solution. Because the vitreous gel is mostly water, you will notice no change between the salt solution and the original vitreous gel.

You will probably be able to return home after the vitrectomy. Some people stay in the hospital overnight. Your eye will be red and sensitive. You will need to wear an eye patch for a few days or weeks to protect your eye. You also will need to use medicated eye drops to protect against infection.

Are scatter laser treatment and vitrectomy effective in treating proliferative retinopathy?

Yes. Both treatments are very effective in reducing vision loss. People with proliferative retinopathy have less than a 5 percent chance of becoming blind within five years when they get timely and appropriate treatment. Although both treatments have high success rates, they do not cure diabetic retinopathy.

Once you have proliferative retinopathy, you always will be at risk for new bleeding. You may need treatment more than once to protect your sight.

Section 41.5

Holmes-Adie Syndrome

Excerpted from "Holmes-Adie Syndrome Information Page,"
National Institute of Neurological Disorders and Stroke,
National Institutes of Health, September 27, 2010.

What is Holmes-Adie syndrome?

Holmes-Adie syndrome (HAS) is a neurological disorder affecting the pupil of the eye and the autonomic nervous system. It is characterized by one eye with a pupil that is larger than normal and constricts slowly in bright light (tonic pupil), along with the absence of deep tendon reflexes, usually in the Achilles tendon. HAS is thought to be the result of a viral or bacterial infection that causes inflammation and damage to neurons in the ciliary ganglion, an area of the brain that controls eye movements, and the spinal ganglion, an area of the brain involved in the response of the autonomic nervous system. HAS begins gradually in one eye, and often progresses to involve the other eye. At first, it may only cause the loss of deep tendon reflexes on one side of the body, but then progress to the other side. The eye and reflex symptoms may not appear at the same time. People with HAS may also sweat excessively, sometimes only on one side of the body. The combination of these three symptoms—abnormal pupil size, loss of deep tendon reflexes, and excessive sweating—is usually called Ross syndrome, although some doctors will still diagnose the condition as a variant of HAS. Some individuals will also have cardiovascular abnormalities. The HAS symptoms can appear on their own, or in association with other diseases of the nervous system, such as Sjögren syndrome or migraine. It is most often seen in young women. It is rarely an inherited condition.

Is there any treatment?

Doctors may prescribe reading glasses to compensate for impaired vision in the affected eye, and pilocarpine drops to be applied three times daily to constrict the dilated pupil. Thoracic sympathectomy, which severs the involved sympathetic nerve, is the definitive treatment for excessive sweating.

What is the prognosis?

Holmes-Adie syndrome is not life threatening or disabling. The loss of deep tendon reflexes is permanent. Some symptoms of the disorder may progress. For most individuals, pilocarpine drops and glasses will improve vision.

Section 41.6

Multiple Sclerosis

Vision problems are relatively common in people with multiple sclerosis (MS); however, rarely do these problems result in total blindness. These are some types of vision problems affecting people with MS.

Optic Neuritis

Optic neuritis is the inflammation of the optic nerve, the nerve that transmits light and visual images to the brain and is responsible for vision.

According to the National Multiple Sclerosis Society, 55 percent of people with MS will have an episode of optic neuritis. Frequently, it's the first symptom of the disease. Although having optic neuritis is very suggestive of MS, it does not mean that a person has or will get MS.

The symptoms of optic neuritis are the acute onset of any of the following:

- Blurred vision

- Graying of vision

- Blindness in one eye (usually)

It's rare that both eyes are affected simultaneously. And pain is rare. Loss of vision tends to worsen over the course of a few days before getting better. This usually takes about four to twelve weeks.

Treatment may include intravenous and/or oral steroids to control the inflammation.

Double Vision

Double vision occurs when the pair of muscles that control a particular eye movement are not coordinated due to weakness in one or more of the muscles. Although annoying, double vision usually resolves on its own without medical treatment.

Uncontrolled Eye Movements

Uncontrolled eye movements or vertical eye movements, called nystagmus, is another common symptom of MS. Nystagmus may be mild or it may be severe enough to impair vision. Some drugs and special prisms have been reported to be successful in treating the visual deficits caused by nystagmus.

Temporary Blindness

Temporary blindness in one eye may occur at the time of an acute exacerbation of MS. An exacerbation—also known as a flare—is a sudden worsening of an MS symptom, or the appearance of new symptoms, which lasts at least twenty-four hours and is separated from a previous exacerbation by at least one month.

Temporary blindness is most often due to optic neuritis.

Section 41.7

Ocular Rosacea

What Is Ocular Rosacea?

Ocular rosacea is associated with a chronic skin condition known as acne rosacea. The problem usually affects those with light skin, and is characterized by redness and bumps concentrated on the forehead, nose, and cheeks. One of the earliest symptoms of rosacea (often experienced during puberty) is facial flushing brought on by changes in body temperature, emotion, or hot drinks. Eventually, the skin may become chronically red, irritated, and inflamed.

Approximately 60 percent of patients with rosacea develop related problems affecting the eye (ocular rosacea). Patients with ocular rosacea most commonly experience irritation of the lids and eye, occurring when the oil-producing glands of the lids become obstructed. Styes, blepharitis, episcleritis, and chronically red eyes are also typical conditions. Ocular rosacea may also affect the cornea, causing neovascularization (abnormal blood vessel growth), infections, and occasionally ulcers.

Signs and Symptoms

Acne Rosacea

- Red, flushed skin

- Breakouts or papules concentrated on the nose, forehead, and cheeks

- Facial flushing after drinking alcohol, eating hot or spicy foods, or events that increase body temperature

- Dry, flaking skin

Ocular Rosacea

- Chronically red eyes and lid margins
- Irritated eyelids (blepharitis)
- Styes (chalazion)
- Dry, irritated eyes
- Burning
- Foreign body sensation

Detection and Diagnosis

Those with ocular rosacea are frequently under the care of a dermatologist and are referred for treatment when the patient develops related eye conditions. However, the ophthalmologist may also make the initial diagnosis with a routine eye exam and evaluation of the skin.

Treatment

Patients with this condition should avoid hot drinks, spicy foods, alcohol, or activities that cause the body temperature to become elevated. Care should be taken to protect the skin from ultraviolet light exposure by using sunscreen with a high sun protection factor (SPF) and wearing hats and sunglasses when outdoors.

Controlling skin inflammation may give marked relief of the eye conditions. Because of this, the eye physician and dermatologist often work together to treat the problem. Eye-related symptoms can often be relieved with warm (not hot) compresses on the lids, eyelid scrubs, and artificial tears. Topical and/or oral antibiotics may also be prescribed to reduce symptoms.

About half of rosacea patients will have ocular rosacea. To what degree the eyes are affected appears to bear little relation to the severity of inflammation of the face. For instance you may have severe rosacea on the face and little or no problems with the eyes. Similarly severe ocular rosacea may accompany mild rosacea.

Common complaints are a dry and gritty feeling in the eyes. These symptoms may be alleviated by over-the-counter eye drops but this is not treating the condition. You must see your doctor and perhaps take some literature with you that shows the connection between facial rosacea and ocular rosacea, as the condition remains underdiagnosed.

Symptoms of Ocular Rosacea May Include

- blepharitis, an inflamed, dry, and crusty eyelid probably at its worse in the morning;.

- conjunctivitis, which feels like grit in the eyes, caused by inflammation of the white part (conjunctiva) of the eye.

More serious problems arise in about 5 percent of those with ocular rosacea:

- iritis, inflammation of the iris causing pain;

- keratitis, ulceration of the cornea.

This may lead to visual dysfunction, rarely blindness. Treatment will be to reduce the inflammation of the affected part of the eye. Steroid eye drops may be prescribed. Tetracycline antibiotics also used to treat facial rosacea have been shown to reduce inflammation and with early intervention can prevent blindness. Your doctor may refer you to an ophthalmic specialist at a hospital, essential with the more severe forms of ocular rosacea. Check to see if there is an eye casualty department at your hospital that you could visit if your eyes are causing you problems.

Section 41.8

Thyroid Eye Disease

"Thyroid Eye Disease," © North American Neuro-Ophthalmology Society (www.nanosweb.org). Reprinted with permission. The full text of this document can be found online at http://www.nanosweb.org/14a/pages/index.cfm?pageID=3282; accessed March 27, 2011.

Your doctor thinks you have thyroid orbitopathy. This is an autoimmune condition where your body's immune system is producing factors that stimulate enlargement of the muscles that move the eye. This can result in bulging of the eyes, retraction of the lids, double vision, decreased vision, and ocular irritation. This is often associated with abnormalities in thyroid gland function (either too much thyroid (Graves disease) or too little (Hashimoto thyroiditis)). The eye findings of thyroid orbitopathy may be independent of treatment of your thyroid abnormalities and may not resolve in spite of the fact that the thyroid is now "controlled." These symptoms may be present even if your thyroid has no apparent problems.

Anatomy

There are six muscles that move your eye.

Four of these, the inferior rectus, superior rectus, lateral rectus, and medial rectus, are most frequently involved. These muscles originate behind the eye at the peak of the eye socket and attach to the eye just behind the cornea (the clear portion of the eye overlying the colored part of the eye). The muscles cannot be seen on the surface as they are covered by a thin layer of tissue (the conjunctiva) but may become visible as the blood vessels over their anterior portion become very prominent. The immune system singles out the fibroblasts, support cells within the muscles, causing the muscles to enlarge. With muscle enlargement the globe (eyeball) is pushed forward, leading to the characteristic "stare." In addition, the muscles become stiff and the upper lid tends to retract, pulling away from the colored portion of the eye. The eyes may become red due to difficulty closing as well as increased prominence of the blood vessels. If the muscles get large enough, they may press on the optic nerve, causing damage to the nerve.

561

This dysfunction within the optic nerve, which transmits information from the eye to the brain, results in decreased vision. This, fortunately, occurs only in about 5 percent of the patients with thyroid orbitopathy and may be reversible if the pressure on the optic nerve is relieved.

Physiology

We aren't sure how or why the immune system attacks the muscles. The result is enlargement of the muscles. As the muscles get larger, three things can happen. The eyeball gets pushed forward, the muscles themselves become stiff (the eye may not move normally), or the muscles may press on the optic nerve. The inferior rectus muscle (located beneath the eye) tends to be more often affected than others. When it becomes stiff, the globe cannot move up normally. This often results in double vision, with one image seen on top of the other. If the optic nerve is compressed, the patient is usually aware of blurred, dark, or dim vision. There may be blurring or distortion related to surface problems due to the exposure and drying. It is important for your physician to sort out whether or not there is any evidence of optic nerve dysfunction. This is detected by carefully checking vision, pupillary reactivity, visual fields, and the appearance of the optic nerve head.

Although thyroid orbitopathy is usually preceded by thyroid abnormalities, sometimes the eye symptoms may come first or the thyroid may appear to be normal. The connection between the eyes and the thyroid is through the immune system. The same conditions that lead to the immune system attacking the eye muscles often precede an attack on the thyroid gland. Most frequently this makes the thyroid gland overproduce thyroid hormone that in turn can lead to tremors, shakes, weight loss, rapid heartbeat or palpitations, nervousness, and sensitivity to heat. Less commonly the attack on the thyroid gland leads to low thyroid production or even normal thyroid levels. We may see antibodies in your blood that can be identified as attacking thyroid tissue.

Symptoms

Patients with thyroid orbitopathy often notice blurred or double vision. As the eye is pushed forward it frequently results in irritation, redness, tearing, and a gritty sensation. Pain is not usually a major finding in thyroid patients, although patients will be aware of fullness within the orbit and sometimes a mild irritation, light sensitivity, or ache. The double vision is most frequently one image on top of the other or offset although it may be side to side. Double vision will often change with direction of gaze, seeming worse when looking up and to the side. Sometimes patients will only be aware of symptoms related to thyroid overaction (nervousness, tremors, rapid or irregular heartbeat, increased sweating and intolerance to heat, weight loss, and diarrhea) or underaction (fatigue, weight gain, constipation, thickening of the skin). These symptoms may precede eye symptoms by months or even years.

Signs

Thyroid orbitopathy is suspected based on the patient's external appearance.

Upper lid elevation, particularly when looking down, is very characteristic of thyroid orbitopathy. The eyes frequently bulge forward and the blood vessels on either side of the pupil tend to become dilated. The lids often don't close completely at night and there is resistance to pushing the globes posteriorly within the orbit. The pupils may not react normally and the eyes may be limited in their movement. Pressure inside the eye may be high particularly while looking in one direction.

Prognosis

Thyroid orbitopathy, like other autoimmune diseases, often comes and goes on its own. There is frequently only one acute inflammatory episode but unfortunately the effects may persist for years or even permanently. Even when the inflammation resolves, things usually do not go back to normal. Thus, although there may be some reduction of the prominence of the globe, eye movements will often not return to normal. Lid position will also likely remain elevated, possibly with persistent problems with closure.

Treatment

Treatment is aimed at improving the symptoms of orbital involvement. In patients with mild involvement, irritation and foreign body sensation may improve with artificial tears and the use of lubricating ointment at night. If the lids are not closing completely, they may be taped closed at night. With more severe corneal problems, lid surgery to help partially close the lids or to raise the lower lids may be necessary. In severe retraction of the upper or lower lid, surgery to reduce the effects of the lid retractors, either without or with spacer placement (such as a piece of tissue removed from the roof of the mouth) can help the lids to close. Smoking may worsen symptoms and should be discontinued.

There is no medicine that improves the ability of muscles to move (and thus relieves double vision). Recent studies suggest that controlling the thyroid function may be beneficial in decreasing the chance of worsening but is unlikely to restore normal motility. Covering one eye immediately relieves double vision. It doesn't matter which eye is covered. It may be possible to optically realign eyes with the use of prisms either applied to glasses or ground into the lens although this may not be effective until things stabilize. When double vision cannot be corrected with prisms, eye muscle surgery may be necessary. In most cases, physicians choose to wait until the double vision is stable. If we operate on a patient who is undergoing progressive change, we may correct them now but have things change within the next few months. Often multiple muscle operations are necessary. It is sometimes not possible to completely remove double vision, but the goal is to remove double vision looking straight ahead and in reading position, as these are the most important directions of sight.

Fortunately, optic nerve problems resulting in decreased vision are uncommon. When it occurs, treatment is aimed at shrinking the muscles, usually by the use of high-dose steroids (prednisone). For those patients who will not tolerate steroids, radiation therapy may be of benefit. If the muscles cannot be made small enough to relieve the compression of the optic nerve (resulting in decreased visual acuity) then the orbit can be made larger. This is usually done surgically by removing one or more of the bony walls of the orbit. Since the optic nerve is usually compressed at the very back of the orbit, removing the posterior medial wall of the orbit is most critical. This may be done directly (through the soft tissues or skin around the eye), through the sinus under the eye, or through the nose. To further reduce the eye bulge the floor, lateral wall, or even the roof of the orbit may be removed. One of the problems with surgical decompression is that this often affects eye movements, thus changing the pattern of double vision (if it already exists) or potentially producing double vision in those patients who don't have it before surgery.

Frequently Asked Questions

The doctors tell me they fixed my thyroid and that it is now normal. Why are my eyes acting up?

In Graves disease the thyroid gland is stimulated by the immune system to secrete too much hormone. This excess hormone results in nervousness, palpitations, weight loss, diarrhea, tremors, and a feeling of being hot all the time. Treatment is aimed at limiting the thyroid gland's ability to make thyroid hormone. This may be done with medications, surgery, or radioactive iodine, usually resulting in normalization of thyroid production (occasionally requiring thyroid replacement). This does not, however, affect the primary autoimmune process and the immune system may continue to target other tissues, in particular the extraocular muscles. Orbital symptoms may even worsen following treatment with radioactive iodine. The eye and orbit changes must be treated separately as outlined.

The steroids made my eyes much more comfortable. Can't I just continue taking them?

Steroid therapy may be effective in halting the inflammatory phase of thyroid orbitopathy and partially shrinking the muscle swelling. Steroid side effects are very common with continued treatment. If there are still problems with eye movements (double vision), exposure problems (irritation and foreign body sensation), or decreased vision then surgery should be considered.

Why can't you fix my eyelids now?

Eye muscle surgery on the vertically acting muscles may change the eyelid position. Thus we don't want to do eyelid surgery until we have done any possible muscle surgery.

Can't you just put my eyes back?

We can reduce the bulging of your eyes by doing orbital decompressive surgery. If you already have tight muscles, decompressing the orbit may produce double vision. This is usually treatable with eye muscle surgery but if you don't have double vision now and your central vision is normal we may be able to deal with the bulged appearance with lid surgery alone without the risk of double vision.

Why do you want to operate on my "good" eye?

Eye muscle surgery may release a restricted muscle but the muscle is often incapable of moving normally due to its enlargement and fibrosis. Thus if we operate only on the more affected eye that eye will have very limited movement and you will have double vision whenever you look away from straight ahead. By limiting the movement of the other eye we can maximize the area over which you can see singly.

Part Seven

Living with Low Vision

Chapter 42

Defining Vision Impairment

Chapter Contents

Section 42.1

What Is Low Vision?

Few people are totally without sight. Most individuals today classified as "blind" actually have remaining sight and, thanks to developments in the field of low vision rehabilitation, can be helped to make good use of it, improving their quality of life.

Anyone with noncorrectable reduced vision is visually impaired, and can have a wide range of problems. The World Health Organization uses the following classifications of visual impairment, using vision in the better eye with best possible glasses correction:

- 20/30 to 20/60 is considered mild vision loss, or near-normal vision;

- 20/70 to 20/160 is considered moderate visual impairment, or moderate low vision;

- 20/200 to 20/400 is considered severe visual impairment, or severe low vision;

- 20/500 to 20/1,000 is considered profound visual impairment, or profound low vision;

- less than 20/1,000 is considered near-total visual impairment, or near total blindness;

- no light perception is considered total visual impairment, or total blindness.

There are also levels of visual impairment based on visual field loss (loss of peripheral vision).

In the United States, any person with vision that cannot be corrected to better than 20/200 in the best eye, or who has twenty degrees or less of visual field remaining, is considered legally blind.

Visual impairments take many forms and exist in varying degrees. It is important to understand that visual acuity alone is not a good predictor of the degree of problems a person may have. Someone with relatively good acuity (e.g., 20/40) can have difficulty functioning, while someone with worse acuity (e.g., 20/200) might not be having any real problems.

Section 42.2

What Is Legal Blindness?

Question: What Does It Mean to Be Legally Blind?

Answer: A person is considered to be legally blind if he or she has a best corrected vision of 20/200 in their best seeing eye.

Many people feel that they are legally blind because when they remove their glasses or contact lenses, they cannot see a foot in front of their face. However, when they put on their vision correction, they can see 20/20. As long as you can be corrected to 20/20 with some visual aid, you are not considered legally blind.

The true definition of "legal blindness" is based upon the best level of vision that you can achieve or the best vision you can be corrected to. Most government agencies and health care institutions agree that legal blindness is defined as one of the following:

1. Legal blindness is defined as visual acuity of 20/200 or worse in the best seeing eye.

2. A visual field that is limited to only 20 degrees.

What Does "Legally Blind" Really Mean?

Being legally blind means that your best seeing eye cannot be corrected with glasses or contact lenses any better than 20/200. The best way to understand this is to think about a normal person with 20/20 vision. This person has the ability to stand 200 feet away from an object and see the finest detail, whereas the legally blind person would have to move all of the way up to 20 feet to see the same detail. A legally blind person has difficulty seeing objects very far away or very close.

If a person has a visual field of only 20 degrees, considered tunnel vision, he or she can be considered legally blind. A normal person has a visual field of 180 degrees. People with a limited visual field can see central detail but can't see someone standing right next to their own shoulder. These people have difficulty with mobility, as safe driving is nearly impossible. Walking into a dark movie theater can also be a major problem.

The definition of legal blindness was developed to help people receive government assistance. Also, as you can imagine, the department of motor vehicles (DMV) has to have some way of measuring vision in order to keep our roads and highways safe.

Source

Lavine, Jay B. *The Eye Care Sourcebook*, pp 24–25. Contemporary Books, 2001.

Section 42.3

What Is Night Blindness?

Excerpted from "Vision: Night Blindness," © 2011 A.D.A.M., Inc. Reprinted with permission.

Night blindness is poor vision at night or in dim light.

Considerations

Night blindness may cause problems with driving at night. People with night blindness often have trouble seeing stars on a clear night or walking through a dark room, such as a movie theater.

These problems are often worse just after a person is in a brightly lit environment. Milder cases may just have a harder time adapting to darkness.

Causes

The causes of night blindness fall into two categories: treatable and nontreatable.

Treatable causes:

- cataracts;
- nearsightedness;
- use of certain drugs;
- vitamin A deficiency (rare).

  Nontreatable causes:
- birth defects;
- retinitis pigmentosa.

Home Care

Take safety measures to prevent accidents in areas of low light. Avoid driving a car at night, unless you get your eye doctor's approval.

Vitamin A supplements may be helpful if you have a vitamin A deficiency. Ask your doctor.

When to Contact a Medical Professional

It is important to have a complete eye exam to determine the cause, which may be treatable. Call your eye doctor if symptoms of night blindness persist or significantly affect your life.

What to Expect at Your Office Visit

Your healthcare provider will examine you and your eyes. The goal of the medical exam is to determine if the problem can be corrected (for example, with new glasses or cataract removal), or if the problem is due to something more serious.

The eye exam will include:

- color vision testing;
- pupil light reflex;
- refraction;
- retinal exam;
- slit lamp examination;
- visual acuity.

  Other tests may be done:
- electroretinogram (ERG);
- visual field.

Alternative Names

Nyctanopia; nyctalopia; night blindness

References

Tomsak RL. Vision loss. In: Bradley WG, Daroff RB, Fenichel GM, Jankovic J, eds. *Neurology in Clinical Practice. 5th ed*. Philadelphia, Pa: Butterworth-Heinemann; 2008:chap 14.

Sieving PA, Caruso RC. Retinitis pigmentosa and related disorders. In: Yanoff M, Duker JS, eds. *Ophthalmology. 3rd ed*. St. Louis, MO;Mosby Elsevier; 2008:chap 6.10.

Section 42.4

Do You Have Low Vision?

Reprinted from the National Eye Institute, National Institutes of Health, May 2011.

There are many signs that can signal vision loss. For example, even with your regular glasses, do you have difficulty:

- recognizing faces of friends and relatives?
- doing things that require you to see well up close, like reading, cooking, sewing, or fixing things around the house?
- picking out and matching the color of your clothes?
- doing things at work or home because lights seem dimmer than they used to?
- reading street and bus signs or the names of stores?

If you answered "yes" to any of these questions, vision changes like these could be early warning signs of eye disease.

Regular eye exams should be part of your routine healthcare. However, if you believe your vision has recently changed, you should see your eye care professional as soon as possible. Usually, the earlier your problem is diagnosed, the better the chance of keeping your remaining vision.

Chapter 43

Tips for People with Low Vision

Chapter Contents

Section 43.1

Coping with Vision Loss

Some experts have likened initial reactions to vision loss to the "stages of grief," defined by Dr. Elisabeth Kubler-Ross, after the loss of a loved one—taking one from denial to anger and depression, and finally, acceptance. Navigating the various stages successfully begins with understanding how they affect you and those around you. With understanding comes the ability to straightforwardly address conflicts, allay fears, and move forward.

To help with this process, here are a few points to keep in mind at all times:

- **You are not alone:** Vision loss affects more than 6.5 million people in the United States aged fifty-five and over from all walks of life. Don't be afraid to reach out to others experiencing vision loss as well as vision loss professionals for information, advice, and encouragement.

- **You can continue to lead a full, rewarding life:** Again, if you're willing to make adjustments, there is no reason you cannot continue to enjoy your favorite hobbies and activities, participate in family activities, do volunteer work, or travel. Indeed, the challenges of vision loss are consistently overcome each day by individuals who have simply chosen to participate fully in society.

- **You don't have to stop working:** With technical assistance and a few basic adjustments, most people who develop vision loss are able to remain in the workforce—many even continue in their current jobs. There are exceptions, of course, but far fewer than you may realize. Indeed, it's quite possible that the person who processed your recent electric bill, the person who upgraded your car transmission, or the person who oversaw your last stock trade all live with some degree of vision loss.

- **You can remain independent:** Whether you are experiencing a modest vision decline or are facing total vision loss, affordable and accessible solutions and tools exist to help you to safely cook your meals, navigate your home, pay your bills, and perform other essential tasks on your own. Better still, new advances in technology designed for people with vision loss, such as a scanner that can read text out loud, are entering the marketplace almost daily, while mainstream products such as computers and home appliances can be adapted for your use with simple techniques.

Section 43.2

Devices to Help Low Vision

There are many different products currently in the market to assist people with low vision, and more are being developed. Here is an overview of what is available, what it does, and what types of vision they can benefit.

Handheld Magnifiers

Often known as "magnifying glasses," handheld magnifiers come in many shapes and sizes, and provide magnification between 1.5 and 20 times. Some styles can be folded up for easy transport in a pocket or handbag, and some are equipped with battery-operated lights. Handheld magnifiers may be difficult to use if your hands tire easily or tend to shake.

Stand Magnifiers

Stand magnifiers can be helpful for weak or shaky hands. They are mounted on stands and must sit flat above the page being viewed. These devices can magnify between 2 and 20 times, and can be moved across the page to see each line. Illuminated stand or handheld magnifiers can be plugged into an electrical outlet or fitted with batteries.

Monoculars/Telescopes

Monoculars are mini telescopes used for seeing things at a distance. Magnification ranges from 2.5 to 10 times, depending on the telescope's size.

Binoculars

Binoculars are similar to monoculars, but allow you to use both eyes to view things at a distance. Many sizes and strengths are available.

Spectacle-Mounted "Magnifiers"

Spectacle-mounted telescopes for distance, or spectacle-mounted microscopes for close-up, can significantly improve visual abilities. These devices protrude from the spectacle frame, and can be used with one or both eyes. When using spectacle-mounted microscopes, objects must be held much closer to your eyes than normal. This type of spectacles are somewhat like bifocals in that they allow a person to switch to the telescope lens for improved distance vision, and back to the spectacle lens for general orientation. These are prescribed by low vision specialists.

Video Magnifiers (CCTVs)

A video magnifier or closed-circuit television (CCTV) uses a stand-mounted video camera to project magnified objects onto a video screen. These devices are very useful for reading, writing, looking at photographs and catalogs, or doing crafts.

Magnification varies with the model and manufacturer. CCTVs are available in black-and-white as well as color models, and come in various sizes. Some include special features such as underlining and shadow masking for easier reading. Others can be used with your personal computer.

Reading Machines with Voice Output

Reading machines (scanners with voice output) can be used to transform printed material into spoken words. Typewritten text placed on the device's scanning surface is read aloud. Some devices can be hooked to a personal computer. Optical character recognition (OCR) software can be used to turn a personal computer into a "reading machine."

Absorptive Lenses

Absorptive lenses regulate the amount of light transmitted through to the eye, and can often be worn over prescription glasses. By eliminating harmful sunrays, reducing glare, increasing contrast, and helping with the transition between light and dark surroundings, these lenses can increase both comfort and safety.

Other Adaptive Devices

There is an impressive range of adaptive devices available. Devices with large print, high-contrast colors, or "talking" features that say information out loud are designed to make life easier for people with impaired vision. Other items include talking watches, large-print phones, writing guides, and magnified makeup mirrors.

Chapter 44

Home Modifications for People with Low Vision

Chapter Contents

Section 44.1

Adapting Your Home

Excerpted from "Room by Room: Evaluate and Modify Your Home Environment," reprinted with permission. Copyright © 2011 American Foundation for the Blind (www.afb.org). All rights reserved. This article originally appeared on http://www.visionaware.org/room_by_room.

Steps and Stairways

Try to keep your stairways free from clutter and don't use your steps and stairs as storage areas.

Use nonslip treads on step surfaces.

If you have low vision, mark the leading edge of the first and last steps with bright paint or light-reflecting tape that contrasts with the background color of the flooring.

If you use tape, change it frequently and keep it in good repair.

A brightly colored and/or textured advance-warning strip can also indicate the presence of steps.

Please note: In many instances, it is not necessary to adapt each step. Placing a mark or indicator on the first and last steps is usually sufficient to indicate where a staircase begins and ends.

Cover the landing areas at the top and bottom of the stairs with carpeting or nonslip material that provides contrast with the texture of the stair treads.

If you have low vision, you can paint staircase handrails in a bright color that contrasts with the walls and flooring.

If possible, try to make handrails continuous on both sides of all staircases and make sure that they extend from the top step to the bottom step.

Place a tactual mark, such as a piece of masking tape or a rubber band, on the handrail at the top and bottom of the staircase to give advance warning of steps or stairs.

Use solid, brightly colored, and/or textured hallway or stair runners to clearly define walking spaces.

Keep runners in good repair, since frayed or uneven edges can create potential tripping and falling hazards.

Lighting, Glare, and Windows

Try to maintain continuous lighting levels throughout your home. If possible, install supplementary lighting in entryways, hallways, and at the top and bottom of each staircase to eliminate shadows or excessively bright areas.

Whenever possible, try to use a combination of fluorescent and incandescent lighting.

Install fluorescent ceiling fixtures for general room lighting, supplemented with incandescent, light-emitting diode (LED), or halogen lighting in desk lamps, table lamps, and floor fixtures.

Please note: Use precautions and follow the manufacturer's instructions when positioning halogen lights or lamps close to your body, curtains, or furniture. Halogen bulbs produce intense heat and can cause fire, severe burns, and personal injury if used incorrectly.

Use flexible-arm lamps for close work, such as reading, meal preparation, and writing.

Use nightlights to create a lighted pathway that can help you move from one room to another at night.

The position of each light source is also important to note. Since cutting the distance in half between the light source and the task creates approximately four times more light on the task or activity, examine your existing light sources and determine whether any can be moved closer to your workspace or activity.

Install dimmer switches on incandescent lamps and ceiling fixtures to control illumination levels and glare.

Use mini-blinds or vertical shades to control direct sunlight and adjust for changing lighting conditions, according to the weather and time of day. They can also be used in combination with sheer or lace window coverings.

Try to avoid using light fixtures with uncovered light bulbs. Instead, use lampshades that are light-colored and translucent; generally, this type of shade allows the maximum transmission of light.

Room by Room Hints and Suggestions

Kitchen and Dining Areas

Use white plates on a dark tablecloth, or place dark dishes on a white or light-colored cloth. If possible, avoid using clear glass cups and dishes.

Use brightly colored fluorescent tape to increase the visibility of drawer pulls and the edges of cabinet doors.

Use a large-print timer with bold, black numerals on either a white or bright yellow background.

Paint cupboard or cabinet doors in a solid bright color to make them stand out against the walls and counters. Replace cabinet hardware with brightly colored contrasting handles.

Use brightly colored raised marking dots on the stove, oven, and microwave controls to allow you feel and adjust them more easily. These markings can also create contrast with the background color, if you have low vision.

Wrap brightly colored contrasting electrical tape around pot handles to make them more visible.

If you're ready to buy new pots and pans, select them in colors that contrast with your stovetop.

Reduce glare by using a nonglare floor wax, installing mini-blinds in windows, using nonglossy placemats and tablecloths, and placing rugs (with the edges secured) over glare spots on high-gloss floors.

Use a reversible black-and-white cutting board to provide contrast. For example, onions, potatoes, and yellow squash will show up more clearly on the black side, while the white side will provide greater contrast with tomatoes and green vegetables.

In the Bathroom

When towels, washcloths, and bath mats need replacing, purchase solid colors that contrast with the tub, floor, and wall tile.

Select a toothbrush with a dark handle that contrasts with the white or light-colored sink and countertop.

Float a brightly colored sponge in the bathtub to help determine the water level and avoid overflow.

Transfer soap, shampoo, and other bath products to brightly colored plastic bottles or wall-mounted containers that contrast with the tub and wall tile.

Use soap-on-a-rope or a wash mitt with a soap pocket to help you locate your soap more easily and prevent you from slipping on it or dropping it in the tub or shower.

Place a contrasting nonskid mat in the shower or tub to prevent falls. It can also provide a cue for judging depth perception. Check the mat regularly for signs of wear.

Drape a dark towel over the seat of a light-colored bath chair to make it easier to see.

Use a contrasting, nonslip rug immediately outside the tub or shower and keep nonskid slippers nearby.

Drape a contrasting bath mat over the edge of the tub or apply a strip of contrasting colored tape along the entire edge of the tub to make it easier to see.

For additional safety and security, install grab bars by the toilet and in the shower and tub area. Wrap them with brightly colored nonslip contrasting tape to make them more visible in case you need to reach out quickly.

Don't use the soap dish, towel rack, or toilet paper holder in place of grab bars. They can pull out of the wall if you lean on them too heavily.

Replace a white toilet seat with a brightly colored one that contrasts with the walls and fixtures.

Hint: To adjust the water temperature, turn the cold water on first, and then add hot water until you reach a water temperature that comfortable for you. You can also lower the temperature on your water heater or use a scald-free adapter for the shower or tub.

Hint: Don't store medications or medical equipment in the bathroom. Heat and humidity can affect their safety and reliability.

Bedrooms and Closets

Use a bedside lamp with a "clap-on" feature, or one that you can activate by simply touching the base.

Place a small lamp just inside the door of your bedroom and switch it on to help you find your bedside light.

Install flexible-arm lamps wherever you need them for reading or identifying clothing and medication.

In closets, install battery-operated lights that can be mounted on the wall.

Attach a bed caddy to the side of the bed to hold your eyeglasses, medication, and tissues.

Anchor all of your lamps in place so that you won't knock or pull them over.

Make it a habit to close closet doors or dresser drawers immediately after you use them.

Maintain a clear, clutter- and obstacle-free pathway between the bedroom and the bathroom.

In the Living Room

Is the lighting too dim, too bright, or does it cover too small an area? If so, consider increasing the wattage of your light bulbs (within recommended limits), repositioning lamps, or adding additional lighting.

Add dimmer switches to your lamps so that you can vary their light intensity as needed.

If your living room drapes block natural daylight, consider using adjustable blinds or lighter translucent curtains.

Try rearranging the furniture so that your reading chair is positioned to take advantage of the natural sunlight.

Reposition your television to reduce glare on the screen.

If your coffee table or end tables have glossy surfaces, cover them with a cloth or placemat to minimize glare.

Section 44.2

Home Safety Tips

There are more accidents in the home than anywhere else, even for people with normal vision. So it's vital for everyone to develop and maintain good safety habits in and around the home. This is especially true for people who are beginning to experience vision loss.

Follow these suggestions to eliminate hazards and be safe:

- Eliminate small throw rugs; they can cause tripping.

- Make sure your bath mat has a nonskid backing.

- Keep electrical cords as close to the baseboards as possible and out of walkways.

- Keep floor lamps and small items such as low tables, magazine racks, plants, etc., out of walkways.

- Label cleaning and toxic products to make them easily identifiable, and store them and any flammable or combustible items away from the kitchen or heating units.

- When plugging a cord into an electrical outlet, first determine if the outlet is vertical or horizontal. For a vertical outlet, place the plug at the top of the outlet, then move it down to locate holes. Do *not* use your fingers to do this. If it's a horizontal outlet, place the plug at the side of the outlet and move it sideways to locate the holes.

- Install wall outlets and covers that contrast in color to your walls. This will make them easier to locate. Also, inexpensive standard outlets with recessed slots are preferable to the more expensive designer types that have a flat face.

- Clean up spills immediately. If you forget the spill is there, you might slip on it.

- Close cabinet, closet, and cupboard doors and drawers completely as soon as you've taken out what you need.

- Install smoke, fire, and carbon monoxide alarms and check the batteries regularly to make sure they are still working.

- Know where your circuit breaker box and water turn-off valve are located and learn how to use them safely.

- When visitors call, keep outside doors locked until they have identified themselves to your satisfaction.

- Mark thermostats with brightly colored fluorescent tape at the settings you typically use.

- Pick up shoes, clothing, books, and other items that you could trip over. In fact, put away an object when you are through using it—for the sake of safety and so you can find it easily again.

Chapter 45

Independence and Mobility for People with Low Vision

Chapter Contents

Section 45.1

Driving with Low Vision

Excerpted from "Driving When You Have Macular Degeneration" and "Driving When You Have Glaucoma," National Highway Traffic Safety Administration, June 2003. Despite the date of these documents, the information provided here is still relevant for readers seeking guidance in driving with low vision.

Driving when You Have Macular Degeneration

For most people, driving represents freedom, control, and competence. Driving enables most people to get to the places they want to go and to see the people they want to see when they want.

Driving is a complex skill. Our ability to drive safely can be challenged by changes in our physical, emotional, and mental condition.

The goal of this section is to help you, your family, and your health-care professional talk about how macular degeneration may affect your ability to drive safely.

How can having macular degeneration affect my driving?

Macular degeneration can distort your central vision and can lead to loss of sharp vision. Macular degeneration also can make it difficult to see road signs, traffic, and people walking, and may affect your ability to drive safely.

Can I still drive with macular degeneration?

If your eye care expert has told you that you have macular degeneration, there are certain things that you should know and do to stay a safe driver.

People experience the visual effects of macular degeneration in different ways. In the early stages of macular degeneration, you may only have small central areas of vision loss or distortion that may not affect your driving. In fact, you may not even notice any change in your eyesight. As macular degeneration progresses, it may become harder for you to see clearly. This may make you worry about your vision and make it harder to drive safely.

What can I do when macular degeneration affects my driving?

If you have a family history of macular degeneration or have any changes in your central vision, you should immediately contact your eye care expert. After a definitive diagnosis of macular degeneration, how often you visit your eye care expert depends on your doctor's advice, the type of macular degeneration that you have, and your symptoms.

Although there is not much that can be done to stop the disease from getting worse, the use of antioxidant vitamins may help retard its progression. Additionally, there are surgical procedures that may help if they are done in the early stages of the disease.

Your eye care expert may refer you to a specialist who can go on a drive with you to see if macular degeneration has affected your driving. The specialist also may offer training to improve your driving skills. Improving your skills could help keep you and others around you safe. To find a specialist near you, contact the Association of Driver Rehabilitation Specialists. You also can call hospitals and rehabilitation facilities to find an occupational therapist who can help with the driving skills assessment.

Driving when You Have Glaucoma

How can having glaucoma affect my driving?

Glaucoma can cause partial vision loss or total blindness. Glaucoma usually affects your peripheral vision—the part of your eyesight that lets you see things "out of the corner of your eye." Because glaucoma often affects your peripheral vision, individuals may not be aware of their vision loss until its advanced stages, when substantial changes in vision have occurred. If you have glaucoma and you drive, you may not see other cars, bicyclists, or pedestrians that are outside of your central field of view.

Can I still drive with glaucoma?

Most likely "Yes," if your glaucoma is found early and if you do not have significant visual field loss.

What can I do when glaucoma affects my driving?

Doctors often can treat glaucoma and slow its progression. It is extremely important that you get your glaucoma checked on a regular basis by your eye care expert and you take any prescribed medications.

Your eye care expert can refer you to a specialist, if needed. This specialist can give you on- and off-road tests to see if, and how, your glaucoma is affecting your driving. The specialist also may offer training to improve your driving skills.

Improving your skills could help keep you and others around you safe. To find a specialist near you, contact the Association of Driver Rehabilitation Specialists. You also can call hospitals and rehabilitation facilities to find an occupational therapist who can help with the driving skills assessment.

If You Have to Cut Back or Give Up on Driving

You can keep your independence even if you have to cut back or give up on your driving. It may take planning ahead on your part, but it will get you to the places you want to go and the people you want to see. Consider:

- rides with family and friends;
- taxi cabs;
- shuttle buses or vans; and
- public buses, trains, and subways.

Also, senior centers, and religious and other local service groups often offer transportation services for older adults in your community.

Don't forget: Always wear your safety belt when you are driving or riding in a car. Make sure that every person who is riding with you also is buckled up. Wear your safety belt even if your car has air bags.

Section 45.2

Tips for Independent Travel

Vision loss does not mean that you can no longer travel alone. You will be able to rely on peripheral or remaining vision, hearing, or the white cane to provide guidance.

As with any activity, confidence and skill come with time. Some people who are blind or visually impaired will be more open to the idea of independent travel than others. You may find that after a period of adjustment, you may have come to terms with vision loss and may feel that you can ask your caregiver to let you run errands without their help.

Here are some ways for to manage potentially frustrating situations outside the home.

Independent Travel Checklist

- Use large-print checks and writing guides to make signing easier.

- Identify coins by touch and fold paper money or separate it in the wallet by denomination.

- Take a moment to let the eyes adjust when switching from a bright environment to a dimly lit one.

- Carry a magnifier and/or penlight to read labels, price tags, elevator buttons, or directions.

- Use a mini tape recorder to make a shopping list, instead of struggling with a handwritten list.

- Tell the bus driver in advance which stop you require, and sit at the front of the bus.

Chapter 46

Low Vision and Employment

Chapter Contents

Section 46.1

Losing Vision Does Not Mean Having to Give Up Working

Many older persons who have experienced vision loss may wish to continue working.

Some reasons you may want to work include:

- additional income;

- the chance to be around other people;

- the opportunity to continue to learn new skills;

- health insurance and/or other benefits;

- feeling part of something again;

- wanting to be productive.

What do you have to offer an employer?

- A proven work history and a strong work ethic

- Lifelong work-related skills

- Job-related education and training

- The capacity to learn

- No earnings limitations after age sixty-five

- Typically no dependent children at home who require care

- Interest and attention to safety issues (less likely to take chances which may result in injuries)

What can you do to find out about employment?

Find out about low vision services and devices and vision rehabilitation services which can make it possible for you as the employee to learn adaptive techniques to carry out your job functions. By taking advantage of these services, you can avoid premature and unnecessary early retirement, and the employer can avoid losing a skilled, productive and reliable employee.

What help is available to make work possible?

Accommodations such as:

- additional lighting and/or lighting positioned directly on work tasks;
- low-vision optical devices such as handheld or stand magnifiers;
- devices such as talking clocks and watches, writing guides, large-print rulers;
- adaptive equipment such as screen magnification systems which magnify the image for ease of reading, computers, and other equipment with speech output.

Services such as:

- eye medical care;
- vision rehabilitation services;
- low vision services;
- job site modification;
- individualized orientation to the job and to the worksite;
- job training or retraining.

So keep in mind that you may continue to be a productive employee and still receive satisfaction from your job.

Section 46.2

Know Your Employment Rights

What Is the State Vocational Rehabilitation (VR) Services Program?

Under the Rehabilitation Act of 1973, as amended, federal grants are awarded to assist states in operating a comprehensive vocational rehabilitation program. This program provides VR services to eligible individuals with disabilities, consistent with their strengths, resources, priorities, concerns, abilities, and capabilities, so that such individuals may prepare for and engage in gainful, competitive employment.

Who Is Eligible for VR Services?

To be eligible for VR services, an individual must:

- have a physical or mental impairment that is a substantial impediment to employment;
- be able to benefit in terms of employment from VR services; and
- require VR services to prepare for, enter, engage in, or retain gainful employment that is consistent with the individual's strengths, resources, priorities, concerns, abilities, capabilities, and informed choice.

How Does an Eligible Individual Receive VR Services?

A VR counselor is assigned to each eligible individual. The counselor gathers as much information as possible about the individual's work history, education and training, abilities and interests, rehabilitation needs, and possible career goals. Together, the counselor and the individual develop an Individualized Written Rehabilitation Program (IWRP) that identifies the individual's long-term vocational goals.

The IWRP lists the steps necessary to achieve the individual's goals, the services required to help the individual reach those goals, and evaluation criteria used to determine whether goals have been achieved. The IWRP also contains a description of how the individual was involved in choosing among alternative goals, objectives, services, and service providers.

The state VR counselor provides some services directly to the eligible individual and arranges for and/or purchases other services from providers in the community.

What Are the VR Services an Eligible Individual May Receive?

VR services are those services that an eligible individual may need in order to achieve his/her vocational goal. These include, but are not limited to:

- an assessment to determine eligibility and VR needs;
- vocational counseling, guidance, and referral services;
- physical and mental restoration services;
- vocational and other training, including on-the-job training;
- maintenance for additional costs incurred while the individual is receiving certain VR services;
- transportation related to other VR services;
- interpreter services for individuals who are deaf;
- reader services for individuals who are blind;
- services to assist students with disabilities to transition from school to work;
- personal assistance services (including training in managing, supervising, and directing personal assistance services) while an individual is receiving VR services;
- rehabilitation technology services and devices; and
- supported-employment and job-placement services.

Does Every Eligible Individual Receive VR Services?

If a state VR agency is unable to serve all eligible individuals with the resources available for the VR program, it must establish an order of selection for services, serving first those individuals with the most severe disabilities. Individuals who cannot be selected immediately for services are placed on a waiting list.

Does the Eligible Individual Ever Have to Pay for VR Services?

Based on the individual's available financial resources, the state VR agency may require an eligible individual to help pay for services. However, all eligible individuals who are accepted have access to the following at no cost to them:

- assessments to determine eligibility and VR needs;
- vocational counseling, guidance, and referral services; and
- job-placement services.

What Are Comparable Services and Benefits?

Before providing certain services, the VR counselor must consider the availability of comparable services and benefits for which the individual is eligible through other sources, such as private insurance, Medicaid, and so on. A counselor is not required to consider the availability of comparable services and benefits, however, when such consideration would delay the provision of services to an eligible individual who is at extreme medical risk or whose job placement might be lost as a result of a delay in services.

What Is the Earnings Status of Rehabilitated Persons in the Years After Case Closure Compared to Persons Who Were Not Rehabilitated?

Based on data from the Rehabilitation Services Administration rehabilitated persons were more likely than those not rehabilitated to have had earnings five years after closure. The likelihood of having earnings was more nearly equal in the years before rehabilitation services. Rehabilitated persons were 44 percent more likely than persons not rehabilitated to have had earnings the fifth year after closure, but only 6 percent were more likely to have had earnings the fifth year before closure.

After the delivery of rehabilitation services, the gap in average annual earnings favoring rehabilitated workers over those not rehabilitated rose to about $2,200. Prior to rehabilitation services, the differences in average annual earnings between the two groups of workers was consistently below $1,000.

In the last five post-closure years for which data were available (1984 to 1988), the average earnings differential in earnings favoring rehabilitated workers widened steadily each year, reaching $2,630 in 1988. Rehabilitated workers averaged 31 percent more in annual earnings than workers not rehabilitated. For each case, the typical rehabilitated person (including non–wage earners) amassed $46,684 on the eight post-closure years, nearly twice the per case, or per capita, accumulation of $24,307 for persons who were not rehabilitated. On a per capita basis, rehabilitated persons averaged 87 percent more in annual earnings than persons not rehabilitated.

What Is the Impact on Individuals with Disabilities?

Sixteen million individuals with disabilities have been assisted in acquiring gainful employment over the seventy-five-year history of the state vocational rehabilitation (VR) program. In fiscal year 1994 alone, this program assisted 202,000 individuals with disabilities in obtaining employment, making them tax-paying members of society. On average, it is estimated that only four years are required for a person rehabilitated by the VR program to pay back costs incurred during his/her rehabilitation in the form of federal and state income and sales taxes and reductions in the cost of dependency.

What Is the Uniqueness of the VR Program?

Well-trained professional staff are the key. At the core of the VR program is the relationship between a well-trained counselor and an individual with a disability. The counselor and the individual with a disability forge a partnership whereby a plan is developed and designed to provide those services necessary to achieve the individual's vocational goal consistent with her/his abilities, needs, and informed choices. In this context, the counselor provides the individual with information and guidance about trends in the job market, how the individual's abilities might be best utilized, reasonable accommodations available, training options available, and other services needed to help the individual prepare for and secure work.

State/Private Partnership

Many VR services are purchased through local service providers such as community-based rehabilitation programs, traditional rehabilitation facilities such as those run by the local affiliates of national of national organizations, hospitals, physicians, colleges, technical schools, and a wide range of other nonprofit and for-profit sources. For example, rehabilitation technology and transportation services can be purchased to assist clients as part of their rehabilitation programs. These vendor relationships are well established and are typically based on the knowledge of the counselor and the state agencies regarding long-term histories of success and performance with clients with various types of disabilities.

Established Program Linkage

The VR program has a long and impressive history of cooperation with other federal and state programs. For instance, state VR agencies have developed strong relationships with education agencies at both the state and local levels to coordinate services for students with disabilities transitioning from school to employment-related activities. Without this seamless transitioning, many such students lose the employment-related skills they have gained while in school. The VR program has a long history of cooperation with other programs. For instance, a unique relationship exists between this program and the Social Security Administration to enable recipients of Social Security Disability Insurance (SSDI) and Supplemental Security Income (SSI) to become employed and decrease their reliance on these entitlement programs. The VR program also has a strong relationship with other employment programs (e.g., programs administered by the Department of Veterans Affairs, programs under the Job Training Partnership Act, etc.).

Part Eight

Additional Help
and Information

Chapter 47

Glossary of Terms Related to Eyes and Eye Disorders

accommodating intraocular lens implant (IOL): An implant containing a hinge that allows for both near and far vision, thereby mimicking the movement of the natural lens of a young person.

accommodation: The process by which the natural lens changes shape, allowing it to focus on near or far objects.

adrenergic agonist eye drops: A treatment for glaucoma. The eye drops reduce intraocular pressure by decreasing the production of aqueous humor and increasing its drainage through the uveoscleral pathway.

age-related macular degeneration (AMD): A loss of central vision caused by changes in the macula.

Amsler grid: A diagram of a box subdivided into smaller boxes that is used for self-monitoring by people with AMD.

angiostatic corticosteroids: Drugs being studied for treating AMD and diabetic retinopathy.

antimetabolites: Drugs sometimes used in filtration surgery for glaucoma.

aqueous humor: A watery fluid that is located in front of the lens and provides nutrients to the lens and cornea.

"Vision Disorders Glossary," reprinted with permission from http://www.johns hopkinshealth alerts.com. © 2007 Remedy Health Media, LLC. All rights reserved. Reviewed by David A. Cooke, MD, FACP, December 2011.

astigmatism: Blurred or distorted vision that is common in near-sighted people.

A-scan ultrasonography: A test that uses sound waves to measure the length of the eyeball.

beta-blocker eye drops: A treatment for glaucoma. The eye drops reduce intraocular pressure (IOP) by decreasing the production of aqueous humor.

bifocals: A pair of glasses with lenses that correct both distant and near vision.

body mass index (BMI): A measure of weight in relation to height. To calculate your BMI, multiply your weight in pounds by 704 and divide that by the square of your height in inches. Overweight is defined as a BMI of 25–29.9; obesity is defined as a BMI of 30 or greater.

B-scan ultrasonography: A test that uses sound waves to view structures in the back of the eye.

carbonic anhydrase inhibitors: Medications used to treat glaucoma. These drugs decrease the production of aqueous humor and are available in both oral and eye drop formulations.

cataract: A cloudiness (opacification) of the lens that can lead to visual impairment.

central vision: The middle part of the visual field.

choroids: A layer of the eye inside the sclera. It contains a dark pigment that minimizes scattering of light inside the eye.

ciliary body: A part of the eye that surrounds the lens and produces aqueous humor.

classic AMD: One of two types of neovascular AMD. Classification is based on fluid leakage patterns.

closed-angle glaucoma: A type of glaucoma caused by a blockage near the iris that prevents aqueous humor from reaching the trabecular meshwork. It results in a rapid buildup of extremely high intraocular pressure that can lead to severe, permanent vision damage within a couple of days.

cones: Nerve cells in the retina that are activated only in bright light and by the colors red, blue, and green.

conjunctiva: A thin, lubricating mucous membrane that covers the sclera and lines the inside of the eyelid.

cornea: The transparent, dome-shaped disk covering the iris and pupil.

coronary heart disease: Abnormality of the arteries that supply blood and oxygen to the heart and can lead to chest pain or a heart attack.

cortical cataract: A cataract that affects the lens cortex.

cyclodestructive surgery: A treatment for glaucoma that destroys the ciliary body with a laser.

cystoid macular edema: A specific pattern of swelling of the central retina.

diabetes: A disease characterized by abnormally high glucose (sugar) levels in the blood.

diabetic retinopathy: Damage to small blood vessels in the retina resulting from the chronic high blood glucose levels in people with poorly controlled diabetes. Proliferative retinopathy is the most dangerous form.

drusen: Small accumulations of debris underneath the retina.

dry AMD: See non-neovascular AMD.

endophthalmitis: An infection of the vitreous humor that develops in a small number of people after eye surgery.

extracapsular surgery: Cataract surgery that removes the front of the lens capsule along with the cortex and nucleus of the lens, while leaving the back of the lens capsule intact.

extrafoveal blood vessels: See neovascular AMD.

exudative AMD: See neovascular AMD.

farsightedness: See hyperopia.

filtration surgery: A treatment for glaucoma that uses conventional surgical instruments to open a passage through the clogged trabecular meshwork, allowing excess aqueous humor to drain into surrounding tissues.

floaters: Black spots or shapes that drift through the field of vision.

fluorescein angiography: A diagnostic procedure for age-related macular degeneration and other retinal diseases. A special dye, called fluorescein, is injected into a vein in the arm. Photographs of the retina are taken as the dye circulates through the blood vessels of the eye.

fovea: The small indentation at the center of the macula. It contains the highest concentration of cones and provides the sharpest vision.

ganglion cells: A type of cell in the retina. Damage to these cells is thought to play a role in the development of glaucoma.

glare: Light within the field of vision that is brighter than other objects to which the eyes have adapted.

glaucoma: An eye disease that results in damage to the optic nerve. Contrary to popular belief, it is not always caused by elevated intraocular pressure.

gonioscopy: A technique used to distinguish between open- and closed-angle glaucoma. It involves an examination of the front part of the eye to check the angle where the iris meets the cornea.

hemorrhage: Leakage of blood from blood vessels.

hyperopia: Farsightedness. Distant objects can be seen clearly, but close ones do not come into proper focus.

indocyanine green angiography: A test similar to fluorescein angiography, using a different dye.

intracapsular surgery: Cataract surgery that removes the entire lens (the front and back of the lens capsule, the cortex, and nucleus). Rarely performed today.

intraocular lens implant (IOL): A plastic lens that replaces the lens removed during cataract surgery.

intraocular pressure (IOP): The pressure exerted by the fluids inside the eyeball.

IOL: See intraocular lens implant.

iridectomy: A treatment for closed-angle glaucoma that involves removing part of the iris.

iridotomy: A treatment for closed-angle glaucoma that creates a hole in the iris with a laser.

iris: The colored circle in the middle of the eye that controls the amount of light that enters the eye.

juxtafoveal blood vessels: See neovascular AMD.

LASEK: Laser-assisted subepithelial keratomileusis, a refractive surgery procedure that reshapes the cornea.

laser trabecular surgery: A treatment for glaucoma that involves making 80 to 100 tiny laser burns in the area of the trabecular meshwork. The procedure increases the drainage of aqueous humor.

LASIK: Laser-assisted in situ keratomileusis, a refractive surgery procedure that reshapes the cornea.

legal blindness: Vision that is 20/200 or worse in both eyes (20/200 vision is the ability to see at twenty feet what a normal eye can see at two hundred feet).

lens: A transparent, dome-shaped disk that is responsible (along with the cornea) for the eye's ability to focus light.

lens capsule: The outermost structure of the lens.

lens cortex: The second innermost structure of the lens, it surrounds the nucleus, and its outer edge is lined with a layer of cells called the epithelium.

lens epithelium: Cells that line the outer surface of the lens cortex.

lens nucleus: The center structure of the lens. Surrounded by the cortex.

low vision aids: Items that can help people with poor vision. Examples include closed-circuit televisions, magnifying glasses, telephones with large numbers, and large-print reading materials.

macula: A small area at the center of the retina that is responsible for central and fine-detail vision.

macular edema: A swelling of the macula caused by leakage and accumulation of fluid. More common in people with diabetes than in the general population.

macular nonperfusion: Closure of small blood vessels that supply the macula.

microaneurysms: Weak spots that bulge outward from blood vessels, including those of the retina.

miotic eye drops: Used to treat glaucoma, these eye drops increase the outflow of aqueous humor through the trabecular meshwork by constricting the pupil.

monofocal IOL: A single-focus lens used after cataract surgery to provide clear distance vision.

monovision: A process in which one eye is corrected for distance and the other for near vision. Achieved with an IOL in cataract surgery, in refractive surgery, or even with contact lenses.

multifocal IOL: A type of lens used after cataract surgery. It contains several rings with a common center that focus and adjust for either near or far vision. This allows the eye to be in focus for near and far vision simultaneously.

myocilin: A protein in trabecular meshwork cells. Mutations in the myocilin gene have been identified as a cause of glaucoma.

myopia: Also called nearsightedness, a vision deficit in which close objects can be seen clearly, but distant ones do not come into proper focus.

neovascular age-related macular degeneration (AMD): A form of AMD in which new blood vessels grow in the choroid layer of the eye. The blood vessels are classified according to their location: sub-foveal blood vessels occur at the fovea, extrafoveal blood vessels are farthest away from the fovea, and juxtafoveal blood vessels are in between.

neovascularization: The growth of new blood vessels.

nonexudative AMD: See non-neovascular AMD.

non-neovascular age-related macular degeneration (AMD): A form of AMD characterized by the breakdown or thinning of tissues in the macula and the formation of drusen and shrinkage of tissues in the retina. This form of AMD often does not impair vision.

normal tension glaucoma: A type of glaucoma that results from damage to the optic nerve although intraocular pressure is normal.

nuclear cataract: A cataract affecting the nucleus of the lens.

occult AMD: One of two types of neovascular AMD, classified by fluid leakage patterns. Occult AMD is common but difficult to treat.

opacification: The process of becoming opaque or less penetrable to light. Common in the cornea and lens of the eye in people with glaucoma.

open-angle glaucoma: The most common form of glaucoma. It usually produces no obvious symptoms until late stages.

ophthalmologist: A physician who specializes in the diagnosis and treatment of eye diseases.

ophthalmoscopy: Examination of the interior structures of the eye, especially the retina, using a specialized instrument called an ophthalmoscope.

optic nerve: A nerve at the back of the eye that carries visual information from the retina to the brain.

optineurin: A protein found in the trabecular meshwork and retina. Its role is not fully understood, but defects in the gene that directs its production have been associated with glaucoma.

pegaptanib: A recently approved drug used to treat neovascular AMD. Sold under the name Macugen.

perimetry: A test used to determine a person's visual fields. While the person looks straight ahead at a bowl-shaped white area, a computer generates a light in fixed locations around the bowl. The patient indicates each time he or she sees the light.

peripheral vision: The ability to see objects at the edges of the visual field.

phacoemulsification: A type of extracapsular surgery that is performed with an ultrasonic device that nearly liquifies the nucleus and cortex so that they can be removed by suction through a tube.

photocoagulation: The standard treatment for neovascular AMD when the new blood vessels are outside the center of the retina. The procedure involves closing the new blood vessels with a laser. It is also used to treat diabetic retinopathy. Focal laser photocoagulation targets individual blood vessels; panretinal photocoagulation creates a grid-like pattern across a larger area of the retina.

photodynamic therapy: A newer treatment for AMD that involves the intravenous administration of a special drug to sensitize blood vessels in the eye to light. A low-power laser, directed at the new blood vessels, activates the drug and closes the vessels in a way that causes less damage to the retina than standard laser treatment.

posterior subcapsular cataract: A cataract in the rear of the lens capsule.

presbyopia: An inability to focus on near objects that commonly develops after age forty-five.

PRK: Photorefractive keratotomy, a refractive surgery procedure that reshapes the cornea.

pupil: The opening in the center of the iris that resembles a large black dot.

retina: The innermost layer of the eye that consists of light-sensitive nerve tissue.

retinal detachment: A vision-threatening condition in which the retina becomes separated from the underlying layers of the eye.

retinal pigment epithelial cells: A layer of cells that contribute to the function of the retina.

rods: Nerve cells in the retina that are sensitive to dim light.

rubeosis iridis: New blood vessel growth on the iris that usually occurs in people with diabetes.

sclera: The white outer layer that covers and protects most of the eye.

scotoma: A blind spot in the visual field.

shunt: A device that creates a new passage to drain excess aqueous humor. It is used in the treatment of glaucoma when filtration surgery is unsuccessful.

slit lamp: A table-mounted microscope that enables an eye specialist to get a three-dimensional view of the optic nerve.

subfoveal blood vessels: See neovascular AMD.

subfoveal surgery: A procedure for age-related macular degeneration in which abnormal blood vessels beneath the retina are surgically removed.

tonometry: A method of measuring intraocular pressure by determining the amount of force needed to make a slight indentation in a small area of the cornea.

topical prostaglandin eye drops: A treatment for glaucoma. These eye drops reduce intraocular pressure by increasing the outflow of aqueous humor through the uveoscleral pathway.

trabecular meshwork: A spongy network of connective tissue through which aqueous humor drains from the eye. Blockage of the meshwork causes a buildup of intraocular pressure.

trabeculectomy: See filtration surgery.

uveitis: Inflammation of the uvea, the part of the eye that contains the iris, ciliary body, and choroid.

uveoscleral pathway: An alternative drainage system for aqueous humor located behind the trabecular meshwork.

vascular endothelial growth factor (VEGF): A protein that promotes the growth of new blood vessels in the eye and elsewhere in the body.

verteporfin: A drug used in photodynamic therapy and sold under the name of Visudyne.

vitrectomy: A surgical procedure that removes the vitreous humor and replaces it with saline solution.

vitreous humor: A thick, gel-like substance that fills the back of the eyeball behind the lens.

wet AMD: See neovascular AMD.

YAG laser: A type of laser that contains yttrium, aluminum, and garnet used to clear blurred vision that may occur after extracapsular surgery for cataracts.

Chapter 48

Directory of Resources Related to Eye Disorders and Vision Loss

General

All About Vision
Website:
http://www.allaboutvision.com

American Academy of Ophthalmology
655 Beach Street
San Francisco, CA 94109
Phone: 415-561-8500
Fax: 415-561-8533
Website: http://www.aao.org
E-mail: eyesmart@aao.org

American Association for Pediatric Ophthalmology and Strabismus (AAPOS)
P.O. Box 193832
San Francisco, CA 94119-3832
Phone: 415-561-8505
Fax: 415-561-8531
Website: http://www.aapos.org
E-mail: aapos@aao.org

American Foundation for the Blind (AFB)
2 Penn Plaza
Suite 1102
New York, NY 10121
Toll-Free: 800-AFB-LINE
(800-232-5463)
Phone: 212-502-7600
Toll-Free Fax: 888-545-8331
Website: http://www.afb.org
E-mail: afbinfo@afb.net

American Optometric Association (AOA)
243 North Lindbergh Boulevard
St. Louis, MO 63141
Toll-Free: 800-365-2219
Website: http://www.aoa.org

Resources in this chapter were compiled from several sources deemed reliable. All contact information was verified and updated in December 2011.

615

EyeCare America
Foundation of the American
Academy of Ophthalmology
P.O. Box 429098
San Francisco, CA 94142-9098
Toll-Free: 877-887-6327
Fax: 415-561-8567
Website:
http://www.eyecareamerica.org

*Eye Surgery Education
Council (ESEC)*
Website: http://www
.eyesurgeryeducation.com

*Foundation Fighting
Blindness*
7168 Columbia Gateway Drive
Suite 100
Columbia, MD 21046
Toll Free: 800-683-5555
Phone: 410-423-0600
Website:
http://www.blindness.org
E-mail: info@FightBlindness.org

Junior Blind of America
5300 Angeles Vista Boulevard
Los Angeles, CA 90043
Toll-Free: 800-352-2290
Phone: 323-295-4555
Fax: 323-296-0424
Website:
http://www.juniorblind.org
E-mail: info@juniorblind.org

Lighthouse International
111 East 59th Street
New York, NY 10022-1202
Toll-Free: 800-829-0500
Phone: 212-821-9200
TTY: 212-821-9713
Fax: 212-821-9707
Website:
http://www.lighthouse.org
E-mail: info@lighthouse.org

National Eye Institute
Information Center
31 Center Drive, MSC 2510
Bethesda, MD 20892-2510
Phone: 301-496-5248
Website: http://www.nei.nih.gov
E-mail: 2020@nei.nih.gov

*North American Neuro-
Ophthalmology Society
(NANOS)*
5841 Cedar Lake Road
Suite 204
Minneapolis, MN 55416
Phone: 952-646-2037
Fax: 952-545-6073
Website:
http://www.nanosweb.org
E-mail: info@nanosweb.org

*Optometric Physicians of
Washington*
555 116th Avenue NE, #166
Bellevue, WA 98004-5205
Phone: 425-455-0874
Fax: 425-646-9646
Website: http://www.eyes.org
E-mail: info@eyes.org

Prevent Blindness America
211 West Wacker Drive
Suite 1700
Chicago, IL 60606
Toll-free: 800-331-2020
Website: http://www
.preventblindness.org

St. Luke's Cataract and Laser Institute
43309 U.S. Highway 19 N
Tarpon Springs, FL 34689
Toll-Free: 800-282-9905
Phone: 727-938-2020
Website:
http://www.stlukeseye.com

University of Illinois Eye and Ear Infirmary
Department of Ophthalmology and Visual Sciences
1855 West Taylor Street, m/c 648
Room 3.138
Chicago, IL 60612
Phone: 312-996-6590
Fax: 312-996-7770
Website:
http://www.uic.edu/com/eye
E-mail:eyeweb@uic.edu

Your-Eye-Sight.org
Website: http://www
.your-eye-sight.org

Achromatopsia

Achromatopsia.info
Phone: 317-844-0919 (Indianapolis Office); 260-432-0575 (Fort Wayne Office)
Website:
http://www.achromatopsia.info

The Achromatopsia Network
Website:
http://www.achromat.org

Anophthalmia

International Children's Anophthalmia Network (ican)
c/o Center for Developmental Medicine and Genetics
5501 Old York Road
Genetics, Levy 2 West
Philadelphia, PA 19141
Toll-Free:
800-580-ican (800-580-4226)
Website:
http://www.anophthalmia.org
E-mail: ican@anophthalmia.org

Choroideremia

Choroideremia Research Foundation, Inc.
23 East Brundreth Street
Springfield, MA 01109-2110
Phone: 413-781-2274
Website: http://www
.choroideremia.org

Disorders of the Cornea

Cornea Research Foundation of America
9002 North Meridian Street
Suite 212
Indianapolis, IN 46260
Phone: 317-844-5610
Fax: 317-814-2806
Website: http://www.cornea.org

National Keratoconus Foundation (NKCF)
622 Wilshire Boulevard
Suite 260
Los Angeles, CA 90048
Toll-Free: 800-521-2524
Phone: 310-623-4466
Fax: 310-623-1837
Website: http://www.nkcf.org
E-mail: info@nkcf.org

Sjögren's Syndrome Foundation (SSF)
6706 Democracy Boulevard
Suite 325
Bethesda, MD 20817
Toll-Free: 800-475-6473
Phone: 301-530-4420
Fax: 301-530-4415
Website: http://www.sjogrens.org

Stevens Johnson Syndrome Foundation
P.O. Box 350333
Westminster, CO 80035-0333
Phone: 303-635-1241
Fax: 303-648-6686
Website:
http://www.sjsupport.org
E-mail: SJSupport@aol.com

Diabetic Eye Disorders

American Diabetes Association
Attn: Center for Information
1701 North Beauregard Street
Alexandria, VA 22311
Toll-Free: 800-DIABETES
(800-342-2383)
Website: http://www.diabetes.org
E-mail: AskADA@diabetes.org

Glaucoma

Children's Glaucoma Foundation (CGF)
2 Longfellow Place
Suite 201
Boston, MA 02114
Phone: 617-227-3011
Fax: 617-227-9538
Website: http://www
.childrensglaucoma.com
E-mail:
info@childrensglaucoma.com

Glaucoma Research Foundation
251 Post Street, Suite 600
San Francisco, CA 94108
Toll-Free: 800-826-6693
Phone: 415-986-3162
Website:
http://www.glaucoma.org
E-mail: question@glaucoma.org

The Glaucoma Foundation (TGF)
80 Maiden Lane
Suite 700
New York, NY 10038
Phone: 212-285-0080
Website: http://www
.glaucomafoundation.org
E-mail:
info@glaucomafoundation.org

Keratoconus

National Keratoconus Foundation (NKCF)
6222 Wilshire Boulevard
Suite 260
Los Angeles, CA 90048
Phone: 310-623-4466
Fax: 310-623-1837
Website: http://www.nkcf.org
E-mail: info@nkcf.org

Macular Degeneration

AMD Alliance International
International Offices
6th Floor, City Gate East
Tollhouse Hill
Nottingham NG1 5SF
United Kingdom
Phone: +44 115 935 2100
Fax: +44 115 935 2001
Website:
http://www.amdalliance.org
E-mail: info@amdalliance.org

Macular Degeneration Partnership
6222 Wilshire Boulevard
Suite 260
Los Angeles, CA 90048
Phone: 310-623-4466
Fax: 310-623-1837
Website: http://www.amd.org
E-mail: ContactUs@AMD.org

Optic Nerve Disease

International Foundation for Optic Nerve Disease (IFOND)
P. O. Box 777
Cornwall, NY 12518
Phone/Fax: 845-534-7250
Website: http://www.ifond.org
E-mail: ifond@aol.com

Retinoblastoma

National Cancer Institute (NCI)
National Institutes of Health
Office of Communication and
Education
Public Inquiries Office
6116 Executive Boulevard
Suite 300
Bethesda, MD 20892-8322
Toll-Free: 800-4-CANCER
(800-422-6237)
Toll-Free TTY: 800-332-8615
Phone: 301-435-3848
Website: http://www.nci.nih.gov

Retinoblastoma International
18030 Brookhurst Street
Box 408
Fountain Valley, CA 92708
Website:
http://www.retinoblastoma.net
E-mail: info@retinoblastoma.net

Uveitis

American Uveitis Society

Website:
http://www.uveitissociety.org

Ocular Immunology and Uveitis Foundation (OIUF)

Massachusetts Eye Research
and Surgery Institution
348 Glen Road
Weston, MA 02493
Phone: 617-494-1431 x 112
Fax: 617-621-2953
Website: http://www.uveitis.org

Uveitis Information Group (UIG)

South House
Sweening, Vidlin
Shetland Isles ZE2 9QE
Phone: 0845 604 5660
Website: http://www.uveitis.net
E-mail: info@uveitis.net

Index

Index

Page numbers followed by 'n' indicate a footnote. Page numbers in *italics* indicate a table or illustration.

A

623

Health Reference Series